Plant-Based Diet Cookbook

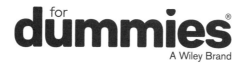

for dummies®

A Wiley Brand

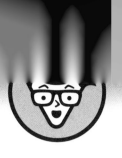

Plant-Based Diet Cookbook

by Jenn Sebestyen
with Marni Wasserman

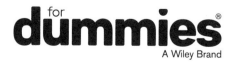

Plant-Based Diet Cookbook For Dummies®

Published by: **John Wiley & Sons, Inc.**, 111 River Street, Hoboken, NJ 07030-5774, www.wiley.com

Copyright © 2022 by John Wiley & Sons, Inc., Hoboken, New Jersey

Published simultaneously in Canada

For general information on our other products and services, please contact our Customer Care Department within the U.S. at 877-762-2974, outside the U.S. at 317-572-3993, or fax 317-572-4002. For technical support, please visit https://hub.wiley.com/community/support/dummies.

Wiley publishes in a variety of print and electronic formats and by print-on-demand. Some material included with standard print versions of this book may not be included in e-books or in print-on-demand. If this book refers to media such as a CD or DVD that is not included in the version you purchased, you may download this material at http://booksupport.wiley.com. For more information about Wiley products, visit www.wiley.com.

Library of Congress Control Number: 2021952569

ISBN 978-1-119-84634-5 (pbk); ISBN 978-1-119-84635-2 (ebk); ISBN 978-1-119-84639-0 (ebk)

SKY10032302_010422

Contents at a Glance

Recipes at a Glance

Breakfasts

Appetizers and Snacks

Salads

Soups

Main Courses

Side Dishes

Sauces and Dressings

Desserts

Beverages

Table of Contents

Introduction

You're intrigued about plant-based eating. You've been hearing about it, and you may be wondering, "How is this different from vegetarianism or veganism? Is this something I can do? How do I do it?" Maybe you've been thinking about how it can benefit your health. This book gives you the road map for a plant-based way of living.

Don't fret and think you have to immediately give up everything you're eating. This book uses a step-by-step approach to transitioning to a plant-based diet by gradually adding more veggies into your diet — not suddenly taking away everything you eat now. That doesn't sound all that bad, does it?

Maybe you're already mostly plant-based, but you're running out of ideas or you don't have the resources, tools, and concepts you need to keep going. Maybe you're feeling undernourished. Whatever your reason for reading this book, we promise that you'll get countless ideas on how to get to know your fruits, veggies, whole grains, beans, nuts, and seeds a whole lot better. These foods will become your friends, not your enemies.

These foods help you succeed at any stage or age in life. Whether you're looking to stay healthy and prevent disease, raising plant-based children, or wondering how to stay plant-based in your golden years, this book gives you a comprehensive look at these phases and provides guidance on how to master them by adopting the most nutritious way of eating.

One of the biggest challenges that people face when deciding to take up a plant-based diet is mental resistance. In fact, maybe you're thinking that it's too difficult or that it's just another diet that won't last or yield the results you're looking for. Eating a plant-based diet isn't a fad or something you do just to lose weight or gain short-term results. This book is about leading a more healthful lifestyle with plants as your fuel. At the end of the day, you need to eat, so let those meals and snacks work for you by providing you with the nutrition, health, and energy you need to live your best life.

We truly believe that with the knowledge found in this book, along with a keen interest in living healthfully, you can discover that eating a plant-based diet isn't difficult and that anyone at any stage can implement a plant-based diet — even you!

About This Book

Part of leading a healthy life is setting general expectations about how you're going to approach and achieve it. This book helps you do exactly that. It provides you with the what, when, where, why, and how to start eating more plant-based foods today.

Of course, as you immerse yourself in this world and learn the basics and beyond of eating plant-based foods, you'll probably start to feel more confident. As you journey through these pages and learn about the ins and outs of eating this way, you'll discover just how easy it is.

This book gives you tools, techniques, tips, and ideas on how to fill your plate every day with plant-based foods to reach your health goals. It gives you an idea of how a plant-based diet benefits your health and what it consists of. It breaks down how much of which foods to eat and where to get your protein. It even explains how to dine out and make healthy choices in unique situations like parties and special events.

The great thing about this book is that we let you know exactly what information is vital and what's nonessential. We've packed the main body with all the stuff we think you really need to know, but you can skip things like sidebars (text in shaded boxes). To tell you the truth, you don't have to read anything you don't want to read, because this book is designed to make every section accessible, regardless of whether you read anything else.

We've also included lots of plant-based recipes that you can start incorporating into your diet as soon as you're ready. Although we've categorized recipes as breakfasts, lunches, dinners, desserts, and so on, if you have a taste for something, pay no mind to the time of day — just eat it! We often eat dinner leftovers for breakfast and breakfast foods at dinnertime!

Within this book, you may note that some web addresses break across two lines of text. If you're reading this book in print and want to visit one of these web pages, simply key in the web address exactly as it's noted in the text, pretending the line break doesn't exist. If you're reading this as an e-book, you've got it easy — just click the web address to be taken directly to the web page.

Foolish Assumptions

We make a few assumptions in this book about you as a reader:

>> You know how to be resourceful to find new information about healthy eating.

>> You're not afraid to try new plant-based foods.

>> You're willing to increase your knowledge about nutrition.

>> You aren't too afraid of what others think about your eating habits.

>> You're eager to try new recipes.

>> You want to take control of your health and you're looking for a new solution that's based on lifestyle, not just diet.

Icons Used in This Book

Look for these familiar *For Dummies* icons to offer visual clues about the kinds of information you're about to read.

TIP

The Tip icon indicates some quick, good advice that's relevant to the topic at hand. Skimming these paragraphs gives you some seriously good information that can help you implement this new diet and make your life just a little easier.

REMEMBER

When you change your diet and lifestyle, there's a lot of information to retain. To make sure that you notice the big stuff, we call it out with the Remember icon. Consider these the "extra-important" paragraphs you want to remember.

WARNING

Read these sections to avoid pitfalls and mistakes that could result in poor health or in ostracizing yourself or others. Figuring out how to eat well involves a lot of detective work to make sure you don't get tricked by confusing labels and powerful marketing. When you see the Warning icon, it means there's something that may lead you to veer off the plant-based path — or endanger your health.

Beyond the Book

In addition to the material in the print or e-book you're reading right now, this product also comes with some access-anywhere goodies on the web. When you want some quick pointers about plant-based eating, simply go to www.dummies.com and type **Plant-Based Cookbook For Dummies Cheat Sheet** in the Search box. You'll find a list of plant-based foods to keep on hand, suggestions for eating plant-based foods at each meal, and a pep talk about how to maintain your new lifestyle.

Where to Go from Here

Each chapter in this book is self-contained, meaning you don't have to read one chapter to understand the next one.

We've organized this book so you can jump in wherever you want, so if you want to skip to the end and read the Part of Tens first, go right ahead. There you can find lots of good information presented in easy-to-digest nuggets.

Suppose you just want to find out about celebrating holidays while on a plant-based diet. If so, head to Chapter 17. Start with Chapter 3 if you want to learn about the macro and micro essential nutrients of a plant-based diet. If you want to cut right to the chase and try some new recipes, head to Chapters 9 through 16. If you're totally new to a plant-based way of eating, start with Chapter 1.

The easiest way to use the book, though, is just to start turning pages and reading the content. Because the true value is in how you apply this information to real life, don't be shy about making notes in the chapters, highlighting information, and putting flags on the pages.

1

Getting Started with a Plant-Based Diet

Discover what eating a plant-based diet means and how to start transforming your diet today.

Find out how eating a plant-based diet can help boost your energy and aid in the fight against diseases like cancer, diabetes, and heart disease.

Get familiar with the different nutrients in a plant-based diet, from protein, carbs, and fats to vitamins and minerals.

Check out the new foods you'll add to your diet, including superfoods and sea vegetables.

Chapter **1**

What Is a Plant-Based Diet?

The goal of a plant-based diet is to eat more plants. Sounds simple enough — or maybe it doesn't. Eating nothing but plant-based foods is intimidating for a lot of people. Most people are comfortable with their current way of eating and are unsure about what to do with plants: Which ones should you eat and when? Can you get full on plants alone? All kinds of questions and concerns come up, and we address some of the common ones in this chapter.

In this chapter, we also give you an overview of life on a plant-based diet and outline what you will and won't eat. We explain how eating this way can benefit so many aspects of your life — mainly your health. At the end of the day, it's all about feeling better, looking better, and just being better, and this way of eating can help you do just that.

What Does Plant-Based Mean?

Eating a plant-based diet simply means the majority of your diet is made up of plants. No matter where you are or what you eat right now, you can eat more plants (everyone can). Of course, our goal and the goal of this book is to get you to eat predominantly (and, ideally, exclusively) plant-based all the time, but you'll likely have a transitional phase, and it starts with eating more of the stuff that the earth has so deliciously and naturally provided.

We get to the "meat" of eating plant-based later in this chapter and explain what this really looks like on your plate on a day-to-day basis, but first we want to compare this approach to some other popular veggie-minded trends.

There are other diets that are similar to the plant-based diet, which focus on different food choices. That doesn't mean you have to label yourself and stick with only one way of eating; these diets include different ways of eating and help you understand what kinds of food choices fall within a certain category. The following breakdown can help you understand how a plant-based diet fits into the bigger picture:

» **Plant-based:** A way of eating based on fruits, vegetables, grains, legumes, nuts, and seeds with few or no animal products. Ideally, a plant-based diet is a vegan diet with a bit of flexibility in the transitional phases, with the goal of becoming 100 percent plant-based over time.

» **Vegan:** A way of eating that doesn't include anything that comes from an animal, be it fish, fowl, mammal, or insect. Vegans refrain from consuming not only animal meats but also any foods made by animals (such as dairy milk and honey). They also abstain from purchasing, wearing, or using animal products of any kind (for example, leather). Veganism is a lifestyle, not just a diet. The vegan way of eating includes the following subsets:

  • **Fruitarian:** A vegan diet that consists mainly of fruit.

  • **Raw vegan:** A vegan diet that is uncooked and often includes dehydrated foods.

» **Vegetarian:** A plant-based diet that may include animal products like dairy and eggs but doesn't include animal meat. The vegetarian diet includes the following subsets:

  • **Lacto-vegetarian:** A vegetarian diet that includes dairy products (for example, milk, cheese, butter, and yogurt) but not eggs.

  • **Ovo-vegetarian:** A vegetarian diet that includes eggs but not dairy.

  • **Lacto-ovo vegetarian:** A vegetarian diet that includes dairy and eggs.

  • **Pescatarian:** A vegetarian diet that includes dairy, eggs, and fish.

» **Flexitarian:** A plant-based diet that includes the occasional consumption of meat or fish.

PLANT-BASED VERSUS WHOLE-FOODS PLANT-BASED

A plant-based diet tends to rely on minimally processed whole foods, but you can find plenty of prepackaged, processed vegan items that aren't necessarily healthy but are technically made from plants and are, therefore, considered plant-based. Items like vegan burgers, vegan sausages, vegan cheese slices or shreds, vegan mayonnaise, vegan butter, and vegan ice cream can mimic the tastes and textures you're familiar with. We don't recommend relying on these foods for the majority of your meals, but they can make the transition to a plant-based diet easier and more convenient. In Part 3, we include a handful of recipes using these plant-based meat and dairy alternatives for those times when you're craving those familiar flavors.

If you choose to follow a whole-foods plant-based diet, on the other hand, you won't be indulging in *any* of those store-bought packaged items. Most people following a whole-foods plant-based diet don't consume oils, refined flours (like all-purpose flour), or refined sugars (like white sugar). A whole-foods plant-based diet is one of the healthiest ways of eating, and we recommend sticking to it the majority of the time. But we don't want you to stress about enjoying a store-bought vegan burger or indulging in a scoop of creamy vegan ice cream on occasion. Just don't make a habit of it.

Getting to the Root of a Plant-Based Diet

A core group of foods makes up a plant–based diet. When you really understand these foods, you have a strong foundation that you can continuously build upon. You'll find so many wonderful foods to explore and try, but in this section, we introduce you to the basics and tell you what foods to avoid.

What's included

The big question is, "If I'm not eating anything from an animal, what is there to eat?" We begin this section by exploring the wonderful plants that we hope you get to know quite well on this journey. You'll find all sorts of diverse foods to enjoy. If you're new to this way of eating, prepare to be pleasantly surprised by what you find!

Valuable vegetables

You'll discover a whole array of veggies that you'll likely get to know quite well while eating plant–based. If you're new to this diet, you'll probably stick to tried-and-true, familiar veggies in the beginning because they'll feel safe — and that's okay! But over time, we encourage you to expand into new areas and pick up that funny-looking squash or try that wild, leafy bunch of something. You'll find a vibrant world of valuable vegetables, but for now, here's our starter kit:

>> Beets

>> Carrots

>> Herbs, including basil and parsley

>> Kale

>> Peppers

>> Spinach

>> Squash

>> Sweet potatoes

Fantastic fruits

Ahhh, the sweet juiciness of fresh fruit. We all love it! If you don't, you need to get on this train, because fruits are delicious; sweet; full of fiber, color, and wonderful vitamins; and so, so good for you. Throughout this book, we encourage you to try new ones, but here are some of our top picks to start with:

>> Apples

>> Avocados

>> Bananas

>> Blueberries

>> Coconuts

>> Mangos

>> Pears

>> Pineapples

>> Raspberries

>> Strawberries

Wonderful whole grains

Consuming good-quality whole grains is a healthy part of a plant-based diet. Don't worry — you can still have your breads and pastas, but *whole* is the key word here. You don't want refined or processed — you want the real thing. When you buy these items, make sure the grain itself is the only ingredient. Although it's possible to buy proper whole grains off the shelf in packaging, double-check the label to confirm that it is, indeed, a whole grain (and only a whole grain). Here are some of our favorites (more in Chapter 3):

>> Brown rice

>> Quinoa (technically a seed, but classified as a grain)

>> Rolled oats

>> Sprouted-grain spelt bread

Lovable legumes

Learning to love beans on a plant-based diet is key, because they're a great source of sustenance, protein, and fuel. It may take you and your body a little while to get used to them, but soon enough, they'll be your friends — especially when you discover how great it is to eat them in soups, salads, burgers, and more. Here are some of the best to start with:

>> Black beans

>> Chickpeas

>> Edamame

>> Kidney beans

>> Lentils

>> Split peas

>> Tempeh

>> Tofu

Notable nuts and seeds

Most people love a good handful of nuts! But the thing about eating them on a plant-based diet is making sure that they're unsalted, unoiled, and raw. As long as you enjoy them in their natural state, feel free to eat them in moderation along-side your other wonderful plant-based foods. Here are the best ones to start with:

- » Almonds
- » Cashews
- » Chia seeds
- » Flaxseeds
- » Hempseeds
- » Pumpkin seeds
- » Sunflower seeds
- » Walnuts

TIP

Try munching on a few nuts or seeds straight up or adding them to salads or other recipes. And if you can't decide which one you have a taste for, toss them all in a trail mix!

The extras

This group of foods isn't really a category per se, but these foods are still part of a plant-based diet. This group includes such things as exotic superfoods, sea vegetables (see Chapter 4), condiments, and natural sweeteners. The following are some specific examples:

- » **Cacao:** The pure form of chocolate.
- » **Honey:** The raw stuff, not the kind in bear-shaped plastic bottles. If you're a vegan, you'll have to skip the honey.
- » **Maple syrup:** Again, the real stuff — no pancake syrup here!
- » **Nori:** A delicious and nutritious sea vegetable.
- » **Nutritional yeast:** A deactivated yeast that has a savory, mildly nutty flavor. It's an excellent source of vitamins, minerals, and high-quality plant protein.
- » **Tamari:** A versatile fermented soy sauce.

What's off limits

As you can imagine, all things that aren't plants are off limits; however, as we mentioned earlier, you may need or want a transitional period during which you wean yourself off these foods one at a time until you can avoid all things from the animal world — including meat, poultry, fish, eggs, milk, and other dairy products.

Of course, this is the ideal — you have to find your own place on the spectrum of plant-based eating and do what works for you. Often, making something off limits just makes you want it more, so you have to strike a balance between being tough on yourself and being practical.

Common Questions and Answers about a Plant-Based Diet

As with anything new, considering a plant-based diet can bring up all sorts of questions and concerns. This book most likely addresses pretty much everything that has you worried. But to nip the fretting in the bud, here are five of the most common questions about a plant-based diet.

Can I get full eating only plants?

Absolutely! The wonderful thing about eating plants is that you're eating lots of fiber, and fiber makes you full! Also, the more wholesome the plants are (in other words, not processed), the more nutrients you're eating, which helps make you feel more satisfied. As the nutrients load your cells with vitamins and minerals, this helps make you feel pleasantly full, but not stuffed.

Also, the diversity of texture can help make you feel full. Because so many plant foods require you to chew more, you actually spend more time getting through the meal. So, a big bowl of salad with lots of stuff in it may not seem that heavy, but it can fill you up quite fast. We promise, after trying just a few recipes in this book, you'll be quite full!

In the beginning, fiber will not be your friend. When you first introduce all the roughage, skins, seeds, and other textures of plants, your gut may have a not-so-fun time getting used to it all. Stick it out. You may feel gassy, bloated, or just "full" all the time, but your gut needs to get used to your increased fiber intake and figure out how to pass these new foods along. When it starts working properly, you'll find that you depend on natural fiber from whole foods, not store-bought powders, to keep you going every day.

Because fiber draws water out of your body, drink lots of water when you eat fibrous foods to help it move through your body.

How will I get protein?

This is always the big question. Well, we have a big answer: from so many different places! A plant-based diet has so much protein, you may not even believe it. Although it may not seem like the grams of protein add up to the amount of protein you find in meat, what you soon realize is that it's not about the quantity but the quality. The standard American diet often provides too much protein, which can contribute to many chronic illnesses. Plant-based protein sources like legumes, nuts, seeds, quinoa, tempeh, avocado, and green leafy veggies all have their own breakdown of amino acids, which build up inside your body to make a complete protein. The best part is, they absorb into your body much better than animal-based protein. You won't feel that same heaviness eating plant-based protein.

What about calcium?

What about calcium, you ask? Well, did you know that plant-based foods like sesame seeds, hempseeds, bok choy, carob, and figs are extremely rich in calcium? Almost more so than a glass of dairy milk. We know this may be hard to wrap your head around, but it's actually proven in most cultures that the less dairy is consumed, the more calcium is absorbed by the body.

WARNING

Oxalates in some foods can bind to minerals like calcium in the gut and decrease their absorption. This can also lead to a possible increased risk of kidney stones. If you have a history of kidney stones, speak with your doctor about whether a low-oxalate diet is necessary. However, most healthy individuals can consume oxalate-rich foods without issue, and, in fact, avoiding them means you could be missing out on many of their health benefits.

So, fret not — just because you have "grown-ups" thinking you need a glass of milk to get your daily dose of calcium, that doesn't mean the so-called experts are right. Turns out, you can eat almonds, seeds, and greens and get the same amount of calcium in your body. You won't feel bloated, either, because these sources of calcium are loaded with vitamins and minerals, making the nutrients much easier to absorb.

How do I get iron? Won't I become anemic?

Iron is definitely an area of concern for anyone not eating meat, so you need to be a bit more cautious to make sure you're consuming enough plant-based sources of iron, such as the following:

» Dark leafy greens

» Dried fruit

>> Legumes

>> Nuts

>> Seaweeds

>> Seeds

If you still feel like you aren't getting enough, you may want to consider taking a good-quality, plant-based iron supplement — even just for a short period of time to boost your stores. It's a good idea to have your iron levels checked regularly by your doctor to make sure they're where they need to be.

Many people — even athletes — survive and even thrive without meat!

Does eating a plant-based diet help people lose weight?

We're adamant that people should never choose to eat a specific way solely for weight loss. This can lead to calorie restricting, which can deprive your body of essential nutrients and slow down your metabolism.

The good news is that by following a whole-food plant-based, healthy lifestyle, you're more likely to feel great and lose weight naturally. When you focus on eating well-balanced and nutrient-dense meals for fuel, your body isn't deprived, and it starts to function efficiently. Deprivation is not an option.

A Quick Guide to Making a Plant-Based Diet Part of Your Everyday Life

You can start with simple ways to make the transition to eating plant-based foods. Here are a few suggestions to help you get started today:

>> **Replace one to three meals a week with plant-based ones.** Use some of the recipes in this book (flip to Part 3) or search for others that appeal to your palate.

>> **Include healthy meat alternatives in place of meat in your meals.** Try beans, legumes, nuts, and fermented soy.

>> **Choose healthy alternatives to dairy.** For example, instead of dairy milk, try rice milk, almond milk, or hempseed milk; instead of cheese, try avocados and cashews.

>> **Explore new vegetables.** Go beyond your usual suspects and experiment with new colors and different green leafy vegetables.

>> **Have a smoothie for breakfast.** Swap out bacon and eggs for a nutritious blended fruit smoothie to get you going in the morning.

>> **Pack power snacks.** Don't lurk around the vending machines, which are filled with non-plant-based ingredients. Instead, bring trail mix (nuts, seeds, and dried fruit) to work, or keep a small container of it handy at all times.

>> **Make a simple veggie dinner at least one night a week.** If you're just getting started, change up at least one of your meat-centered meals to something plant-based yet familiar, like a vegetable stir-fry, hearty soup, or pasta.

FIVE CONVENIENT AND VERSATILE STORE-BOUGHT PROTEIN OPTIONS

As we mention earlier, store-bought packaged items should be used sparingly. Consider them a treat, not something to consume every day or even every week. Different brands have slightly different textures and tastes, so experiment to find which ones you like best. Here are some options to try:

- **Vegan ground "meat":** Use just as you would animal-based ground meat. Try our recipe for Vegan Sloppy Joes (see Chapter 12).

- **Vegan burgers:** These are ready to pan-fry or grill. Top them off with your favorite burger toppings, and you won't know the difference. Try our recipe for Vegan Burgers with Apricot Jalapeño Jam (see Chapter 12).

- **Vegan sausages:** Italian, hot, brats, breakfast . . . there is no shortage of vegan sausages on the market today. Try our Vegan Sausage and Roasted Vegetables Sheet-Pan Meal (see Chapter 12).

- **Vegan cheese slices:** For those times when you just need something cheesy! Try our recipe for Pickled Onion Pesto Grilled Cheese (see Chapter 11).

- **Vegan mayonnaise:** Sometimes you just can't beat the creamy, tangy flavor of mayo. Try our recipe for Coleslaw Pasta Salad (see Chapter 10).

» Managing weight, staying energized, and sleeping well on a plant-based diet

» Preventing and treating diseases with plant-based foods

Chapter **2**

Seeing the Benefits of a Plant-Based Diet

The plant-based diet isn't just about food — it's a framework for your well-being. Think of it as preventive health care. The money and time you invest now to better yourself through your diet pays off in leaps and bounds both sooner *and* later. How? So glad you asked. This chapter outlines the benefits of following a plant-based diet, from getting a better night's sleep to managing your weight management and fighting disease. When you opt to transition to a plant-based diet, you make not only a positive lifestyle choice but also a smart health choice.

Eating According to a Plant-Based Food Guide

We've all seen some version of a food guide — a graphic representation of food categories divided into segments. The more space a food group takes up, the more of it we're supposed to eat in order to maintain a healthy diet. Many traditional food guides include meat or protein, fruit, vegetable, grain, and dairy categories. Vegetarian food guides are also available to help guide your dietary choices.

This way of grouping foods to provide a one-size-fits-all way of eating is not necessarily ideal for or relevant to everyone. Our goal is to encourage you to take all food guides in stride. How much you eat and what you choose to eat need to apply directly to you and your lifestyle, activity level, and health concerns.

The guidelines in this book follow a plant-based food guide. The plan can be adjusted in cases of disease or food sensitivities, but for the most part this is an excellent foundation for superior health. Here's how this breakdown looks on a daily basis:

>> **Fruits and vegetables**

- These should make up most of your overall food intake, approximately 40 percent to 60 percent, with an emphasis on leafy green veggies.

- Include at least five servings of vegetables, focusing on a mixture of leafy greens and cruciferous vegetables and starchy, colorful veggies, such as beets, carrots, or sweet potatoes.

- Focus on fresh vegetables first, but frozen vegetables are also healthy and can be convenient in a pinch.

REMEMBER

Many frozen vegetables are even *more* nutritious than fresh vegetables because they're frozen at their peak ripeness, which means they maintain their nutrients.

- Include sea vegetables, such as arame, dulse, and nori (see Chapter 4 for more information on sea vegetables).

- Have at least one to two servings of fresh fruit, preferably in season and organic.

>> **Whole grains**

- Eat two to five servings.

- Focus on whole grains, such as brown rice, buckwheat, millet, quinoa, and rolled oats.

- Choose alternatives to whole wheat (such as barley, kamut, oats, spelt, and rye) when you can for variety.

- Choose sprouted-grain products as often as you can.

>> **Legumes**

- Have two to three servings.

- Choose from beans, lentils, tempeh, and tofu.

Protein supplements aren't usually necessary to get enough protein on a plant-based diet because plant protein is abundant from many sources, such as fruits, nuts, seeds, vegetables, and whole grains. So, be careful not to consume too much protein. Focus on the quality of the protein you get, not the quantity.

>> **Fats and oils**

- Eat two to three servings of healthy fats per day, depending on your calorie goals.

- Eat one serving (approximately ½ cup) of nuts or seeds.

- Have 1 to 2 tablespoons of nut or seed butters.

- Enjoy one or more servings of whole fatty fruits, such as avocados, coconuts, and olives. This can be in the form of ¼ avocado, ¼ to ½ cup fresh coconut meat, or four olives.

- Use 1 tablespoon of oil for cooking or in salads. Chia seed, coconut, flaxseed, grapeseed, hempseed, and olive oil work great for salads. Don't cook with chia seed, flaxseed, or hempseed oil, though — these oils should be used only with foods that don't require heating.

If your goal is weight loss, be mindful of the caloric density of oils. You may choose not to use these at all.

These are just general guidelines and suggestions to help get you started with your new plant-based lifestyle. As you become accustomed to these guidelines, adapt them to what works best for you.

We don't get too caught up in exact amounts or measurements of food or servings. We believe that as long as you're eating a well-rounded and balanced diet, your body will get what it needs. It's important to follow some general guidelines to get started, but in time you'll start to trust yourself because your body knows best.

Feeling Good with Food

Although it sounds simple, feeling good is really important. When you don't feel good, all other aspects of your life get out of balance — you can't be your optimal self, either personally or professionally. Luckily, you have an ace up your sleeve: proper nutrition. You have control over your diet every day, and you can choose what goes into your mouth. Choosing a plant-based diet can be extremely powerful in your quest to stay healthy. You may find that after you make the switch to this diet, you'll start to feel better, lose weight, have more energy, and sleep better. The following sections detail these benefits of a plant-based diet.

Managing your weight

Changing over from animal foods to plant foods means you consume far less saturated fat and fewer dense, low-nutrient calories that can lead to weight gain. The calories and nutrients that come from plant-based foods do so much more for you in terms of helping with metabolism and many functions in the body. By eating more fiber and nutrient-dense foods, you generally don't eat as much in one sitting. This may encourage you to eat more frequent meals, which is incredible for weight loss. Meat and dairy products are heavy and filled with saturated fat, and they pack on the calories. A plant-based diet is lean and efficient, preventing you from taking in food that just turns into fat.

People sometimes get hung up on the fact that following a plant-based diet means consuming more carbohydrates. That may be true, but it doesn't necessarily mean you'll gain weight. The key is to choose carbs that are high in fiber and have lots of other nutrients. Your body will digest them well and use them for energy. You gain weight from carbs when you eat beyond your needs or you eat simple carbohydrates, like refined sugar and refined grains.

TIP

When eating a plant-based diet, be sure to choose complex carbs (such as apples, quinoa, rolled oats, and sweet potatoes) that are rich in vitamins, minerals, and protein, and enjoy them in moderation. Stay away from simple carbs (such as sugars, as well as breads and pastas made with refined grains). If you follow those general guidelines, you can still reach your weight goals.

Having energy and vitality

Within days of consuming more green leafy veggies and fruits, you'll feel more energized. This is a result of the water content of these foods, which hydrates your body, providing your cells with more oxygen (as compared to meat), and it's also because of the life force running through these foods. They're filled with vitamins and minerals that go directly into your blood system, helping your body detoxify and rejuvenate itself. Heavy animal-based foods, such as meat and dairy, can weigh you down, decrease your energy, and make you tired. Plant-based foods are lighter and better for digestion.

Getting better sleep

When you eat better, you sleep better. We know this sounds too simple to be true, but it is. Consider this: When you nourish your body during the day with regular plant-based meals, you may find, in time, that the quality of your sleep is better. Many plant foods, such as green leafy vegetables, which are rich in magnesium and calcium, can help the body relax for a peaceful sleep. Other plant foods, such as whole grains, which are full of fiber, help the body produce serotonin, which has a calming effect. Eating a plant-based diet doesn't necessarily mean you get more sleep — just better sleep. In fact, you may find that you need *less* sleep.

In addition to increased energy, better sleep can lead to a decreased risk of cardiovascular disease as well.

TIP

If you have problems sleeping, try having a banana, some oatmeal, or some almond butter on toast. These foods tend to help the body and the nervous system relax at night by causing the body to release the hormones required for a restful sleep. You can also try drinking herbal tea, such as chamomile, kava root, or valerian root, because it has a sedative effect on the body and can aid in falling asleep.

Becoming a Wellness Warrior

By committing to a plant-based diet, you become a warrior of your own wellness. A plant-based diet may help to prevent many diseases. Common diseases like cancer, diabetes, heart disease, and osteoporosis have all been known to be lessened or even reversed with a high-quality plant-based diet that is rich in fiber, phytonutrients, and protein.

The following sections explain how to prevent, minimize, or eliminate certain health conditions by following a plant-based diet. However, be sure to talk to your doctor or health-care practitioner before making any significant dietary changes.

Cancer

Plant-based diets are effective against cancer because they're jam-packed with *phytonutrients* — the chemicals in plants that help prevent disease and infection. The more phytonutrients you eat, the better you feel, and the more you help yourself beat the odds of cancer.

If you want to prevent or fight cancer, focus on a diet that is rich in

>> **Colorful fruits and vegetables,** such as blueberries, cucumbers, grapes, mangos, squash, and tomatoes

>> **Green leafy vegetables,** such as bok choy, collards, kale, and Swiss chard

>> **Whole grains,** such as amaranth, brown rice, millet, and quinoa

>> **Legumes,** such as lentils, mung beans, and split peas

>> **A variety of healthy nuts and seeds,** such as almonds, pumpkin seeds, and sunflower seeds

Diabetes

Diabetes is becoming one of the leading diseases and causes of death in North America. With fast food, sugary snacks, and soda pop at our fingertips, it's no wonder that this blood sugar disorder has become so prevalent. Before you inject yourself with insulin or go on medication, understand that a plant-based diet has been known to dramatically shift and even reverse type 2 diabetes. For the most part, people living with type 2 diabetes can control their disorder through their food choices.

Those living with type 1 diabetes will never eliminate their need for insulin. However, by adopting a plant-based lifestyle, they may be able to keep their insulin doses to a minimum and reduce the risk of complications.

Type 2 diabetes occurs when the pancreas doesn't produce enough insulin or the body doesn't properly use the insulin it makes. As a result, glucose (sugar) builds up in the blood instead of being used for energy.

Here's a quick rundown of plant-based foods that have special properties for maintaining a healthy blood sugar level:

>> **Avocado** contains a sugar that depresses insulin production, which makes it an excellent choice for people with hypoglycemia (low blood sugar). Try adding some slices of avocado to a piece of toast, blend it into a smoothie, or toss it in a salad. Guacamole is delicious, too (see Chapter 14 for a great recipe). Ideally eat ¼ of an avocado several times per week.

>> **Soybeans and other legumes,** such as black-eyed peas, chickpeas, kidney beans, lentils, and lima beans, slow the rate of absorption of carbohydrates into the bloodstream because of their high protein and fiber content. Ultimately, this can reduce spikes in blood sugar. Try making a dip with different kinds of beans or tossing them into a salad. They even make great veggie burgers (see the recipe in Chapter 12). Eat at least ½ to 1 cup of legumes a day.

>> **Other blood-sugar-controlling foods** include berries (especially blueberries), celery, chia seeds, cucumbers, green leafy vegetables, ground flaxseeds, lemons, oat bran, parsley, psyllium, radishes, sauerkraut, sprouts, squash, string beans, sunflower seeds, and watercress. Many of these items can be combined into a smoothie, breakfast cereal, or colorful salad or grain dish.

TIP

Beyond knowing *what* foods are good to eat, knowing *how* and *when* to eat them can be vital in keeping your diabetes in check. Here are some additional tips for naturally regulating your blood sugar levels with plants:

» **Eat a balanced plant-based breakfast every day.** It helps kick your metabolism into gear, which is needed for proper sugar and insulin processing.

» **Don't go more than two hours without food.** Eat six to eight small meals throughout the day. Even eating a small snack before bed may help. Eating more frequently helps keep blood sugar levels in balance. You don't want to consume large, heavy meals because they can be hard for the body to digest. Plus, excess food means excess calories, which can increase blood sugar levels in the body and cause weight gain.

» **Eat a diet high in fiber.** Fiber doesn't raise blood sugar levels, and it helps with digestion and elimination. Choose whole grains and legumes, and include large amounts of vegetables, especially dark leafy greens, green beans, squash, sweet potatoes, tofu, and whole fresh fruits.

» **Use natural low-glycemic sweeteners, such as stevia or monk fruit — but only infrequently and in very small amounts.** These sweeteners have a low impact on blood sugar levels and don't cause them to spike as much as white sugar, which should be avoided completely.

» **Stay away from highly fatty and fried foods.** They typically contain excess processed oils, which are highly inflammatory, increase caloric intake, and can inhibit proper functioning of insulin and glucose regulation. Instead, choose healthy fats, oils (avocado, coconut oil, olive oil, or other cold-pressed natural oils), raw nuts, and seeds.

» **Skip alcohol, processed foods, saturated fats, soft drinks, table salt, white flour, white sugar, and foods with artificial colors and preservatives.** These foods are extremely refined and have little to no nutritional value. They can contribute not only to an increase in sugar intake but also to weight gain because these are all forms of empty calories. People with diabetes should focus on foods that are rich in vitamins, minerals, and nutrients and are beneficial to their blood sugar levels and overall well-being.

Gastrointestinal illnesses

Plant-based eating can help with a wide variety of gastrointestinal conditions. A diet high in fiber, vitamins, and minerals can help prevent the onset and progression of these common diseases.

» **Acid reflux:** In this condition, some of the acid content of the stomach flows up into the esophagus. Eating more plants reduces acid levels by decreasing or eliminating animal protein (which is more difficult to digest) from the diet.

A plant-based diet also improves elimination of waste from the body by increasing fiber intake and removing foods that may cause an increase in acid levels in the stomach. The more veggies in your diet, the less inflammation of the upper digestive tract you get because plants (especially green ones) neutralize acid levels.

>> **Celiac disease:** Celiac disease is an autoimmune disorder of the small intestine that occurs in genetically predisposed people of all ages. It's associated with pain and discomfort in the digestive tract. Consuming plants and gluten-free grains can help someone with celiac disease prevent flare-ups, discomfort, and bloating. When you eliminate gluten from your diet, it's essential to find substitutes and alternative grains that are healing. Eliminating milk products and meat — which are inflammatory — is also critical for intestinal healing. Plant foods are also rich in enzymes that aid digestion — an extra bonus for people with celiac disease.

>> **Irritable bowel syndrome (IBS) and inflammatory bowel disease (IBD):** IBS is characterized by chronic abdominal pain, discomfort, bloating, and alteration of bowel habits. IBD is a group of inflammatory conditions of the colon and small intestine. Plant-based eating can be healing to the bowels. It can help stabilize blood sugar, thus promoting stable insulin levels and lowering inflammation. It allows for a more balanced intake of essential fatty acids (more omega-3s and omega-9s than omega-6s), which decreases inflammation in the body. Increased fiber in a plant-based diet improves elimination of wastes from the body, which promotes the flushing of harmful toxins. Plant-based eating is often alkalinizing (as opposed to dairy, grains, meats, and sugar, which are acid-forming), which also helps lower inflammation and creates an environment in which harmful bacteria starve and beneficial bacteria thrive.

Heart disease and high blood pressure

When it comes to heart health, a plant-based diet is really the only way to go. Animal-based foods contain fat and cholesterol that build up in arteries, causing high blood pressure. Worse, you need to avoid them if you're at risk for or have heart disease. Luckily, plenty of plant-based foods can provide your heart with maximum nutrition. These foods are all from whole sources. A diet rich in these foods not only helps your heart but also promotes an overall state of optimal health and well-being. Tables 2-1, 2-2, and 2-3 outline foods that are especially beneficial for your heart.

TABLE 2-1   # Heart-Friendly Proteins, Grains, Nuts, and Seeds

Food	Vitamins and Minerals	Ways to Enjoy
Almonds	Fiber, heart-favorable mono- and polyunsaturated fats, magnesium, omega-3 fatty acids, phytosterols, and vitamin E	Mix a few raw organic almonds into coconut milk yogurt, trail mix, or fruit salads.
Black beans or kidney beans	B-complex vitamins, calcium, folate, magnesium, niacin, omega-3 fatty acids, and soluble fiber	Stir some beans into your next soup or salad.
Brown rice and quinoa	B-complex vitamins, fiber, magnesium, and niacin	Cook up a pot and make pilafs or soups, or top with a colorful vegetable stir-fry.
Flaxseeds (ground)	Fiber, omega-3 fatty acids, and phytoestrogens	Hide ground flaxseeds in all sorts of foods — coconut yogurt parfaits, cereal, homemade muffins, or cookies.
Oats	Calcium, folate, magnesium, niacin, omega-3 fatty acids, potassium, and soluble fiber	Top hot oatmeal with fresh berries for a heart-healthy breakfast. Oatmeal and raisin cookies also make a hearty treat.
Pumpkin seeds	B-complex vitamins, calcium, iron, omega-3 fatty acids, phosphorus, protein, vitamin A, and zinc	Eat them raw in trail mixes, salads, and granola, or toast them lightly for an extra boost of flavor.
Tofu and tempeh	Calcium, folate, niacin, magnesium, and potassium	Thinly slice firm tofu or tempeh and marinate for several hours before baking, grilling, or stir-frying.
Walnuts	Fiber, folate, heart-favorable mono- and polyunsaturated fats, magnesium, omega-3 fatty acids, phytosterols, and vitamin E	Add them to salads, pastas, cookies, muffins, and pancakes for a flavorful crunch.

TABLE 2-2   # Heart-Friendly Vegetables

Food	Vitamins and Minerals	Ways to Enjoy
Acorn squash	B-complex vitamins, beta-carotene, calcium, fiber, folate, lutein, magnesium, potassium, and vitamin C	Serve with sautéed spinach, pine nuts, or raisins.
Asparagus	B-complex vitamins, beta-carotene, and folate, and lutein	Grill or roast, then dress with lemon.
Beets	B-complex vitamins, calcium, iron, magnesium, phosphorous, and vitamins A and C	Shred some raw into salad or roast and cut into slices.
Broccoli	Beta-carotene, calcium, fiber, folate, potassium, and vitamins C and E	Chop fresh broccoli and add it to soup or dip into hummus.

(continued)

TABLE 2-2 *(continued)*

Food	Vitamins and Minerals	Ways to Enjoy
Carrots	Alpha-carotene and fiber	Cut into snack-size pieces to munch on. Use in recipes such as stir-fries, salads, and soups, or sneak shredded carrots into spaghetti sauce or muffin batter.
Red bell peppers	B-complex vitamins, beta-carotene, lutein, fiber, folate, and potassium	Grill or oven-roast until tender. Delicious in wraps, salads, and sandwiches.
Spinach	B-complex vitamins, calcium, fiber, folate, lutein, magnesium, and potassium	Choose spinach over lettuce for nutrient-packed salads and sandwiches. Tastes great when added to cooked dishes.
Sweet potato or butternut squash	Beta-carotene; fiber; and vitamins A, C, and E	Steam in a steamer basket, bake, roast in oven, or boil in a pot of soup.
Tomatoes	Alpha-carotene, beta-carotene, fiber, folate, lutein, lycopene, potassium, and vitamin C	Try fresh tomatoes on sandwiches, salads, pastas, and pizzas.

TABLE 2-3   **Heart-Friendly Fruits**

Food	Vitamins and Minerals	Ways to Enjoy
Blackberries, blueberries, cranberries, raspberries, and strawberries	Anthocyanin, beta-carotene, calcium, ellagic acid, fiber, folate, lutein, magnesium, potassium, and vitamin C	Add to trail mixes, muffins, and salads.
Cantaloupe	Alpha-carotene, B-complex vitamins, beta-carotene, fiber, folate, lutein, potassium, and vitamin C	A fragrant, ripe cantaloupe is perfect for breakfast, lunch, or potluck dinners. Simply cut and enjoy.
Dark chocolate	Cocoa phenols and resveratrol	A square of dark cocoa is great for blood pressure, but choose varieties that have 70 percent or higher cocoa content.
Oranges	Alpha-carotene, beta-carotene, beta-cryptoxanthin, fiber, flavones, folate, lutein, potassium, and vitamin C	Make your own orange juice with freshly squeezed organic oranges. Use the zest in marinades, chutneys, and salad dressing. You can even use it in baking.
Papaya	Beta-carotene, beta-cryptoxanthin, calcium, folate, lutein, magnesium, potassium, and vitamins C and E	Mix papaya, pineapple, scallions, garlic, fresh lime juice, salt, and black pepper.

Osteoporosis

Osteoporosis is the deterioration of bone mass in the body. This condition can happen as a result of aging, lifestyle, and diet. Many people have grown up thinking that a glass of milk will prevent osteoporosis. Although the dairy industry wants you to believe that, overall health is improved when getting calcium from plant sources (specifically dark leafy greens and seeds) in your diet. Be sure to get plenty of vitamin D in order for your body to absorb the calcium.

WARNING

Dairy foods are rather acidic, and consuming large amounts can leach calcium from your bones, causing bones to break down instead of building up. Plant foods, on the other hand, are rich in calcium and magnesium and directly nourish the bones, giving them the minerals they need to thrive and help prevent breakdown.

Plant-based foods provide your body with calcium while tasting delicious. There is no need to worry about exact measurements of calcium when you're getting it from whole-food sources. Just be sure to get a variety of items in your diet on a daily basis, and you'll be loaded with the right kind of calcium that your body will love.

TOP NUTRIENTS FOR YOUR HEART

You may know which nutrients are good for your cardiovascular health, but you may not know *why* they're good. Here's a quick rundown of the most commonly mentioned heart-healthy nutrients and what good they do for you:

- **B-complex vitamins:** Help reduce plaque buildup in the heart.
- **Folate or folic acid:** Helps reduce and prevent hardening of arterial walls.
- **L-arginine:** Helps rid the body of ammonia and helps release insulin. It's also used to make nitric oxide, which is a compound that helps relax blood vessels.
- **Magnesium and calcium:** Help regulate electrical impulses of the heart, lowering cholesterol and blood pressure.
- **Omega-3 fatty acids:** Has anti-inflammatory properties and helps strengthen heart tissue.
- **Potassium:** Helps the heart pump and move blood through the body by pushing sodium out of the system and relaxing blood vessel walls, thereby lowering blood pressure.
- **Vitamins A, C, and E:** Help with overall cardiovascular health.

Top bone-building foods include the following:

>> Beans and legumes (peas and lentils)

>> Beet greens

>> Bok choy

>> Carob

>> Collards

>> Hempseeds

>> Kale

>> Sesame seeds

See Chapter 3 for more sources of calcium-rich plant-based foods.

The news that your calcium intake doesn't have to come from dairy may be difficult to digest, because most people believe that dairy is the only source of calcium. However, from our perspective, the foods you need to focus on are ones that not only give your body its calcium requirements, but also are easy to digest and allow your body to soak up many other beneficial minerals and nutrients.

Other conditions that benefit from a plant-based diet

The nutrients available in plant-based foods can drastically improve your health, no matter which disease you're suffering from or trying to prevent. Plants are nature's medicine! In case you need more convincing, here are some other chronic conditions that benefit from a plant-based diet.

Alzheimer's disease

Glial cells, which provide support and protection for neurons in your brain and parasympathetic nervous system, are believed to help remove debris and toxins from the brain that can contribute to Alzheimer's disease. For example, accumulation of aluminum in the body has been linked with the development of Alzheimer's disease.

Many plant-based foods, especially those that are rich in antioxidants, such as green tea and dark berries, may help protect glial cells from damage. When glial cells are damaged, they lose their ability to function properly, which can affect brain function. Additionally, the increased fiber intake in a plant-based diet helps rid the body of toxins via elimination of wastes. Increased consumption of heavy-metal *chelators* (foods that help remove toxins from the body, such as chlorella, cilantro, and parsley) also helps to remove aluminum from the body.

Autoimmune diseases

An autoimmune disease is a condition in which a person's immune system attacks itself. This class of diseases includes many different disorders that bring on a variety of symptoms. Some common autoimmune diseases include

>> **Graves' disease:** A hyperthyroid condition that causes the thyroid to enlarge to twice its size

>> **Multiple sclerosis:** An inflammatory disease in which the insulating covers of nerve cells in the brain and spinal cord are damaged

>> **Rheumatoid arthritis:** An inflammatory disorder that affects tissues, organs, and joints

>> **Vitiligo:** A condition that causes skin depigmentation

For people with autoimmune diseases, plant-based foods can help minimize symptoms, boost energy, prevent the development of other diseases, and stop the disease from progressing any further. Meat and dairy have been known to have negative effects on people living with autoimmune diseases because they can aggravate the condition, so simply removing such foods from your diet and switching to plant foods can be very helpful.

Gout

Gout is characterized by sudden, severe attacks of pain, redness, and tenderness in joints, often the joint at the base of the big toe. Obesity, unstable blood sugar, and — yes — a meat-based diet can increase the risk of developing gout. To combat it, eat fresh veggies, whole grains, nuts, seeds, and healthy fats. Plant-based eating aids blood sugar management, helping you keep gout at bay. Because you fill up on whole foods, you have fewer cravings for and less dependence on refined grains and sugars and processed foods.

WARNING

When treating gout, limit your consumption of dried beans and lentils. These items are high in purines, which can increase the levels of uric acid in the body. Gout results from a buildup of uric acid.

PLANTS BENEFIT OUR PLANET, TOO

Because the planet is made up mostly of plants and the elements, the choice to eat a plant-based diet has a direct positive impact on the environment.

The resources used in the meat and dairy industries negatively affect the quality of soil and water, the welfare of animals, and, of course, our health. A 2006 United Nations report revealed that the livestock sector accounts for the creation of 18 percent of all greenhouse gases, more than the entire transportation sector combined.

The cost of meat isn't entirely reflected by the price you pay at the checkout stand; the real price goes all the way back to how animals are handled on the land — and how the land itself is handled, including the water resources used for industrial livestock farming and in processing facilities. Add transportation costs, packaging, and advertising, and the cost really starts climbing.

By making the choice to eat less meat and more plant-based foods, you're helping the land, the animals, and your health.

Chapter **3**

The Macro and Micro Essentials of a Plant-Based Diet

The food you consume is composed of chemical compounds that are divided into two main categories: macronutrients and micronutrients. *Macronutrients* are the compounds you consume in the largest quantities, and they include protein, carbohydrates, and fat. *Micronutrients*, on the other hand, are nutrients required in small quantities to orchestrate a range of physiological functions; they include vitamins and minerals. This chapter details what macronutrients and micronutrients are and where to find them; it also mentions some you should stay away from.

Making the Most of Macronutrients

The macronutrient category is the catch-all for protein, carbohydrates, and fats. These nutrients are the main building blocks you require from your diet to help you thrive, feel satisfied, have enough energy, and build muscle and overall health.

If you're missing any one of these major categories, it can set you up for cravings, malnourishment, chronic illness, and an overall yearning to stock up on what your body is missing.

WARNING

Sometimes people overcompensate by overconsuming a particular macronutrient when one is missing. For example, consuming a high-protein diet when you're missing carbs can be dangerous. Eating a lot of protein isn't necessarily better; the body needs a healthy ratio of all three macronutrients to thrive and survive.

Pondering protein in the plant-based world

Protein. You eat a lot of it so you can get big muscles, right? But wait, can you only get enough protein if you eat meat? Most people think they understand protein and that it's pretty straightforward. The truth is, there's a lot more to know about this macronutrient than you may realize.

Protein is the major building block the body uses to produce things like muscles, hair, and nails and to help with growth and regeneration of tissue. Plus, it's essential to pretty much all major functions of the body. Without it, your body would totally break down.

There are two types of proteins:

>> **Complete:** To be considered complete, a protein must comprise all nine *essential amino acids* (the molecules that combine to form protein). Essential amino acids are those that your body can't produce and that you must get from your diet. We list some great plant-based complete proteins in the "Examining plant proteins" section, later in this chapter.

>> **Incomplete:** Proteins that are low in some essential amino acids are considered incomplete. But the good news is that if you eat a variety of incomplete plant-protein foods together, they act as a complete protein — for example, brown rice and chickpeas or almond butter on toast. Even better news is that these foods don't have to be eaten in the same day — the body has an amino-acid bank that accumulates over a couple days, after which it combines and assembles the single amino acids to make complete proteins.

Understanding what a healthy body requires

As the World Health Organization (WHO) has researched this topic, it has discovered that people need less protein than previously thought. The U.S. Department of Agriculture (USDA) Recommended Dietary Allowance (RDA) recommends that 10 percent to 35 percent of calories come from protein. Dr. T. Colin Campbell, who has a PhD in nutrition and biochemistry and is the author of *The China Study*, believes that number should be closer to the 10 percent mark. (Go to https:// nutritionstudies.org for more information about Dr. Campbell's work.)

You don't have to go too crazy trying to measure everything out. The type and *combination* of protein you consume throughout the day is far more important than the quantity.

Examining plant proteins

Plant protein is loaded with benefits: It's relatively alkaline-forming compared to animal protein (meaning it has a nourishing effect on the blood), low in fat, free of growth hormones, easy to digest, and better for the environment. And despite common misconceptions, the plant world offers plenty of sources of protein. In fact, complete plant-based proteins are found in foods like hemp, nutritional yeast, quinoa, and soybeans. Truth be told, many plant-based proteins are pretty complete, so as long as you eat a variety of them, you get what your body requires.

Here are some sources of plant-based protein:

>> **Beans:** Fresh or canned organic beans, black beans, chickpeas, green and yellow split peas, lentils, navy beans, white beans

>> **Butters:** Almond, cashew, pumpkin, sunflower

>> **Greens:** Brussels sprouts, chard, kale, spinach, spirulina

>> **Nuts:** Almonds, Brazil nuts, cashews, macadamia nuts, pecans, walnuts

>> **Protein powders:** Brown rice, hemp, pea

>> **Seeds:** Chia, flax, pumpkin, quinoa, sesame, sunflower, tahini

>> **Soy:** Edamame, sprouted tofu, tempeh

>> **Sprouts:** Adzuki, lentil, mung bean, pea, sunflower

Some particularly protein-packed plant foods include spinach, which is 41 percent protein; mushrooms, weighing in at 30 percent to 45 percent protein, depending on the variety; black beans, which are 26 percent protein; and oatmeal, which is 14 percent protein.

KNOWING PROTEIN SOURCES TO AVOID

If you're committed to eating a plant-based diet, you probably won't be getting your protein from animal sources. However, you may be wondering why plant-based sources are so much better for you. Animal proteins (such as eggs, fish, meat, and whey) place quite a bit of stress on the body — much more than plant-based proteins do — because they're highly acidic (especially dairy and red meat). It also takes much longer for your body to digest and assimilate them into usable protein.

Animal protein also lacks fiber, which aids in digestion and is strongly associated with a lower risk of heart disease. (Turn to Chapter 22 for a more in-depth look at why eating meat is bad.)

Aside from naturally occurring protein found in animals and plants, protein also comes in synthetic forms, which can be damaging to your health.

Be sure to read labels and watch out for products containing these unnatural or highly processed forms of protein:

- Soy isolates

- Textured vegetable protein

- Whey protein powders

Considering carbo-riffic plants

Carbohydrates are long chains of carbon that provide energy in a time-release fashion to ensure a steady blood sugar level. Contrary to what many people believe, high-carbohydrate foods are not inherently fattening. You may think that carbs are fattening because they're made up of sugars, and eating refined sugars (such as fructose) in excess can make you gain weight. In reality, carbohydrates have less than half the calories found in fat. Additionally, carbohydrates have high concentrations of protein and essential vitamins and minerals, including B vitamins, calcium, folate, iron, magnesium, selenium, vitamin E, and zinc. So, hooray! Bring on the bread.

TIP

Research shows that women who eat carbohydrates recover more quickly from symptoms of premenstrual syndrome (PMS). Carbs can act as natural tranquilizers and are beneficial for people with seasonal affective disorder (SAD) and depression.

The main function of carbohydrates is to provide a source of energy for your body. Each gram of carbohydrate provides approximately 4 kilocalories of energy. You need a constant supply of carbohydrates in the form of glucose for all metabolic reactions to happen properly. Complex carbs also help the amino acids in protein to be absorbed and used properly.

WARNING

If you don't consume enough carbs, your body can turn to fat or protein for energy. This situation isn't ideal because the conversion of fat to glucose can happen only so quickly and can cause a buildup of acid in the blood, creating a condition known as *ketosis.* The keto diet may be all the rage right now, but it can have negative side effects, like headache, nausea, fatigue, muscle aches, mental fog, and bad breath. Cutting out an entire macronutrient is never a good idea.

Comparing simple and complex carbs

You need to understand the different kinds of carbs and how to identify them. The simple ones are the ones you want to minimize so you can focus on the complex.

SIMPLE CARBS

There are two types of simple carbohydrates:

>> **Monosaccharides:** Monosaccharides consist of only one sugar. Examples include fructose, galactose, and glucose.

>> **Disaccharides:** Disaccharides consist of two chemically linked monosaccharides. They come in the form of lactose, maltose, and sucrose.

Foods that contain simple carbohydrates include table sugar, products made with white flour, dairy products, whole fruit, fruit juice, jam, soda, and packaged cereals. So, it's pretty obvious that simple carbohydrates should be ditched (except for the whole fruit, of course, because it contains fiber and many other wonderful nutrients).

COMPLEX CARBS

Complex carbohydrates have a higher nutritional value than simple carbohydrates because they consist of three or more sugars that are mostly rich in fiber, vitamins, and minerals. Because of their complexity, they take a little longer to digest, and they don't raise blood sugar levels as quickly as simple carbohydrates do. Complex carbohydrates act as the body's fuel; they contribute significantly to energy production. They're important in the absorption of certain minerals and the formation of fatty acids.

Foods that contain complex carbohydrates include brown rice, legumes, oats, and sweet potatoes.

Getting enough of the right carbs

Ancient grains are some of the oldest foods on the planet. They have been used for thousands of years and are an excellent source of complex carbohydrates, which help curb appetite. These grains also contain phytonutrients, which can help lower cholesterol and prevent cancer and other diseases (more on phytonutrients in Chapter 4). When combined with legumes and vegetables, whole grains provide complete nourishment!

TIP

Here are some handy grain how-tos:

>> **Consume one to two servings each day.** ½ cup cooked or one slice of bread is equivalent to one serving of grain.

>> **Focus on gluten-free whole grains (such as amaranth, brown rice, buckwheat, millet, and quinoa).** These types of grain are generally much easier to digest and contain a variety of nutrients. They also cook quickly.

>> **Choose alternatives to wheat (such as barley, kamut, oats, rye, and spelt).**

>> **Choose sprouted-grain products.** We like Ezekiel 4:9 breads and wraps because they're full of fiber and protein, are easy to eat, and make great sandwiches.

>> **Use these grains in their whole form or as ground flours, in pastas, breads, wraps, and crackers.**

Table 3-1 runs down what the different grains are and how to prepare and store them. Many of the recipes in Part 3 use grains mentioned here, so refer to this table if you need additional cooking tips.

A category of similar foods called pseudo-grains are actually seeds but have grain-like characteristics. Table 3-2 shows you more about the pseudo-grains you should add to your plant-based diet, as well as how to cook and store them.

TABLE 3-1 **Ancient Grains**

Grain	Health Benefits	How to Use It	How to Store It
Barley: A rich and chewy grain	Barley is an incredible source of soluble fiber and B vitamins. Both are essential for lowering cholesterol and protecting against heart disease.	After rinsing, add 1 part barley to 3½ parts boiling water or broth. After the liquid returns to a boil, reduce the heat to low, cover, and simmer for 45 minutes.	Store barley in a tightly covered glass container in a cool, dry place. You can also store it in the refrigerator.
Brown rice: A grain that's more wholesome than white rice; the unhulled and unmilled version	Brown rice is light, gluten-free, and an incredible source of long-lasting carbohydrates for energy. It is also high in fiber and contains several vitamins and minerals, as well as protein.	After rinsing brown rice, add 1 part rice to 2 parts boiling water or broth. After the liquid returns to a boil, reduce the heat to low, cover, and simmer for about 45 minutes.	Because brown rice still features an oil-rich germ, it's more susceptible to becoming rancid than white rice and should, therefore, be stored in the refrigerator. Stored in an airtight container, brown rice will keep fresh for about six months.
Kamut: A type of ancient wheat that's high in protein	Kamut has 20 percent to 40 percent more protein than wheat and is richer in several vitamins and minerals, such as calcium and selenium.	Soak 1 cup kamut overnight. Then add 3 cups water and bring to a boil, add a pinch of salt (if needed), reduce the heat to low, cover, and simmer for 40 to 45 minutes or until tender.	Store kamut in a tightly sealed glass container in a cool, dry place.
Oats: A category that includes oats, oat bran, and oatmeal	Oats contain fiber, which helps lower cholesterol levels. Oats are also beneficial for stabilizing blood sugar levels and contain antioxidants, which reduce the risk of cardiovascular disease.	For all types, it's best to add oats to cold water and then simmer for 10 to 30 minutes, depending on the variety. For raw porridge, soak rolled oats overnight for a ready-to-go breakfast in the morning.	Store oatmeal in an airtight container in a cool, dry, dark place. It will keep for approximately two months.
Rye berries: Rye berries look like wheat but are a little longer and more slender.	Rye berries help with weight loss, gallstone prevention, and diabetes management.	After rinsing them, bring ½ cup rye berries, ¼ teaspoon sea salt, and 1¾ cups water to a boil. Reduce the heat to low, cover, and simmer for about an hour.	Store rye berries in a cool, airtight container. They will keep up to six months in the pantry or a year in the freezer.

(continued)

TABLE 3-1 *(continued)*

Grain	Health Benefits	How to Use It	How to Store It
Spelt: An ancient grain with a nutty flavor	In addition to being an amazing source of fiber and niacin, spelt is easier to digest than wheat.	After rinsing, soak spelt in water for 8 hours or overnight. Drain, rinse, and then add 3 parts water to 1 part spelt. Bring to a boil, reduce the heat to low, cover, and simmer for about an hour.	Store spelt in an airtight container in a cool, dry, dark place. Keep spelt flour in the refrigerator to best preserve its nutritional value.
Wheat berries	Wheat berries are an excellent source of fiber, folic acid, protein, and other nutrients.	After rinsing wheat berries, soak them overnight. For 1 cup berries, use 2 to 2½ cups water. Bring to a boil, reduce the heat to low, cover, and let simmer for 1 to 1½ hours.	Store wheat berries in an airtight container and keep in a cool, dark place. Food-grade storage pails are a good option.

TABLE 3-2   ## Pseudo-Grains

Grain	Health Benefits	How to Use It	How to Store It
Amaranth: The seed of a plant from Central America that has a nutty flavor and can be combined well with other grains	Higher in protein than many other grains, amaranth also contains the essential amino acid lysine, which is hard to find in plant-based foods. It's a good source of calcium and iron, which are important for bone health.	Use 1 part seeds to 2½ parts water. Bring to a boil, reduce the heat to low, cover, and simmer for 20 minutes.	Keep amaranth fresh in a tight-fitting container with a lid. It's best stored in a cool, dry, dark place.
Buckwheat: A fruit seed that's related to rhubarb and sorrel, making it a suitable grain substitute for people who are sensitive to wheat or other grains that contain gluten	Buckwheat is rich in flavonoids, which are phytonutrients that protect against disease by extending the action of vitamin C and acting as antioxidants. It's a great source of manganese, protein, and vitamins B and E. Buckwheat helps balance and lower cholesterol levels while also protecting against heart disease.	After rinsing, add 1 part buckwheat to 2 parts boiling water or broth. After the liquid returns to a boil, reduce the heat to low, cover, and simmer for about 30 minutes.	Place buckwheat in an airtight container and store it in a cool, dry place. Always store buckwheat flour in the refrigerator; keep other buckwheat products refrigerated if you live in a warm climate.

Grain	Health Benefits	How to Use It	How to Store It
Millet: Millet is a varied group of small-seeded grasses, central to the diet in India, Africa, and parts of Europe. It has a corn flavor and is good for people with celiac disease or other wheat allergies	Millet is high in B-complex vitamins, iron, and phosphorus.	Toast 1 cup of millet in a skillet over medium heat for 4 to 5 minutes to bring out the nutty flavor. Add 2 cups water or broth and bring to boil. Reduce the heat to low, cover, and simmer for about 15 minutes. Remove from the heat and let stand, covered, for 10 minutes.	Store millet in an airtight container in a cool, dark place. It can be kept up to two years if stored properly.
Quinoa: A seed that has a fluffy, creamy, slightly crunchy texture and a somewhat nutty flavor when cooked	Quinoa is a complete protein, providing all nine essential amino acids. It's also high in fiber, calcium, and iron.	Add 1 part quinoa to 2 parts liquid in a saucepan. After bringing the mixture to a boil, reduce the heat to low, cover, and simmer. One cup of quinoa cooked this way usually takes 15 minutes to prepare.	Store quinoa in an airtight container. It will keep for three to six months if you store it in the refrigerator.
Teff: A grain that appears purple, gray, red, or yellowish brown; the seeds range from dark reddish brown to yellowish brown to ivory	Teff leads all the grains by a wide margin in its calcium content, with 1 cup of cooked teff offering 123 milligrams. It's also an excellent source of vitamin C, a nutrient not commonly found in grains. It's a source of dietary fiber that can benefit blood sugar management, weight control, and colon health.	Cook teff for about 20 minutes, with 1 cup of teff in 3 cups of water.	Store teff seeds or flour sealed in a container in a cool, dark place on your shelf for up to one year.
Wild rice: An aquatic seed found mostly in the upper freshwater lakes of Canada, Michigan, Minnesota, and Wisconsin; when cooked it has a nutty flavor	Wild rice is a source of B vitamins and lysine (an essential amino acid). It has almost twice the protein content and almost six times the amount of folic acid as brown rice.	Put the grains in a sauce-pan with warm water to cover, and stir the rice around to allow any parti-cles to float to the top. Skim off the particles and drain the water. Repeat the rinsing one more time before cooking. Use 1 cup dry wild rice to 3 cups water. Cover and bring to a boil over high heat. Reduce the heat to medium-low and steam for 45 minutes to 1 hour.	Seal wild rice in a dark glass or opaque container and store in a cool, dark place for up to three years.

THE ART OF BUYING AND STORING GRAINS

Believe it or not, there's an art to buying and storing grains. It makes sense if you think about it — after all, who goes through a whole bag of rice in one sitting? We usually use a small amount for a specific recipe, and then the rest of it sits around in the cupboard for a while. Try these tips for keeping your grains great:

- When buying prepackaged grains, make sure that the package is tightly sealed.

- When buying bulk grains, shop at stores that have a high inventory turnover to ensure the freshest supply.

- Instead of stocking up, buy small amounts often.

- Look for grains that are dry, clean of debris, and fresh-smelling.

- Store whole grains properly to avoid spoilage (when their natural oils become rancid).

- Seal grains tightly to avoid attacks by insects and mold.

- Store grains in the refrigerator to give them a longer shelf life (up to five months).

Now, grains aren't the only game in town. Other beneficial sources of complex carbohydrates include

>> **Fruits:** Organic, seasonal, low-glycemic fruits, such as apples, berries, and pears

>> **Legumes:** Black beans, chickpeas, kidney beans, lentils, pinto beans, and split peas

>> **Starchy vegetables:** Beets, carrots, squash, sweet potatoes, and yams

Planning meals with complex carbohydrates

Carbs are a big nutrient category and tend to be where many people get most of their calories. Because carbohydrates make up such a healthy and large part of a plant–based lifestyle, we've listed some quick ideas here for meal planning (more recipes in Part 3 of this book).

>> **Breakfast**

- Porridge: Scottish or steel-cut oats soaked in water overnight and cooked in the morning on gentle heat for 5 to 10 minutes; add rice milk and some pure maple syrup and cinnamon (and soaked dried fruits)

- Fresh, seasonal fruit with homemade granola and coconut yogurt or cashew cream

- Whole-grain sprouted bread or rice crackers with nut butter

- Whole-grain pancakes with fresh fruit and cashew cream

>> **Lunch or dinner**

- Spelt or rye bread or wrap with hummus, beans, raw or grilled veggies, avocado, and tempeh or tofu

- Brown rice with lentils or beans and steamed veggies

- Grain salads and pilafs (barley, quinoa, wild rice) with vinaigrette

- Baked yam or winter squash with a green leafy salad, steamed veggies, and beans or tempeh

>> **Minimal-appetite meals**

- Soaked oats or porridge with raw honey or coconut nectar

- Plain brown rice with olive oil and steamed veggies

- Quinoa with flax oil, olive oil, or tahini

Avoiding the bad carbs

In addition to making sure that you consume complex carbohydrates as part of your balanced plant–based diet, you should avoid the three really bad carbohy–drates entirely: refined sugars and flours and artificial sweeteners. They not only directly impact your blood sugar levels by triggering sharp spikes and drops but also are "empty" in terms of nutrients and extremely addicting.

Refined sugar and flour are the most processed form of carbs you can consume, and unfortunately they're everywhere. Refined sugars hide in plain sight, so you have to really be on your game to dodge them! In addition to avoiding the obvious white granulated and powdered sugars, steer clear of ingredients like the following:

>> Enriched flour

>> High-fructose corn syrup

>> Sugar

>> Wheat flour

FIGURING OUT FIBER

Everybody needs fiber to ensure a well-functioning digestive tract and lower the risk of cancer, diabetes, heart disease, and high blood pressure. Fiber resists digestion by human enzymes, which means it reaches the colon in the same form it was eaten. This has a beneficial effect on gastrointestinal function, allowing your body to eliminate waste more thoroughly and efficiently.

Fiber comes in two main types:

- **Soluble fiber:** Attracts water and forms a gel, which slows down digestion. Soluble fiber delays the emptying of your stomach and makes you feel full, which helps you control your weight. Slower stomach emptying may also affect blood sugar levels and have a beneficial effect on insulin sensitivity, which may help control diabetes. Soluble fiber can also help lower LDL (bad) cholesterol by interfering with the absorption of dietary cholesterol. Sources of soluble fiber include apples, beans, blueberries, carrots, celery, cucumbers, dried peas, flaxseeds, lentils, nuts, oat bran, oat cereal, oatmeal, oranges, pears, psyllium, and strawberries.

- **Insoluble fiber:** Increases the size and weight of feces through water absorption, increases the frequency of bowel movements, stimulates *peristaltic movement* (the wavelike muscle contractions that move food through the digestive tract), and reduces the time it takes for food to travel through the digestive tract. A diet rich in insoluble fiber is associated with decreased risk of colon and rectal cancer, decreased constipation, and a reduction in blood pressure. Sources of insoluble fiber include barley, berries, broccoli, brown rice, cabbage, carrots, celery, corn bran, cucumbers, dark leafy vegetables, grapes, green beans, nuts, onions, raisins, root-vegetable skins, seeds, tomatoes, wheat bran, whole grains, and zucchini.

Artificial sweeteners are chemically made-up sugars that can work against you. They can trick your body into thinking you're getting some form of sugar, but instead they make you crave more refined carbohydrates. Plus, they're extremely toxic to your blood, liver, and nervous system. Artificial sweeteners include sucralose, aceulfame potassium, and aspartame, which are common in diet drinks and foods.

Eating fatty plants: Gotta love 'em, gotta have 'em

Fat gets a bad rap. You probably think of it as the enemy. You may even try to avoid it at all costs. Or you may believe it's the source of all evil (and increasing waistlines), but here's a newsflash: You need fat. Fats are your friends. Or at least some of them — in moderation — are. In the following sections, we separate friend from foe.

The important ones you should know: Saturated, monounsaturated, and polyunsaturated

Saturated, monounsaturated, and polyunsaturated fats are the three most common forms of fat that you encounter in the plant world. Fats are classified by their density and the number of carbons in a chain. Without getting too complicated, the more carbons a fat has, the more saturated it is. Here's a little breakdown, starting with the most saturated of fats:

» **Saturated fats:**

- Don't normally go rancid, even when heated for cooking

- Constitute at least 50 percent of cell membranes, giving cells stiffness and integrity

- Are needed for calcium to be effectively incorporated into the skeletal system

- Protect the liver from alcohol and other toxins

- Enhance immune function

- Are needed for the proper use of essential fatty acids (EFAs)

Plant-based sources of saturated fats tend to be solid or semisolid at room temperature and include coconut oil and palm oil.

» **Monounsaturated fats:**

- Tend to be liquid at room temperature

- Don't go rancid easily and can be used in cooking at moderate temperatures

Plant-based sources of monounsaturated fats include almonds, avocados, cashews, olive oil, peanuts, and pecans.

» **Polyunsaturated fats:**

- Contain omega-3 and omega-6 fatty acids

- Are liquid even when refrigerated

- Should never be heated

Plant-based sources of polyunsaturated fats include chia seeds, hempseeds, flaxseeds, and walnuts.

Most politically correct nutrition (meaning what the government wants you to eat) is based on the assumption that you should reduce and ideally eliminate your intake of fats — particularly saturated fats — from animal sources because they're to blame for things like heart disease. But don't let your plant-based diet lull you into a false sense of security. More and more, scientists are finding that it's not so much the *saturated* fats that are to blame but rather the processed foods of today's modern industry and all of those trans fats hidden in most products. That means even though you're eating plant-based, you're still at risk for heart disease and other health complications if you consume too much margarine, shortening, refined oils and sugars, and processed foods in general.

Essential fats versus fats to avoid

You need to consume a number of fats on a daily basis from a wide variety of sources. The nutrition they provide is essential to your body and your health.

ESSENTIAL FATS

Essential fats are fats that your body needs but is unable to manufacture, so you have to get them from dietary sources. These fats fall into two groups — omega-3 and omega-6 — which are made up of both monounsaturated and polyunsaturated fats.

>> **Omega-3:** Omega-3 fatty acids are vital to the development of a child's brain and nervous system and for the maintenance and repair of the adult brain and nervous system; they're also anti-inflammatory. In the plant-based world, omega-3 fatty acids are found in chia seeds, flaxseeds, leafy greens, and walnuts. Lack of omega-3 fatty acids can result in behavioral and learning disorders.

  On average, you should consume 1 or 2 tablespoons of oil or seeds per day, or a few walnuts.

>> **Omega-6:** Omega-6 fatty acids can be helpful to many inflammatory conditions and diseases. In the plant-based world, they're readily available in avocados, grain products, nuts, seeds, and many commonly used cooking oils, such as safflower, sesame, and sunflower.

  On average, you should consume ¼ avocado, ¼ cup of nuts or seeds, or 1 to 2 tablespoons of one of these cooking oils per day.

The ideal ratio of omega 6 to omega 3 is thought to be somewhere between 1:1 and 4:1.

The tricky thing about essential fats is that most people get enough in their diet already, but they come from the wrong sources, such as products made with refined sugars and trans fats, which can actually *cause* inflammation. All the processed foods in the standard American diet have increased the amount of omega-6 fatty-acid consumption drastically, causing an imbalance.

An overall imbalance between omega-3 and omega-6 fatty acids can contribute to Alzheimer's disease, arthritis, asthma, attention-deficit hyperactivity disorder (ADHD), cancer, chronic inflammatory disorders, depression, diabetes, heart attack, insulin resistance, lupus, obesity, postpartum depression, schizophrenia, and stroke.

Focus on getting more omega 3, like chia seeds, hempseeds, and walnuts, and getting less of omega 6, like processed vegetable oils, which are mostly found in fried foods, packaged baked goods, and most other junk foods.

Your body also needs omega-9 fatty acids, but they're considered nonessential because your body can synthesize this fat on its own. You don't have to depend on dietary sources to obtain it. Olive oil is the best known source of omega-9s, so keep it on hand at home for an extra boost — assuming that it's extra-virgin olive oil and that you use it in moderation.

FATS TO AVOID

The main group of fats to avoid entirely is trans fatty acids (TFAs). Avoiding TFAs is difficult because many processed foods are laden with them, but TFA consumption is linked to heart disease and elevated cholesterol levels. Plus, TFAs impair *lipoprotein receptors* (the place where cholesterol binds) and your body's ability to process LDL (bad) cholesterol, which eventually elevates LDL levels in the blood, generally considered to be unhealthy.

WARNING

Not all vegetable oils are healthy!

When LDL and total cholesterol levels are elevated, many doctors tell people to restrict animal fats, butter, cheese, and eggs, which is appropriate advice. However, they often suggest replacing butter with margarine — which makes the problem worse! Margarine is a vegetable-oil-based product designed to compete with butter in the marketplace. It's notorious for having high levels of TFAs! Margarine is pretty much one molecule away from plastic. Do you want that in your body?

Steer clear of these bad boys:

» Candy bars

» Commercially baked cakes, cookies, doughnuts, and pastries

» Fried foods

>> Packaged snack foods (for example, chips, crackers, and popcorn)

>> Vegetable shortening

TIP

Watch out for hidden forms of fat, like lard, that are animal-based.

Healthy fat consumption

TIP

Okay, so how do you easily digest all this information into usable practice? So glad you asked. Here's a rundown of basic tips to help you make sure you're consuming fat in a way that helps, not harms, you:

>> **Choose good sources of high-quality fat.** Examples include avocados, coconuts, olives, raw organic nuts, and seeds (especially flaxseeds).

>> **Always choose organic foods for safe fats.** Many industrial chemicals and commercial farming chemicals are fat soluble and stored in the fats of animals, fish, fowl, and plants.

>> **Know which fats to avoid.** They include trans fatty acids, hydrogenated or partially hydrogenated oils, vegetable oils (the high temperatures used to produce such oils destroys the nutrients in the oil), and fats from conventionally raised animals and fish.

>> **If purchasing omega-3 or omega-6 supplements, contact the manufacturer to determine the *carrier oil* (base oil) if it isn't listed on the label.** Soy oil is commonly used because it's cheap. Horrifyingly enough, the carrier oils are often rancid upon arrival and have already drawn the antioxidant qualities out of the good oil in the capsules.

>> **Avoid eating roasted nuts.** The roasting process causes the fats and oils to go rancid, increasing free-radical damage in your body. In other words, they make you age more quickly.

>> **Avoid any and all deep-fried foods unless you prepare them yourself using coconut oil.** Of course, frying and deep-frying should always be kept to a minimum.

>> **Always use heat-stable fats and oils, such as grapeseed and coconut oil, for cooking.** Avoid using polyunsaturated olive oil.

>> **Always use pure, unrefined, organic oils for uncooked items.** Flaxseed oil, hempseed oil, and olive oil are good choices.

>> ***Never* eat *any* food from fast-food restaurants.** They use low-quality foods and fats, many of which are highly processed.

>> **If you have kids, make a special effort to ensure that your growing children get enough omega-3s.** It's worth it.

Meeting the Micronutrients

Micronutrients are the vitamins, minerals, and phytonutrients that help your body absorb macronutrients. A limited (or nonexistent) amount of them can result in poor health. A majority of micronutrients comes from plant-based foods, so being on a plant-based diet virtually guarantees you're getting plenty! In the following sections, we explain more about the top ones you should include in your diet.

Vitamins and the plants you can find them in

The vitamins you get from plant sources are essential for growth, vitality, and health. They're the cornerstones of proper digestion, elimination, and resistance to disease. Here are some of the top ones:

>> **B vitamins:** The family of B vitamins includes B1, B2, B3, B5, B6, B7, B9, and B12. B vitamins have many functions, which means your body needs a constant supply of them. They're helpful for managing anxiety, fatigue, insomnia, nervousness, and stress. The main food sources are the *germ* (the nutrient-dense component of grains) and bran of wheat and rice husks, and the outer portion of whole grains.

   All B vitamins are important, but here are the two you probably hear the most buzz about:

   - **B9 (folate or folic acid):** Essential for bodily functions and the formation of red blood cells. It's also essential for brain development and function. You can find it in green leafy vegetables in abundance — especially in beet greens, kale, and spinach.

   - **B12:** Plays an important role in aiding the nervous system and helps with energy and longevity. It's one of the few vitamins for which you need to take supplements when you're on a plant-based diet because it's not all that abundant in plant-based foods. Fermented foods such as miso and tempeh are sources, but unless you're eating those by the truckload, you probably aren't getting enough vitamin B12 naturally, so be sure to take your B12 supplement. Look for a supplement that provides 10 micrograms daily (your body needs about 2.4 mcg per day, but only a percentage of the supplement will actually be absorbed). As with any supplement, don't take more than the recommended dosage. It's always a good idea to have your levels checked by your physician to make sure that they're where they should be.

>> **Vitamin A:** Great for eyesight and night vision. It's found in a variety of yellow and orange fruits and vegetables, as well as leafy green vegetables.

>> **Vitamin C:** Helpful to the immune system, the building of connective tissue, and adrenal support. It can be found in cabbage, cantaloupe, citrus fruits, green leafy vegetables, peppers, strawberries, and tomatoes.

>> **Vitamin D:** An essential vitamin for the immune system and overall bone health. It's mostly found in animal-based foods, but fear not — this is the "sunshine vitamin," so just get a good 15 to 30 minutes of sunlight a day (depending on your skin type), and that should replenish your stores of vitamin D. In the darker, colder months, you may want to consider taking a supplement.

TIP

If you get enough sun exposure in the spring and summer, your body's reserve of vitamin D should supply your needs during the winter, so you may not need supplements. If you're concerned about your vitamin D levels, ask your doctor to order a vitamin D test next time you have your blood drawn.

>> **Vitamin E:** An antioxidant that's helpful in protecting cells from oxidation and preventing aging and chronic disease. The best sources are grains, nuts, and seeds.

As long as you eat a well-balanced, colorful, and varied diet that is rich in plant-based foods, you should get your daily supply of these nutrients. However, in some cases additional supplementation may be required under the care of your health practitioner. As a general guideline, as long as you're eating at least two to three servings of whole grains, more than four servings of green vegetables, and two or more servings of colorful fruits each day, you should be more than on your way to meeting your vitamin needs.

Minerals and the plants you can find them in

Minerals are naturally occurring substances that come from the earth and eventually return to the earth. They're the basic building blocks of all matter! In essence, they're the life force of most foods, especially plant-based foods, that make everything else work. Without minerals, your body wouldn't thrive or function in an optimal way.

The minerals you should include in your diet

Literally thousands of minerals exist in the world, but we discuss here only the main minerals that plant-based eaters should include in their everyday diets. In the average diet, minerals often come from animal sources, but plants can also be a source of minerals (and, in some cases, plants provide more minerals than animal sources do).

When it comes to minerals, make sure you're taking in four or more servings of green leafy vegetables, other colorful vegetables, and fruits each day. These are the most abundant sources of calcium and iron in a plant-based diet. For zinc and iron, focus on two or more daily servings of nuts, seeds, dried fruits, and whole grains.

CALCIUM

As the most abundant mineral in the human body, calcium is the most important for good health. Calcium is known for the development and maintenance of bones and teeth. In addition, calcium is required for muscle contraction and regulation of the heartbeat. Calcium can be found in many plant-based foods, and the good news is that it's also well absorbed.

Here are some top sources of calcium in the plant world:

>> **Fruits:** Dried apricots and dried figs

>> **Nuts and seeds:** Almonds, Brazil nuts, sesame seeds, and sunflower seeds

>> **Legumes:** Soybeans and tofu

>> **Sweets:** Blackstrap molasses and carob

>> **Vegetables:** Beet greens, bok choy, parsley, and turnip greens

WARNING

Calcium supplements aren't the same as naturally occurring calcium in whole foods. Supplements may pose a risk for heart health, because they can promote the buildup of plaque in the arteries, causing restriction of blood flow to the heart. Be sure to consult a health-care or nutrition professional before taking supplements.

IODINE

Iodine is a trace mineral required for healthy metabolism and thyroid function so the body can produce and regulate hormones. The best source of plant-based iodine is sea vegetables — dulse in particular, which is also low in sodium and a good source of seasoning instead of table salt. (Turn to Chapter 4 for more on sea vegetables.)

You can also get iodine (and other minerals) from unrefined sea salt; in general, unrefined sea salt is lower in sodium than table salt is.

Even with sea salt, you don't want to overdo it. You need so little to reap the benefits and get enough flavor out of your food! A little goes a long way.

IRON

Iron is found in every cell of the body, almost always combined with protein. Its main function is the formation of *hemoglobin* (the essential oxygen-carrying component of red blood cells). You need iron to prevent anemia and fatigue. A variety of plant-based sources are abundant in iron:

>> **Dried apricots and dried figs:** Add them into recipes for baked goods, granola, and trail mix, or eat them on their own.

>> **Lentils and chickpeas:** You can cook all varieties into dips, salads, soups, or stews.

>> **Quinoa and millet:** Cook and make into a breakfast cereal, pilaf, or salad.

>> **Soybeans:** Add edamame, tempeh, or tofu to salads, sandwiches, stir-fries, and whole-grain dishes.

>> **Spinach and kale:** Lightly steam them to eat as a side dish or add them into pasta dishes, sauces, smoothies, soups, or whole-grain dishes.

ZINC

Zinc is vital for many body functions and is part of many enzyme systems. It helps maintain healthy skin and collagen formation and aids in wound healing. Plant-based zinc sources include whole grains, such as rye and oats. Nuts and seeds, such as Brazil nuts and pumpkin seeds, are also great sources of zinc.

Minerals to avoid

Yes, the mineral world contains some bad guys, too. They sometimes dress up like the good guys or hang out completely undetected. Here are three in particular to avoid:

>> **Table salt:** The common table salt with which most people are familiar is a derivative of sea salt, which is made up of sodium chloride and has been processed and, therefore, has lost many of its vital minerals (such as iodine). To make table salt, manufacturers strip sea salt and then often lace it with bleach or anti-coagulating substances to make it "marketable." Ever notice that sea salt likes to clump? Well, that's actually completely natural — the way salt is *supposed* to be. So, ditch the table salt and change over to sea salt.

» **Kosher salt:** Kosher salt is popular, too, but it's made up of sodium chloride just like table salt (and other processed salts). It has fewer additives than table salt, but many varieties contain anti-clumping agents. Stay away from the kosher salt and go straight for the best — sea salt.

» **Monosodium glutamate (MSG):** MSG is a synthetic flavor enhancer that is traditionally used in Chinese food, but these days you can find it in many foods, such as breakfast sausages and potato chips. Understanding the pitfalls of MSG can be confusing. Regular glutamate is a naturally occurring amino acid that the body uses and needs. However, the synthetic manipulation and processing of glutamate produces a form (MSG) not found in nature. Synthetically re-creating a product of nature often produces less-than-desirable results. MSG has been labeled an *excitotoxin* (a chemical that is thought to have the ability to overstimulate cells to death). Many people link headaches, flushing, poor attention, and other symptoms, as well as diseases like fibromyalgia, to a high consumption of MSG.

Chapter **4**

Packing an Extra Punch with Power Foods

W hen it comes to understanding nutrients and maximizing their potential, you'll discover more levels beyond the baseline of macro- and micronutrients (see Chapter 3). For optimal health, you should consume some specific "super nutrients" on a regular basis.

Many people rely on a multivitamin or other synthetically mixed vitamins and minerals to get their daily dose of nutrients. However, plant-based foods contain so many nutrients, you don't necessarily need pills (with the exception of vitamin B12). You can eat almost everything you need to power up your nutrition naturally. In this chapter, you'll discover the world of superfoods, sea vegetables, phytonutrients, bioflavonoids, and antioxidants, and why and how to include them in your plant-based diet.

Enriching Your Diet with Super Nutrients

Countless research studies have shown the positive effects that super nutrients can have on your health. The beauty of plant-based foods is that they offer extra goodness that your body just loves to soak up. Some of these foods are rare, some can be found in abundance, and some even travel long distances to make it onto grocery-store shelves. So, of course, supply and demand can impact your consumption of certain superfoods, such as sea vegetables and acai, but having even a small amount of these foods and the nutrients they contain improves your health by leaps and bounds. What the earth has to offer us in terms of nutrient-rich foods is truly amazing.

It may not be realistic or logistically possible to eat all the foods we name in this chapter. But do the best you can to get at least some — if not many — of these foods into your diet on a regular basis. They're such an important part of establishing good nutrition and upping your health game. Sometimes even just a small serving (such as a tablespoon of goji berries added to your smoothie) can make a world of difference.

These nutrients give you energy, curb cravings, and contain a multitude of vitamins and minerals. Powering up with superfoods and super nutrients takes your well-being to the next level. It's not just about being healthy; it's about maximizing your wellness potential. Do what you can to work these wonders into your regular diet and discover just how good your body will feel.

TIP

These foods can be on the pricier side because they're not as easy to come by. Help yourself out by doing some research ahead of time at health-food stores and farmers markets before you buy so you can budget accordingly. And keep in mind the good news: A little of these power foods tends to go a long way, so your supply should last you a while!

Celebrating Superfoods

Superfoods are superior sources of essential, super-powered nutrients that your body can't make itself. They're extremely nutrient dense, so you don't have to consume very much to reap the benefits, such as a boosted immune system, better skin, increased energy, and much more. Superfoods are the most powerful foods on the planet — powerhouses for the transformation to and maintenance of a healthier you. If you are what you eat, why not be super?

For recipes that use superfoods, flip to Part 3 and check out our recipes for Super Chia Banana Porridge (Chapter 9), Soaked Oats with Goji Berries (Chapter 9), Kale and Cabbage Slaw Salad (Chapter 10), Super Brazil and Goldenberry Trail Mix (Chapter 14), and Chocolate Avocado Pudding (Chapter 16).

What they are and what they do

Superfoods have concentrated nutrients (protein, carbohydrates, and fats; see Chapter 3 for more about these nutrients) and provide an intense amount of nutrition in every bite. Anyone can benefit from eating more superfoods!

Superfoods protect your body from free-radical damage (which contributes to the aging process and illness), give you more energy, promote clear and bright skin, give you mental clarity, help with weight loss, and improve immunity. Some superfoods are common foods, while others are a bit more rare.

As you venture into this new world, start out by trying some everyday superfoods and then work up to the more exotic ones. But before you run off to procure these magical treats, here's more about what you're looking for.

The superfoods you may already know

These are foods that you're most likely familiar with and hopefully consuming on a somewhat regular basis. If not, now's your chance to get more of these items into your everyday diet:

>> **Fruits:** Avocados, blackberries, blueberries, cranberries, kiwis, mangos, papayas, pomegranates, and pumpkins

>> **Veggies:** Beets, broccoli, kale, spinach, squash, and sweet potatoes

>> **Seeds and nuts:** Almonds, cashews, chia seeds, flaxseeds, hempseeds, and walnuts

>> **Pseudo grains:** Seeds that act like grains and are extremely high in protein, fiber, and low-glycemic carbohydrates (such as buckwheat and quinoa)

The green superfoods

Green superfoods have the highest concentration of easily digestible nutrients, fat-burning compounds, and vitamins and minerals to protect your body. They contain a variety of beneficial substances, including proteins; protective phytonutrients (more on those later); and healthy bacteria, which help you build stronger muscles and tissues, aid your digestive system, and more effectively protect you against disease.

Green superfoods are also rich in chlorophyll, the pigment that gives plants their green essence. The molecular structure of chlorophyll is similar to human blood, so it helps build and cleanse the blood, providing cells with more oxygen — which is just one of the reasons it's so good for you!

These green superfoods are especially generous with their healthful properties:

>> **Chlorella:** A single-celled form of green algae.

>> **Dark green, leafy vegetables:** For example, collards, dandelion, kale, and Swiss chard.

>> **Sea vegetables:** See "Considering Sea Vegetables," later in this chapter.

>> **Spirulina:** A *cyanobacteria* (blue-green bacteria) that is a complete protein (for more on complete proteins, see Chapter 3).

>> **Sprouts:** Green living foods that come from seeds. Common varieties of sprouts come from buckwheat, flax, kamut (an ancient wheat that contains significantly more protein than modern wheat), quinoa, and sunflower seeds.

WARNING

Watch out for alfalfa sprouts. Whether homegrown or store bought, they're a known source of foodborne illness. Children, older people, pregnant women, and anyone with a weakened immune system should avoid eating raw sprouts.

The exotics

You may not be as familiar with these superfoods, and you may have a harder time finding them, depending on your location. We include a little description of each, in case you're hearing about these for the first time.

>> **Acai berries:** These are boosted with an array of nutrients, from B vitamins to zinc. Plus, they're loaded with healthy cell-promoting antioxidants. These are great in juices and smoothies.

>> **Cacao:** This is chocolate in its purest state, not heat-treated. It provides antioxidants that are superior to almost anything else in nature. High in magnesium and iron, cacao powder is best in raw desserts, such as avocado pudding or chocolate smoothies, and cacao nibs are great for snacking on or adding to granola bars and trail mix.

>> **Goji berries, mulberries, and goldenberries:** These berries are full of protein and trace minerals, along with vitamin C and vitamin A, and they contain antioxidants and bioflavonoids. They also protect against chronic disease and can help reverse aging. They can be added to cereal, trail mixes, or muffins.

>> **Lucuma:** This fruit can be used as a low-glycemic sweetener and contains many nutrients, including beta carotene, calcium, iron, protein, vitamin B3, and zinc. It has a sweet caramel flavor that's divine in smoothies, baked goods, and raw desserts.

>> **Maca:** This plant root is used to increase energy, improve mood, balance hormones, and enhance the immune system. It can be added to smoothies, cereal, or warm drinks.

WARNING

Buy activated maca powder or gelatinized maca (which isn't actually gelatin at all and is completely vegan). Raw maca tends to have high bacterial and mold concentrations. Plus, its high starch content can be hard to digest, causing gas and bloating. Activated maca is generally sweeter and has better texture than raw maca, as well.

Raw foods: The ultimate superfoods

Raw foods include any natural food that hasn't been heated. Technically (or scientifically) speaking, that means not above 120 degrees. However, different experts have different theories about what constitutes raw food. Raw foods are not only loaded with enzymes (which help you break down food), but also bursting with all their nutrients in their natural state. This is especially true when you choose to eat raw, plant-based foods such as fruits, veggies, nuts, and seeds that are organic and local. You're basically eating food in its most nutritionally dense way. Ultimately, this makes most raw foods the superfoods of the superfoods.

Note: We believe that raw food should be an additional yet abundant part of a cooked plant-based diet. Depending on where you live, raw foods may not be as accessible as in other parts of the world. Also, the climate in your area may not be conducive to eating raw all the time. A warm, cooked plant-based meal is likely what you'll crave in colder climates. Finally, we truly believe in variety and diversity — most people require both to feel balanced and satisfied. That's why the best compromise is to enjoy as many raw additions to your meals as possible, whether you toss them into a smoothie or add sprouts to a cooked stir-fry. The ultimate goal is to try to get as many raw foods as possible for superior health. You'll feel the difference.

TIP

Although adding raw foods into your life is beneficial, you don't have to eat raw all the time. Instead, try to eat just some raw foods with your plant-based cooked foods. This can mean preparing a salad with a cooked meal, drinking a pure vegetable juice, or enjoying a green smoothie.

REMEMBER

When shopping for superfoods, focus on nutrient-dense foods over low-calorie ones. Calories don't determine the amount of vitamins, minerals, enzymes, or overall nutrition in a food item. Also, look for a variety of colors, textures, flavors, and shapes. This makes your meals and snacks exciting. No one wants a boring meal that doesn't taste good!

Considering Sea Vegetables

Sea vegetables are loaded with trace minerals like calcium, chlorophyll, iodine, iron, and magnesium. They're abundant in antioxidants, are alkaline forming and detoxifying, and are an excellent addition to your diet. Whether you eat them as a snack, condiment, or meal, be sure to add some sea veggies into your diet. Sea veggies are particularly beneficial for plant-based eaters because they contain many nutrients that are typically thought to be deficient in vegan and vegetarian diets, such as calcium, chromium, iodine, iron, magnesium, potassium, sodium, vitamin B12, and vitamin K.

WARNING

Sea veggies are meant to be consumed in small amounts because they're so nutritionally dense. Be careful to eat them in moderation! This may sound funny, but if you eat too much, you may feel detox-like effects, such as headaches and stomachaches. Also, it's important to be careful about sourcing your sea veggies through trusted sources. Sometimes they're preserved with other additives that aren't good for you, even in moderation.

What they are and what they do

Sea vegetables are plants from the sea (check out Figure 4-1 to see what some of these veggies look like). They not only carry an amazing array of nutrients, but also are energetically charged, taste amazing, and come in many different forms. Most sea vegetables contain a similar array of nutrients, including iodine, iron, protein, vitamin B12, vitamin C, zinc, and many more. Many of them require rehydration before eating. Here's a little "who's who":

>> **Agar:** Clear, colorless, tasteless, and often used as a natural thickening agent, it's best used to gelatinize foods such as pies, tarts, and puddings. Agar doesn't really have any nutritional value, but it's good for digestion because it's high in fiber.

>> **Arame:** This sea veggie is loaded with calcium and other minerals, such as iodine, iron, and magnesium. It's subtle, soft, and stringy, and it makes a wonderful condiment for soups, salads, stir-fries, sandwiches, and wraps.

- » **Bladderwrack:** This one is packed with vitamin K and mostly used medicinally as an excellent adrenal stimulant. It's commonly used by Native Americans in steam baths for arthritis, gout, and illness recovery.

- » **Dulse:** Sprinkling this red/purple seaweed in your soups and salad dressings is an easy way to add vitamins and minerals to your meals. It's also the key "fishy" ingredient in mock tuna salads and Caesar dressings.

- » **Irish moss:** This sea veggie, also referred to as sea moss, is full of electrolyte minerals, such as calcium, magnesium, potassium, and sodium. It helps you detoxify; boost your metabolism; and strengthen your hair, skin, and nails. It's also traditionally used to treat low sex drive. In nondairy cream and smoothies, it acts as a thickener.

- » **Kelp:** This brown marine plant contains vitamins A, B, D, E, and K; is a main source of vitamin C; and is rich in minerals. Kelp proteins are comparable in quality to animal proteins. Kelp contains sodium alginate (algin), an element that helps remove radioactive particles and heavy metals from the body. Keep a container of kelp flakes on the table mixed with garlic powder and sesame seeds to add extra nutrition as well as seasoning to your food.

WARNING

  Eating too much kelp can cause iodine overload and thyroid dysfunction, so proceed with caution. It may also interfere with some blood-thinning medications. Always discuss any dietary changes with your personal physician if you have concerns.

- » **Kombu:** Kombu is the dehydrated form of kelp. All you need is a 1-inch piece of kombu to put into your soup stock or beans. Kombu adds minerals and natural salt and helps prevent gas and bloating.

- » **Kuzu:** A root starch that is similar to agar, this sea veggie is often used as a natural thickening agent. It can be used in custards, pie fillings, puddings, and sauces. It's the perfect alternative to cornstarch. Kuzu is extremely medicinal and has been used to sooth digestion because of its fiber content.

- » **Nori:** This is one of the most widely known sea vegetables. Most people have it in sushi, but it can also be eaten as a snack or added to miso soup. Nori contains chlorophyll; vitamins A, B, C, and E; and a wide spectrum of minerals.

- » **Sea palm:** This is a brown seaweed that grows only on the Pacific coast of North America. One of our favorites, it has a sweet, salty taste that goes especially well as a vegetable, rice, or salad topping.

- » **Wakame:** Full of calcium, iodine, iron, and magnesium, wakame has a subtly sweet flavor and is often used in soups and salads.

TIP

Having trouble finding these items? Try hitting up Asian markets, where these foods are more common.

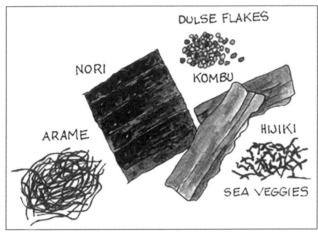

FIGURE 4-1: Keeping a few different sea veggies on hand at all times makes it easy to incorporate them into your meals.

Illustration by Elizabeth Kurtzman

How to use them

When you know what sea veggies are and how to eat them, the next question is this: How the heck do you cook them to make the most of their nutrients? The following tips on preparation and cooking techniques can help you make sure to get them right.

Preparation quick tips

TIP

Use these quick how-tos to get your sea veggies ready:

>> **Arame:** Place it in a small strainer and rinse. Then place it in a bowl of warm water and soak for about 20 minutes. Strain and rinse again. Chop it to the desired size and use it in salads or stir-fries.

>> **Dulse:** You can usually add dulse to your recipe without soaking it first. Just rinse it quickly under cool running water. Using a rocking motion with your chef's knife, chop it to the desired size.

>> **Irish moss:** Irish moss must be thoroughly cleaned before using. Place it in a large bowl, cover with water, and swish it around so that any dirt or debris falls to the bottom of the bowl. Remove the Irish moss to a clean bowl and cover with clean filtered water. Cover and soak at room temperature for 12 to 24 hours. You can use it as is or prepare sea moss gel. To make sea moss gel, remove the soaked Irish moss from the water and transfer to a blender along with 1 cup of the soaking water (use more as needed for consistency). Blend until smooth; then transfer to an airtight jar and place in the fridge to thicken for about 2 hours. ***Note:*** You can also buy sea moss gel instead of making it yourself.

>> **Kombu:** Rinse it first under running water for a short time and then place it in warm water until it's soft. Kombu usually takes 10 to 15 minutes to soften. Chop it and add it to your recipe.

>> **Sea palm:** Soak dehydrated sea palm in a large bowl of cold water for 30 minutes or until softened. It can then be added to salads or stir-fries. Dried sea palm can also be eaten as a snack or crumbled and used as a seasoning.

>> **Wakame:** Rinse your wakame under cool running water for a short time and then soak it in a bowl of warm water. Wakame softens fairly quickly, in 5 to 7 minutes. Chop it and add it to your recipe.

Healthy cooking for sea vegetables

Try these easy ways to cook some of these mysterious-sounding foods. Not so mysterious anymore, huh?

>> **Agar:** Agar is a thickening agent that is usually sold in the form of powder or flakes. To thicken 1 cup of liquid, you'll need about 1 teaspoon of agar powder or 1 tablespoon of agar flakes. Add the agar to cold liquid, bring to a boil, and simmer for 10 to 15 minutes. The mixture will begin to thicken and set as it cools. It's great for making vegan jams, jellies, custards, and pudding.

>> **Bladderwrack:** Bladderwrack can be purchased in dried, powdered, or tea form. To make tea from dried or powdered bladderwrack, add 1 teaspoon to 1 cup of boiling water and let it steep for 10 to 15 minutes.

>> **Irish moss:** ½ tablespoon of soaked Irish moss or 1 to 2 tablespoons of sea moss gel (see the directions in the preceding section on how to make the gel) can be added to smoothies as an incredibly healthy thickener.

>> **Kelp:** Fresh kelp is rarely used, but dried kelp flakes or granules can be used as a seasoning. Simply sprinkle on soups, salads, pasta, stir-fries, or even popcorn!

>> **Kombu:** Kombu takes longer to cook than other sea vegetables, so add chopped kombu to soup and simmer for at least ten minutes before adding any other sea veggies. Cook for at least 20 minutes.

>> **Kuzu:** Like agar, kuzu is a thickening agent. Simply dissolve 1 teaspoon in 2 teaspoons of cold liquid. Add the slurry to gravies or sauces and gently simmer until thickened. If you're making a very thick sauce, use up to 1 tablespoon dissolved in 2 tablespoons cold liquid.

>> **Nori:** You can usually buy nori already toasted. If your nori isn't toasted, you can toast it in a 350-degree oven for 1 to 2 minutes, until the nori changes color from dark purple/black to phosphorescent green. Our preference, however, is to use raw nori to keep all the nutrients intact.

>> **Wakame:** Wakame softens quickly and takes very little time to cook. Chop it and add it to soup, and then cook it for only 5 to 10 minutes.

TIP

The water you use to soak sea vegetables becomes very nutritious and flavorful and can be used in the recipe you're making. To gain maximum flavor and nutrition, use no more water to soak your sea vegetables than can be incorporated into the recipe.

Favoring Phytonutrients

Phytonutrients (also known as phytochemicals) are the major contributors to the color, taste, and smell of many plant-based foods. The word is also an umbrella term for the compounds that plants make that improve a human's health. These gems have natural chemicals that protect plants from germs, fungi, bugs, and other unsavory characters. This brilliance gives us a glimpse of what they can do in our bodies as well, in terms of overall wellness. For more about the specifics, read on.

What they do

Phytonutrients are small compounds that have powerful results. Knowing the different subcategories, such as tannins, bioflavonoids, and alkaloids, may not be as useful as understanding what phytonutrients do. Here are just some of the wonderful benefits they offer:

- » Neutralizing free radicals
- » Inhibiting bacterial formation
- » Preventing cell damage
- » Reducing inflammation
- » Providing immune support
- » Protecting and supporting tissue

You can read more about these benefits in the pages ahead.

Where to find them

Phytonutrients are pretty much everywhere in plant land, which means you probably don't have to go out of your way to buy unfamiliar foods. They exist most prolifically in the following:

- » Beans
- » Fruits
- » Herbs
- » Nuts
- » Seeds
- » Tea
- » Vegetables
- » Whole grains

Biting into Bioflavonoids

Although phytonutrients come in many forms, bioflavonoids (sometimes just called *flavonoids*) are extra important because they're among the most powerful.

What they are and what they do

Bioflavonoids are plant pigments that give color to many fruits and flowers. They were once referred to as "vitamin P." They're the water-soluble companion to ascorbic acid (a form of vitamin C). As a result, they're easily absorbed through the intestines. Although some are stored in the body, most excess bioflavonoids are eliminated via perspiration and urine.

Bioflavonoids act as antioxidants, antibiotics, anti-inflammatories, and even cancer preventives. Another wonderful benefit is that they maintain the health of *collagen*, a protein that strengthens and protects various bodily structures (such as skin, smooth muscle, blood vessels, organs, hair, nails, bone, and cartilage).

Where to find them

Because bioflavonoids are so foundational to plant life, they're easily available. You don't need to make any special trips to special stores; you only need to make sure you have a nice supply of fresh fruits and veggies at all times. Here's a little list of the more bioflavonoid-laden foods to get you started:

>> Apricots

>> Black currants

>> Blackberries

>> Broccoli

>> Buckwheat

>> Cherries

>> Citrus fruits

>> Dark chocolate

>> Grapes

>> Green bell peppers

>> Papayas

>> Rose hips

>> Tomatoes

Acknowledging Antioxidants

When you're on a plant-based diet, you naturally consume large quantities of antioxidants without having to think about it too much. However, they're very important and helpful little guys, so we want to go into a bit more detail so you know why they're so cool — and which foods contain them.

What they are and what they do

Antioxidants are protective compounds that prevent cells and tissues from being damaged by clearing your system of free radicals. Free radicals are chemically unstable oxygen atoms that have one or more unpaired electrons. They steal electrons from other atoms in your body, which can cause damage to your cells, proteins, and DNA.

Because of their ability to shoo away the bad guys, antioxidants have also been known to help in the fight against several degenerative and age-related diseases, such as:

» Alzheimer's disease

» Cancer

» Cardiovascular disease

» Cataracts

» Cognitive impairment

» Macular degeneration

Where to find them

Antioxidants are everywhere! Here are some favorites:

» **Fruits:** Acai berries, apples, apricots, blueberries, goji berries, grapes, mangoes, plums, pomegranates, pumpkin, strawberries, and tomatoes

» **Veggies:** Broccoli, cabbage, carrots, cauliflower, eggplant, kale, red bell peppers, and spinach

» **Roots and shoots:** Garlic, green tea, leeks, onions, and parsley

» **Legumes:** Black beans, kidney beans, and pinto beans

Chocolate is the ultimate antioxidant! Because chocolate is a bean, it counts as an antioxidant — in fact, one of the most concentrated sources of antioxidants, especially in the pure, raw, and natural form known as cacao — so be sure to get your daily dose. Yes, you heard me, daily if you want. Whether it's a tablespoon of pure cacao powder or a square (or two) of dairy-free dark chocolate, go for it!

2

Converting Your Kitchen

Get the details on how to move from your current dietary habits to a plant-based diet.

Explore the foods you can dish up on your plant-based plate and check out some ideas for different meal plans.

Fill your kitchen with plant-based foods and figure out what equipment you may need.

Know where to shop and what to look for when it's time to restock your cupboard shelves.

Chapter **5**

Taking the Plunge into a Plant-Based Diet

Ready to make the move and become a full-fledged "plant-a-tarian"? Well, you're in good company — many people take the plunge every day to join the millions who already enjoy this diet. If you want to move forward with implementing a plant-based diet, the first step is to understand your reasons for doing so and choose a transition method that makes sense and is easy for you. Of course, a big transition may present some unexpected challenges (as anything new does), but you can set yourself up to enjoy the process.

In this chapter, we outline how to approach your transition to a plant-based lifestyle so it works best for you. We also explain some common obstacles and ways to overcome them. In no time at all, you'll be ready to take on this new diet with gusto!

Transitioning to a Plant-Based Diet

Getting started on a plant-based diet can seem a little daunting at first, but the good news is that you can do it relatively easily and at your own pace. Whether you change your lifestyle overnight or over the course of months or years, the main thing is to prepare yourself mentally and physically for the big changes that lie ahead.

Feeling a little overwhelmed or nervous when making big changes is normal. A key part of preparing yourself is remembering why you're making this change. Perhaps you're working through this transition because you want to lead a more ethical or environmentally friendly life. Maybe you want to improve your health or the health of your family. Whatever your personal reasons and goals, keeping those thoughts in mind can help you stay focused and motivated during the tougher moments.

REMEMBER

Your body and mind will reap the benefits of a plant-based diet almost immediately, regardless of how you approach the transition. Sometimes getting started can be the scariest part of a new experience but remembering that you'll see progress quickly can help you take the leap.

In this section, we help you figure out which way works best for you, whether it's jumping into the deep end or slowly getting your feet wet.

Going cold turkey

Removing all meat, poultry, fish, dairy, and eggs at once can feel like a dramatic change, but on the other hand, this method keeps things pretty simple. Some people, when they make a decision, need to hurry up and implement it before they change their minds. Going cold turkey has its benefits and drawbacks.

Benefits to going all in

Switching to a plant-based diet all at once can pay off for your body, mind, and spirit. Check out these advantages:

>> **You'll likely see improvements in your health and overall well-being right away.** Your body will likely respond well to eating more fiber- and nutrient-rich foods.

>> **You'll set a dramatic example for your friends and family.** Not only does it make you publicly accountable (which is great if you're the sort who thrives on external motivation), but your level of commitment may even inspire others to take on a plant-based diet, which means you may have company! Extra bonus: If you're making the switch for animal rights or environmental reasons, your example can set off a positive chain reaction.

>> **You get something to fully focus on and keep your mind (and body) busy with what to eat next, what you need to buy, and what you need to figure out about nutrition.** Going cold turkey gives you the opportunity to really sink your teeth into something!

Drawbacks to the quick switch

When you make a sudden change, you may experience unexpected consequences. In most cases, you can overcome the drawbacks if you just give yourself some time to adjust. Here are some drawbacks to suddenly converting your diet to a plant-based approach:

>> **You may have made the decision to change your lifestyle, but your body may not be ready for it.** Often when people drastically change their diet, they begin to detox. Detoxing may sound good in theory, but it doesn't feel so good when you're experiencing headaches, bloating, and discomfort, so be sure to consult your doctor or naturopath about whether this method is appropriate for you, especially if you have health conditions (more on this later in the chapter).

>> **Your wallet takes a beating.** Not only is replacing your kitchen inventory expensive, but it may end up costing extra because you aren't used to your new food-purchasing patterns. You may aimlessly try to fill in the blanks of your new meals without knowing quite what to buy, which may lead to some expensive mistakes.

>> **You may not really understand what you're doing and why you're doing it.** You may be eating foods that aren't even that healthy or in line with your new philosophy because you haven't done your research yet.

Sometimes abruptly taking a big staple out of your diet can make it more likely that you'll get off track. Before you try the cold-turkey approach, make sure that you have enough resources to get started so you don't feel overwhelmed.

Steps to making the switch

After you've decided to eliminate all foods that aren't plant-based from your diet, you need to have a couple of conversations with near and dear family and friends. Then you need to take some strategic steps to ensure that you maintain your new lifestyle and realize some success quickly:

>> **Tell your family or housemates about your plan and discuss whether the whole household will be going plant-based.** If so, set aside some time to clean out your fridge, pantry, and cabinets together. (Think about donating those items to your local food bank.) If not, talk about distinguishing certain areas of your kitchen or certain pots and pans as "plant-based," if needed.

If you're not sure whether something you have in your kitchen is entirely plant-based, read the labels and "added ingredients" thoroughly. If you're still not sure, search online for unknown ingredients.

>> **Talk to your doctor, naturopath, or dietitian about any health concerns you may have and how to go about the transition properly.**

>> **Go shopping for new plant-based goodies to fill your fridge and pantry.** See our suggestions for pantry, fridge, and freezer staples in Chapter 7.

>> **For your first plant-based meal, plan something easy.** Don't put added pressure on yourself to make an extravagant meal.

Going plant-based gradually

Some people prefer the softer approach of easing into a plant-based diet. We like this approach because, in general, the longer it takes to get into a habit, the longer the habit sticks. You can approach a gradual implementation of a plant-based diet in two ways — you want to focus either on what you can eliminate or what you can add in. We're fans of adding in — it's not as scary as taking something out.

In the next sections, we outline the pros and cons of making a gradual switch. If you decide that a gradual transition is for you, decide whether to eliminate foods or add them. To help you out, we provide some guidelines for both approaches.

Benefits to taking the slow approach

Taking a slow, cautious approach to implementing a plant-based diet means you get the chance not only to absorb the physical and logistical changes that occur but also to slowly digest all the new foods and information along the way. Here are some other advantages:

>> **You're not as likely to feel anxious that familiar foods have to be taken out of your diet right away.** The goal is to focus on adding things in that can help you experience new foods, meals, and recipes and how they impact your body and your overall approach to food.

>> **Your body enjoys the process more as it begins to adjust to fiber, different greens, and seeds.** All these things take time for your body to get used to. Doing it gradually means you won't likely feel harsh detox symptoms, as you might if you went cold turkey.

>> **Your grocery shopping experiences may be more pleasurable and less stressful than with the cold-turkey approach.** You have time to find out about new things, experience them, test them out, and see what sticks and feels right for you. You can also enjoy the process of understanding why plant-based foods are so good for you and your health. It's a whole process, so embrace it with ease.

Drawbacks of a slow process

Sometimes when you strive to create new habits, going too slowly can negatively affect your transition. A move to a plant-based diet is no exception, so here's what you should watch out for:

>> **You may lack accountability.** When you do this process little by little, you may be more likely to fall off the wagon or cheat. Because you're taking a more relaxed approach, it may be easy to say, "Oh, I'll have my plant-based meal *tomorrow*." Find ways to keep yourself focused on your decision to transition, such as making a calendar that you display on the fridge.

>> **You won't feel the expected health benefits right away, and you may give up as a result.** You may be hoping to have more energy, get better sleep, and lose weight — but these things take time! You have to motivate yourself until the physical results eventually start to reveal themselves.

>> **It's hard to form a new habit for the long term if you haven't given it a solid few weeks of immersion.** Experts say it takes 21 days to form a habit. If you go too slowly, you're more likely to deviate from the plan.

>> **If you only buy a few new ingredients at a time to restock your pantry, you may find that it's hard to make new recipes.** For example, if you don't have the right sweeteners or alternative meat options for your meals, it may be more difficult to make them. A total shift in your pantry can help you make sure you have the ingredients needed to keep you on track.

The process of elimination

When you decide to transition slowly to a plant-based diet, you can take two different paths: You can eliminate non-plant-based foods, or you can add plant-based foods. Of the two gradual approaches, choosing to eliminate non-plant-based foods is probably more difficult. Giving things up that you like and are familiar with is definitely a challenge, but having a plan to phase things out makes it a lot more doable.

Everyone is different, and it's important to go with what works for you, but here's the order we recommend for taking foods out of your diet over the course of a few weeks or a few months:

>> **Red meat:** The heaviest of the animal-based foods should only be consumed once in a while. Your body has to work hard to break it down. Look to minimize your intake of red meat every week, working toward total elimination. Try consuming red meat only on weekends and reducing further from there.

- **Chicken and other poultry:** Chicken is a staple in most homes. It's lighter than red meat, so you can start at a higher consumption frequency. Try reducing your poultry intake to three meals a week to start and going down from there.

- **Fish:** This is the lightest of the animal-flesh foods, but it's not as commonly consumed as poultry. Look at reducing your intake to one to two servings per week and then reducing that intake over time.

- **Cheese, milk, and other dairy:** This is usually the hardest for people to give up. Most people have an addiction to dairy. Try to consume dairy foods only once or twice per week until you wean yourself off of them completely.

TIP

Many people still consume dairy on a vegetarian diet. If you're among them, we suggest opting for goat- or sheep-derived milks and cheeses. They're cleaner and higher in nutrients, and they can be digested by the human body much more easily than cow dairy. If you do choose to consume dairy from time to time, do it mindfully. A few pieces of salty feta or strong blue cheese over a salad or pasta can go a long way toward satisfying cravings without overindulging.

- **Eggs:** These tend to be a staple for vegetarians, and all we can say to that is, "Everything in moderation." Eggs shouldn't be consumed every day. Save them for the occasional weekend brunch, if at all. It's best to buy organic, pasture-raised eggs, ideally from a local small farm that you can visit, until you give them up completely.

If you want to eliminate foods meal by meal, you can choose one full day a week to go plant-based or choose a few meals throughout the week. Choose days or meals that work well with your lifestyle. For example, you may want to do your plant-based meals on days when you have time to experiment with new recipes instead of trying to squeeze it in after working late and before the kids' homework time.

The adding-in process

In this process, you focus on adding new items to your diet on a regular basis. Choosing some plant-based essentials helps smooth the transition and gives you a healthy and balanced start. Here are some foods to add:

- **Green leafy vegetables:** I suggest adding one new green vegetable per week. Also, look to add as many leafy greens to as many meals during the day as possible. They nourish you and provide your body with vitamins and minerals. Some examples are spinach, kale, and arugula.

TIP

>> **Nondairy milk, such as almond milk or rice milk:** Sometimes, totally switching the milk you drink or put in your cereal is too drastic. You can start transitioning by doing a mix of dairy and nondairy milk, gradually changing the ratio over time.

You may need to experiment with different types of nondairy milks to find the one you like best. For example, you may prefer rice milk in cereal and almond milk for smoothies. Always look for unsweetened, plain varieties to avoid added sugars.

>> **Beans, tofu, tempeh, and lentils:** Serve these alongside your meat for one or more meals a week so you can get used to them. Work up to including them with one meal a day, and eventually replace your meat with these options.

>> **Whole grains:** Experiment by adding different whole grains, such as brown rice, millet, and quinoa, to the base of burgers or meatloaf.

You Can't Do It Alone: Leaning on Others for Support

You don't have to take on these changes to your lifestyle alone. Getting support from people around you will make the process that much more rewarding and successful. The following sections outline how you can get the support you need to thrive during this transition.

Surrounding yourself with others who support your lifestyle

You're more likely to be successful if you have people around you who are encouraging you and supporting what you're doing. You may want to have one of the following to turn to, so you can transition to a plant-based diet successfully:

>> **Community potlucks and meetups:** Attending these events is a great way to meet people who are on the same journey. They can likely introduce you to new restaurants and markets in the area and to fun activities they participate in as a group. You can find like-minded people online, at vegetarian restaurants, at health food stores, or through community centers.

- >> **Social media groups:** Social media groups provide up-to-date information on plant-based trends and events. Most groups post success stories or highlight role models to follow. This can be a fast avenue to help you get into the plant-based mindset. If you're into hashtags, do a search for #plantbasedliving, #plantpowered, #wfpb (short for *whole foods plant-based*), or #eatplants — just to name a few.

- >> **Cooking classes:** Your local community center or health food store may hold cooking classes at restaurants or other venues. Often, vegetarian websites tell you where local classes are held.

- >> **Friends and family:** Having your family on board or at least interested in your decision can only make the process easier. It's ideal if they're open to trying your new food creations or at least being supportive of your decision, no matter your reasons.

WARNING

You may find that some friends and family members aren't receptive or don't understand what you're up to. Resist the urge to become defensive; instead, just trust that you've made a choice that's going to benefit you and your health, and let them worry about the rest. Inspire by example — as you lead, even the naysayers may eventually jump on board to try your new, fun recipes.

Enlisting the help of a nutritionist, naturopath, or medical doctor

When you first make the switch to a plant-based diet, getting some support from professionals may be a good idea. They can make sure you're adopting the new lifestyle correctly, answer any questions, and help you see (and celebrate) the changes that take place in your body as a result of eating better. Consider contacting one of these professionals in your area:

- >> **Nutritionist:** A nutritionist can help you with food and meal planning. Many nutritionists can even provide tips on how to overhaul your pantry and fridge and set you up with grocery lists to restock your kitchen. Depending on the nutritionist, you may be able to get customized meal plans and recipes that can help you map out your meals during the week.

  Many nutritionists also work with your overall goals for choosing this lifestyle, whether for weight loss, increased energy, or better sleep. Some can help with natural supplementation to make sure you're getting the nutrients you need to thrive on this diet

- >> **Naturopath:** Working with a natural medicine doctor can help you address the potential health concerns of changing your diet. Some naturopaths can help with dietary suggestions and meal recommendations, make suggestions regarding allergies and food sensitivities, and even work according to your blood type.

>> **Medical doctor:** You may choose to enlist a medical doctor, which is especially helpful if you're taking any prescription medications. Your doctor can help you monitor your dosage as you change your diet. You may find that after several months of eating a wholesome, plant-based diet, you need less of your medication, but only a doctor can help you with this. Never alter or eliminate your medications without consulting your doctor.

REMEMBER

Several medical conditions, such as arthritis, high cholesterol, diabetes, and heart disease, may improve as a result of eating more vegetables. (See Chapter 2 for more details.)

WARNING

If you're an insulin-dependent diabetic, talk with your health-care practitioner before making any dietary changes. Taking the prescribed dose of insulin when that amount is no longer needed can be very dangerous.

Overcoming Common Pitfalls

Part of making a big change in your eating habits is facing challenges and overcoming them. Although everyone is different and has their own struggles, it may help to consider these common obstacles and how to tackle them. Half the battle is knowing what to expect and being ready when the time comes. There's nothing you can't surmount!

Having little or no experience in the kitchen

Many people feel like they need a culinary education to start eating more healthfully. You can easily get overwhelmed at the idea of eating more meals at home when you're not used to that. Don't let this feeling stop you! When you start anything new — especially when you're taking full responsibility — it can present a challenge. However, you just need to start. We promise it'll get easier as you go!

TIP

Enlist a friend or family member to be your partner, and make a cooking date to start tackling some recipes together. You don't even need a partner who is plant-based — all you need is someone who knows their way around a kitchen and may even enjoy giving you some basic help. Make it fun by hosting a group at your home, where everyone can share cooking tips, strategies, and even favorite utensils and tools. Work together and create a meal as a group so you can watch and learn — take notes if you want! Keep it low-key and social by making sure that the guest list includes your friends and family.

Another option is to go to a cooking class and get to know other people who are in the same boat. As you build a foundation of basic skills and recipes, you start to feel more confident and willing to take on more challenging recipes. Don't forget to find someone who will be an encouraging taste-tester and cheerleader!

Feeling intimidated by new foods

Arame? Quinoa? Swiss chard? These words may feel like a different language to you. That's okay. At one point you didn't know what an apple, tangerine, or tomato was either. The best thing to do is jump right in!

Start by choosing just a couple of new ingredients that you find in this book (or elsewhere) and do some research on them. Look them up, watch videos on how to prepare them, and find restaurants that serve them so you can experience them before you take them on yourself at home. Don't be afraid to ask questions about how the food is prepared! Practice, experiment, and try all sorts of preparations to find ones you like.

When you feel confident with a food, move on to a new one. New foods (which may actually be ancient varieties) are introduced to the market all the time. Get to know them and you may come to love some of them in new favorite recipes!

TIP

Keep your eyes open for "seasonal" or "market" vegetables and fruits on restaurant menus and always order them (especially if you don't know what they are or how to cook them). This is a wonderful, nonthreatening way to expand your veggie repertoire while sampling produce at the height of its deliciousness!

Feeling like the odd man out

It can feel strange when you take on something that no one else seems to understand. Sticking to your guns can be especially challenging in social settings, such as when dining out with friends and family members, eating a meal with work colleagues, or even discussing food topics with your neighbors. If you feel strange or awkward, just remember that you've made the decision to take this on for a reason (or many reasons). Instead of feeling left out, you can be inspiring! Be the trendy, cool person who suggests new restaurants or makes a killer tempeh stir-fry. Leading by example can even cause others around you to join in.

As you host dinner parties or go out to eat, invite a plant-based buddy to join. Maybe it's someone you met in a cooking class or through an online group for vegans or vegetarians, or maybe it's a really good friend who goes plant-based for one night to keep you company. Don't be afraid to reach out and ask for help — you're doing a great thing for yourself, and many of your loved ones will want to support that. Just tell them how they can!

WARNING

Be careful not to preach to others that what you're doing is the "right way." This attitude only ostracizes folks and makes you seem like, well, a know-it-all jerk. And nobody likes that. Instead, be silently content with the way you live and the way you eat. In time, others may come to you with questions, at which time you can answer honestly about what's working for *you*.

Fighting food fatigue and boredom

To keep your meals interesting, continue to add new foods, new recipes, and new preparation methods to your repertoire. Even in the non-plant-based world, getting stuck in a food rut is easy. Expand your horizons. You can't eat brown rice or veggie burgers every day and feel inspired. Keep trying new cookbooks (the library is a great resource for trying out new ones!), new cooking classes, and new restaurants. Go to different stores to do your shopping.

REMEMBER

You don't always have to change up the food itself — you can find different ways to prepare the same ingredient, so experiment with different techniques and seasonings. For example, try steamed kale with garlic and olive oil one night as a side dish, and the next day try baked kale chips with sea salt as a snack! Don't be afraid to go off book — you can use recipes as loose guides but add your own spin to keep your meals lively and interesting.

TIP

Farmers markets and specialty shops usually have a high changeover of product and also work with the season. You're virtually guaranteed to see foods you haven't seen before. This may push you outside your comfort zone, help you reconnect to your plant-based goals, and get you excited about trying new foods!

Chapter **6**

Looking at What's on Your Plate

A plant-based plate may look a bit different from the Standard American Diet meal you're used to, but the macronutrients and micronutrients your body needs are the same no matter which diet you choose. Protein, carbs, healthy fats, vitamins, and minerals are essential for optimal health and well-being.

In this chapter, we give you some specific points to keep in mind about the foods you choose and outline some sample menus to get you started on your new plant-based lifestyle. We also suggest ways to convert some of your favorite foods into plant-based favorites.

Thinking about Your New Plate

When you look at your plate from now on, we hope it's bright and bountiful! Your plate at every meal should be loaded with a balance of wholesome plant-based foods that are both nutritious and delicious. Read on to find out how you can create a plate that satisfies your taste buds and supports your health.

Keeping it whole

Choosing foods that are as wholesome and real as possible is the first step to achieving nourishing meals and should be your focus. What do we mean by "real" foods? Foods that are in their natural forms and not packaged or processed. Processed foods are typically filled with additives, excess salts, sugars, and preservatives, even if they're vegan.

Choosing organic over nonorganic

Choosing organic produce over conventional produce really comes down to personal preference and affordability. There isn't much of a nutritional difference between the two, but if you're concerned with the amount of pesticides you may be ingesting, start by choosing organic varieties of the *Dirty Dozen*, a list of foods, published by the Environmental Working Group (EWG) each year, that are most likely to contain pesticide residues. You can find the list at www.ewg.org/foodnews/dirty-dozen.php.

Always wash produce well before using, regardless of whether you choose organic or not.

REMEMBER

Conventional fruits and vegetables are always a better choice than organic junk food.

Dishing it up in the right proportions

Ideally, you should keep your plate proportionate. Try to maintain certain ratios of different plant-based foods so you get enough protein, carbohydrates, and fats to nourish you at every meal. You want to feel like your meal will sustain you, which means having eaten enough food to feel energized and being able to wait two to three hours before eating your next meal. But don't rule out a healthy snack in between meals if you're truly hungry. At the end of the day (literally), you want to feel satisfied — because you ate from each food category and are nourished from the inside out.

Figure 6-1 shows what your typical plate should look like. A majority of the plate is made up of vegetables because they're the mainstays of a plant-based diet. However, you want to choose the right balance of vegetables so you'll be sustained and full after each meal. Root vegetables and leafy greens should make up most of your plate. Whole grains, legumes, and a bit of healthy fat should fill up the rest of your plate.

REMEMBER

Keep in mind that Figure 6-1 may not represent how every single meal in a day will look. Instead, it gives you an idea of how your meals should be balanced over the course of a day.

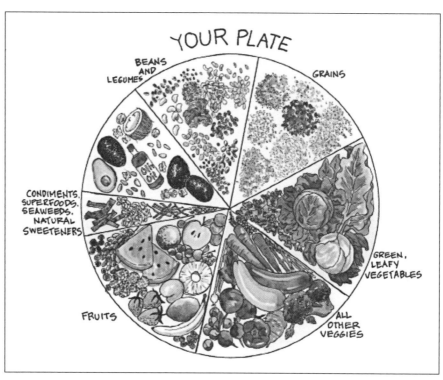

YOUR PLATE

BEANS AND LEGUMES

GRAINS

CONDIMENTS, SUPERFOODS, SEAWEEDS, NATURAL SWEETENERS

GREEN, LEAFY VEGETABLES

FRUITS

ALL OTHER VEGGIES

FIGURE 6-1:
It's all about the right proportions!

Illustration by Elizabeth Kurtzman

Consuming calories that count

Calories. Most people are all too familiar with these little guys as something to count and minimize. But they do serve an actual purpose beyond tormenting you — they measure the approximate amount of energy needed to raise the temperature of 1 gram of water by 1 degree Celsius. This unit of measure is used to understand how food adds up or is stored in the body and how it's metabolized.

When it comes to counting calories, it's not so much about the amount of calories but more about the source of those calories. When you focus strictly on the caloric values of foods, you stop paying attention to what's actually in them (the good and bad nutrients). Now, we're not telling you to completely overlook the caloric content, but we *are* saying that the number of calories isn't as relevant as the actual nutrients. So, let's talk about how to get good calories that are nutritious!

Getting your calories from whole foods is the first step. Whether you're eating beans, fruits, grains, nuts, seeds, or veggies, strive to eat fresh foods from whole sources that don't come out of a package. (Of course, packaged products may find their way into your life from time to time, and that's okay. Many health foods come in a package.) It's your job to look closely at what you're eating, whether it comes in a package or not, and ultimately be conscious about the calories you take in.

It comes down to how your food impacts you nutritionally, not calorically. For example, a single serving of junk food (such as chips, bagels, or cookies) easily contains way more than 200 calories. The nutritional value of these foods is minimal at best. However, if you consume 200 calories in a single serving of plant-based foods (such as avocados, coconut, nuts, quinoa, or seeds), you're much better off. These foods provide your body with nourishment from protein, healthy fat, and complex carbohydrates. So you're likely to feel satisfied more quickly, and you may even consume fewer calories because your body is using the nutrients. With junk food, you can pretty much eat endlessly with nothing to show for it except maybe a pair of jeans that doesn't fit anymore.

Table 6-1 shows how 200 calories of common foods stack up against one another. Notice how much of the plant-based foods you can eat (approximately) compared to a junk-food equivalent.

TABLE 6-1

Comparison of 200 Calories in Plant-Based Food versus Junk Food

Plant-Based Food	Junk Food
2 to 3 apples	1 small blueberry muffin
1 avocado	1 handful of chips
2 heads of broccoli	Half of a chocolate bar
2 bunches of celery stalks	Half of a side serving of french fries

REMEMBER

You need to look at your food calories more critically and decide how you want to gain the most nutrition from your food.

TIP

Try these pointers to make it easier to stick to healthy choices:

>> **Shop with a plan, not with an empty stomach.** When you're hungry, you lose your judgment and basically want to put anything you see in your mouth! So, plan ahead — not only by making a shopping list but also by making sure you have some food in your belly.

>> **Stock up on fiber.** Fiber-rich whole foods fill you up and are the nutritional opposite of refined foods, which have been stripped of their fiber.

» **Swap out sugary drinks for homemade brews.** This is a surefire way to drop calories within moments. Just a few sips of a processed fruit juice or soda can add a significant amount of nonnutritive calories before you've even eaten a meal. Make ginger or peppermint tea, or throw some fresh berries in a bottle of water.

» **Avoid fast foods.** Fast food is quite possibly the worst thing you can eat, because most menus are loaded with fat, calories, and sodium. Set yourself up for success by always having enough food on hand to make quick meals. Plan ahead by making a little extra for dinner so you can have leftovers the next day.

» **Snack healthier.** These common plant-based snacks are wrapped up and ready to go:

- Coconut yogurt
- Dairy-free dark chocolate bars
- Dried fruit and nut bars
- Granola and other whole-grain cereals
- Kale chips
- Organic corn chips
- Trail mixes
- Whole-grain or gluten-free crackers

Maintaining proper hydration

Hydration is an important but often neglected subject. The body is made up of about 60 percent water, and yet many people don't drink nearly as much as they should to keep their bodies well hydrated. Many plants are made up mostly of water, which is good news for plant-based eaters, but you still need to down some good-quality H_2O several times a day.

If you aren't hydrated, your body can't metabolize, process, and function at its best. By the time you feel thirsty, you're already dehydrated. When you're dehydrated, you can experience everything from fatigue and headaches to cramping and false feelings of hunger.

REMEMBER

Drink water throughout the day. Whether it's plain water, lemon water, or herbal tea, just make sure to get it in. Opinions differ on how much you should drink, but a typical recommendation is to drink half your body weight in ounces; if you weigh 150 pounds, you should drink about 75 ounces (about 9 cups) of water a day. This may not be realistic, but at least make sure you're drinking something.

Getting Organized

The first step to meal planning and the one that most people have the most difficulty with is organizing meals for the week. If you don't plan ahead, you can set yourself up for falling off track, eating the wrong foods, or, even worse, missing a meal. To help prevent this, use meal planning to outline successful eating all week. The following sections explain how to plan a week's worth of meals and how to use that meal plan to create a list of ingredients you need from the grocery store.

Meal planning

Meal planning, whether it's just for you or for your whole family, can be challenging and overwhelming. Even if you intend to eat only healthy foods, it's easy for your lifestyle and other excuses to get in the way. Maybe you work late or you forget to pack a lunch. Maybe you just don't have time to grocery shop. At the end of the day, you're hungry and prone to ordering in or going out for dinner, where the choices aren't always as nutritious as what you can cook for yourself.

The best way to get started with meal planning is to make a chart with the days of the week written across the top and the meals listed down the side. You can base the columns on either five days or seven days. (We like to leave days open for leftovers and the occasional night of eating out.) Then create four to six rows to account for breakfast, lunch, and dinner, and one to two snacks in between.

After you've created your chart, select the recipes or foods you want to serve each day and plug them into the plan. Check out the recipes in Part 3 for some great ideas.

You may want to focus on some of the guidelines mentioned in the earlier "Dishing it up in the right proportions" section to create balanced meals. In that case, you need to figure out how many items you need to make per meal or what foods you need to add to make sure to get your beans, grains, and veggies.

In order to keep your grocery list from getting out of control, use some of the same ingredients in multiple recipes each week. For instance, batch-cook a 1-pound bag of dried black beans early in the week, and you'll have enough cooked beans to make three or four meals that week, like Black Bean Quinoa Chili (Chapter 12), Sweet Potato Black Bean Quesadillas (Chapter 11), and Black Bean Cumin Burgers (Chapter 12). If you still have leftovers, throw them in salads or wraps or freeze them for future meals.

In the preceding example, you could also use sweet potatoes several ways: first in the quesadillas and then cut into wedges and roasted for a side of fries for the burgers.

REMEMBER

You don't have to make a new dish every day for every meal. Prepare extra food and use the leftovers to maximize your meals and your time.

TIP

For new ideas and recipes, subscribe to a recipe-focused blog, like www. veggieinspired.com or get a handful of plant-based cookbooks that you can rotate through. Your local library is a great source for trying out new cookbooks!

TIP

Later in this chapter, we provide some simple, delicious meal ideas that can help you prepare for your busy week. But first, try these tips to help you follow a meal plan:

>> Do your grocery shopping on the weekend for easy meal prep through-out the week.

>> Batch-cook beans and grains on the weekend or at the beginning of the week so they'll be ready to add to meals all week long. Roast a few pans of vegetables, whisk up a jar of homemade salad dressing, and/or make a batch of hummus or dip for the week (see Part 3 for all kinds of recipe ideas).

>> Have on hand a variety of on-the-go snacks, such as trail mix, nut and seed bars, cut-up veggies, and bean dip.

>> Get yourself equipped with a cooler or cold pack and to-go containers.

Making your plant-based grocery list

So, how do you make a good grocery list? Well, the first thing you need is pen and paper. No, seriously. To have an effective list, you need to either write it down or create it on your phone or computer (you can find apps to help you do that) — whichever way works best for you. In Chapter 7, we offer a complete list of plant-based items to stock up on, so refer to that for more specifics on what to get. Here we're talking about how to make your list.

First, it helps to determine into which shopper category you naturally fall:

>> **The organizer:** This person likes to be on top of things and knows what to expect. They methodically go through each of the food categories (grains, proteins, vegetables, fruits, oils and fats, and superfoods) every week and write down what they need. Even if they don't think they need anything, they go through the process anyway to make sure nothing is missed.

This approach is good for beginner plant-based foodies, because you can visualize which foods are in which category, and it also helps you navigate the grocery store in an efficient manner.

>> **The shopper by recipe:** This person selects a few recipes they want to make for the week and makes a list based on those recipes specifically. So, in essence, they just buy what the recipes call for.

>> **The on-the-fly shopper:** This person wants to take a chance, walk around, and grab things as they see them. Likely this is someone creative who can work with whatever food items they have on hand.

>> **The list runner:** This person keeps a running list of items they run out of, perhaps on the counter or fridge. They look at and add to the list constantly. They typically have a mental idea of what they need to get and what they already have, and they may just need to make an additional mini list of extras. Likely, their kitchen is well stocked to begin with because of regular grocery store trips, and they just need things like produce or specialty items.

After you determine what type of shopper you are, formulate your grocery list and then hit the grocery store.

Not making a list can set you up for not-so-good results. When you don't make a list, you may buy random, unwanted items that waste your time and money, among other things. Consider these three consequences of not making a good list:

>> **You overbuy on items you already have.** Be sure to take an inventory of items at home; otherwise, you may end up with foods well past their expiration date.

>> **You buy unhealthy or unwanted ingredients.** This is kind of like impulse buying the latest gadget or trendy article of clothing. You may think you want it, but it's not really in your plans for the week — again, just wasted money.

>> **You don't get what you want or anything at all.** Without a proper plan, you may get overwhelmed at the store and be too intimidated to buy anything, resulting in a wasted trip and an empty shopping bag.

Exploring sample meal plans

Now that you have the tools to make a great list (see the preceding section), make sure to get yourself on track every day with a good, solid meal plan. These sample meal plans for breakfast, lunch, dinner, and snacks can help you get started. After that, we go into more-specific plans to help you meet your goals as a new plant-based eater.

Breakfast ideas

Add these ideas to your list to start your day off right (see Chapter 9 for even more):

>> One or two slices of sprouted-grain toast with your nut butter of choice and a sliced banana, along with a glass of rice milk (with or without a scoop of protein powder).

>> Half a cup of cooked whole-grain porridge (buckwheat, oats, quinoa, or spelt) cooked with almond milk or rice milk. Add in dried fruits (such as apricots, cranberries, or raisins), fresh fruits (such as blueberries), nuts (such as almonds, pecans, or walnuts), or seeds (such as chia seeds, hempseeds, flaxseeds, pumpkin seeds, or sunflower seeds).

>> Fresh fruit or green smoothie made of 1 to 2 cups of almond milk, coconut milk, hemp milk, or rice milk. Add in a banana, berries, ground chia seeds or flaxseeds, a scoop of plant-based protein powder, and a handful of kale or spinach.

Lunch and dinner options

Keep your menu (and belly) full with these meal ideas (more recipes in Chapters 11 and 12):

>> Power-packed salad with a base of romaine, leaf lettuce, or arugula. Add in:

- *Veggie protein:* ¼ to ½ cup black beans, chickpeas, kidney beans, lentils, lima beans, or marinated tempeh or tofu

- *Raw or steamed veggies:* Beets, bell peppers, carrots, celery, cucumbers, onions, spinach, sprouts, or tomatoes

- *Healthy fat:* Avocados, hempseed oil, nuts, olive oil, olives, and seeds

- *Soaked or toasted sea vegetables:* Arame, dulse, nori, or wakame (see Chapter 4)

- *Fresh or dried fruit:* Apple, currants, dried cranberries, pear, raisins, raspberries, or strawberries

- *Extras:* ½ cup cooked whole grains, such as barley, brown rice, millet, or quinoa (see Chapter 3)

>> Sandwich with whole-grain, sprouted-grain, or gluten-free bread or a wrap loaded with avocados, hummus, leafy greens, sprouts, and veggies.

>> Soup with chunky veggies or a pureed vegetable soup:

- *Base:* Water and dried herbs, miso paste, or homemade vegetable broth

- *Veggies:* Asparagus, bok choy, broccoli, carrots, cauliflower, celery, kale, onions, spinach, or zucchini

- *Beans:* Black beans, chickpeas, lentils, split peas, or white beans

- *Starchy veggies:* Squash or sweet potatoes

- *Whole grains:* Barley, brown rice, or quinoa

- *Sea veggies:* Arame, dulse, nori, or wakame (see Chapter 4)

Macronutrients plate

You can create an entire meal from nothing but wholesome sides. A good selection of sides can become a full meal that's hearty and nourishing. You may have heard these types of meals referred to as *Buddha bowls*, *power bowls*, or *nourish bowls*. Mix and match foods from the following categories:

>> **Cooked whole grains:** Brown rice, buckwheat, farro, millet, quinoa, or whole-grain pasta

>> **Starchy vegetables (steamed, roasted, or grilled):** Beets, legumes, parsnips, sweet potatoes, or winter squash

>> **Steamed or sautéed veggies:** Asparagus, bell peppers, bok choy, broccoli, collards, eggplant, green beans, kale, mushrooms, onions, snap peas, Swiss chard, or zucchini

>> **Organic tofu, tempeh, beans, or lentils (marinated, baked, grilled, stewed, or steamed)**

>> **Fats:** Avocados, coconut oil, olive oil, nuts, or seeds

>> **Condiments:** Apple cider vinegar, herbs, hummus, lemon juice, olive oil, pesto, seaweed, spices, or tamari

Snacks

In between meals, you'll want to keep yourself fueled with snacks or mini-meals. Try one or two of these suggestions:

>> Whole-grain crackers or brown-rice cakes with nut or seed butter

>> Fresh fruit

>> Trail mix (try the Super Brazil and Goldenberry Trail Mix recipe in Chapter 14)

>> A homemade muffin (see the Apple Cinnamon Mini Muffins recipe in Chapter 9)

>> Hummus or bean dip with brown-rice crackers or sliced veggies (check out the Edamame Hummus recipe in Chapter 14)

>> Guacamole with corn chips (see the Sweet Pea Guacamole recipe in Chapter 14)

>> Homemade energy bar

>> A smoothie (try the Chocolate Banana Super Smoothie recipe in Chapter 14 or the Liquid Nutrition Smoothie in Chapter 9)

Punches of protein

Whether you train hard at the gym or just find that you feel better eating more protein, you may want to follow a meal plan that looks like the one in Table 6-2. However, be sure to rotate these items regularly with other high-protein plant-based foods.

TABLE 6-2   **Protein-Filled Meal Plan**

Breakfast	Lunch	Snack	Dinner
Turmeric Tofu Scramble (Chapter 9) with a slice of sprouted-grain toast and ¼ avocado	Quinoa Tabbouleh Salad (Chapter 10)	Super Brazil and Goldenberry Trail Mix (Chapter 14)	Tangy Tempeh Teriyaki Stir-Fry (Chapter 12) on a bed of brown-rice noodles or wild rice
Liquid Nutrition Smoothie (Chapter 9) with a full scoop of protein	Hearty sandwich with tempeh, avocado, and sprouts, plus a large salad	Happy Hemp Loaves (Chapter 14)	Black Bean Cumin Burgers (Chapter 12) with a Kale and Cabbage Slaw Salad (Chapter 10), sliced avocado, and Garlic Oregano Yam Fries (Chapter 13)
Soaked Oats with Goji Berries (Chapter 9) with additional plant-based protein mixed in	New Age Minestrone (Chapter 10) with a green salad or 1 slice sprouted-grain toast	Chocolate Banana Super Smoothie (Chapter 14)	Maple-marinated tofu, quinoa with spinach and citrus, and steamed broccoli
Super Chia Banana Porridge (Chapter 9)	Kale and Cabbage Slaw Salad (Chapter 10) topped with avocado, sprouts, and chickpeas	Apple Cinnamon Bites (Chapter 14) with 1 cup almond milk or Homemade Hempseed Milk (Chapter 9)	Warm Festive Farro Salad with sautéed collard greens with garlic and olive oil

Foods for energy and endurance

You don't have to be athletic to want energy all day long. The meal ideas in Table 6-3 are balanced and well-rounded to keep you sustained with nutrients to keep you going.

TABLE 6-3   Energy-Boosting Meal Plan

Breakfast	Lunch	Snack	Dinner
Super Chia Banana Porridge (Chapter 9)	Veggie sandwich with Edamame Hummus (Chapter 14)	Chocolate Banana Super Smoothie (Chapter 14)	Arame Soba Noodle Salad (Chapter 10) with Chunky Miso Soup (Chapter 10)
Blueberry Buckwheat Pancakes (Chapter 9) with fresh fruit and 1–2 tablespoons of nut butter	Quinoa Tabbouleh Salad (Chapter 10)	Apple Cinnamon Bites (Chapter 14)	Sweet Potato Shepherd's Pie (Chapter 12) with steamed kale
Soaked Oats with Goji Berries (Chapter 9)	Chunky Miso Soup (Chapter 10) or New Age Minestrone (Chapter 10) with a side salad with olive oil and vinegar	1 apple with Almond Butter and Cinnamon Dip (Chapter 14)	Warm Festive Farro Salad (Chapter 10) on a bed of spinach topped with ¼ cup white beans
Liquid Nutrition Smoothie (Chapter 9)	Sun flower Seed Nori Rolls (Chapter 11) with Kale and Cabbage Slaw Salad (Chapter 10)	1 rice cake topped with tahini, Edamame Hummus (Chapter 14), or Sweet Pea Guacamole (Chapter 14)	Zesty Pesto Pasta with White Beans (Chapter 12) and a green salad

Modifying Your Favorite Recipes to Be Plant-Based

You may be thinking, "It's all well and good to learn about these new foods and how to prepare them, but what about my old favorite comfort foods?" You know the ones we mean — the ones you're afraid you'll miss so much that you'll just have to cheat on your plant-based diet. They're the ones that are so good, you feel certain there isn't a plant-based alternative. Well, we can't think of even *one* food that we haven't been able to modify in the plant-based world. Everything from chili to chocolate cake can be made with wholesome and natural ingredients.

Try these tips for modifying common comfort foods. Chapter 7 gets even deeper into detail on how to swap common non-plant-based ingredients for plant-based ones.

>> **Chili:** Because chili is a vegetable-dense meal, you just have to skip the ground meat. Adding extra protein from beans or lentils is a great choice.

>> **Chocolate cake:** Replace the milk, eggs, and butter with nondairy milk, ground chia seeds, and coconut oil.

>> **Pizza:** Make the crust from whole-grain flour and use toppings such as chopped veggies, pesto, and nutritional yeast — among other creative ideas.

>> **Macaroni and cheese:** Revamp this comforting childhood classic with whole-grain noodles and a sauce made from butternut squash and tahini.

>> **Meat and potatoes:** Make a hearty dish with portobello mushrooms, tempeh, or tofu instead, with a side of Rosemary Cauliflower Mashed Potatoes (see Chapter 13), squash, or sweet potatoes.

Consuming whole foods is always the best choice for health, but using store-bought meat and dairy alternatives can be helpful for those missing certain tastes and textures. Plus, they can be very convenient when you're short on time. We don't recommend making them a staple in your plant-based diet, but we certainly enjoy them from time to time and you can, too. Serve some of these new plant-based dishes alongside your old favorites. This may help you ease the transition to a plant-based lifestyle and show you just how delicious and satisfying plant-based foods can be! (Turn to Chapter 5 for more about transitioning to a plant-based diet.)

Chapter **7**

Overhauling Your Kitchen Contents

I t's time to renovate your kitchen, plant-based style! This chapter guides you through the basics of getting rid of what doesn't belong anymore and restocking with plant-based goodness. Although this undertaking may be a little scary because you have to start letting go of some long-time habits and food friends, it's also a really fun adventure because you get to make a fresh start and buy new things (and who doesn't like buying new things?).

This is all about feeling confident in your kitchen — when you have all the supplies (including food and utensils) you need, you're much more likely to be inspired to spend time in your kitchen to make delicious plant-based meals. This chapter tells you what foods and utensils to keep on hand.

Cleaning Out Your Kitchen

As with any new undertaking, it's out with the old before it's in with the new, so the first step is to clean up your kitchen and make some room for all the new goodies you need to stock! Look at your fridge, your pantry, and any other places where you store unhealthy, packaged, and processed food — and remove anything that doesn't fit into a plant-based lifestyle. Just follow these easy steps:

1. Get rid of the junk.

There's a good chance your pantry is like ours once were — loaded with a wide variety of chips, crackers, cookies, and cereals that need to be expelled because they're loaded with sugar, salt, and fat. Although some of those things may actually be plant based, your focus should be on whole foods. Then move on to your fridge, where you probably have condiments, salad dressings, and fruit juices, all of which can be discarded. As hard as it is, letting go of your ties to these foods is super important — not just so you can more easily adjust to a plant-based diet but also so you can live better! Although you may think your old-faithful foods make your life happier or healthier, we can assure you that most things in your cupboard are only sabotaging you.

The bottom line is that you want to get rid of any foods that don't naturally come from the ground, meaning they're as wholesome as possible. This includes all meats (look in your freezer), eggs, and dairy products, as well as refined flours and pastas and processed cooking oils, such as canola oil and generic vegetable oil.

2. Dump or donate.

Anything that is open needs to go directly into the garbage. Unopened, unexpired food can go to a food bank — use your discretion on what to donate. Otherwise, just dump it! If it's not good for you, chances are it's not better for anyone else to consume. Junk food is junk food! That doesn't mean you can't treat yourself every now and then, but don't keep it in your kitchen — that's just setting you up for temptation and an unhealthy choice down the road. Take initiative and dump it.

3. Get over it.

After detoxing your cupboards, you may be a bit sad and worried that you have nothing left to eat. We can assure you that's absolutely not true. You can find a healthy, wholesome, and tasty alternative to everything you got rid of. Trust us, we don't believe in tasteless food or dieting. We believe in whole, fresh, and delicious food, which is what you need from now on. You'll be satisfied and content when you have a kitchen that's loaded with incredibly delicious food. Just keep reminding yourself that it's all going to be okay — we promise!

4. Restock.

Now is the time to get to the market and stock back up. You can find pretty much everything you need at your local grocery store. Most stores now have sections that are just bursting with natural, fresh, and organic products. Look for cereals that are high in fiber and low in sugar, cookies that are sweetened with fruit juice, and crackers with sea salt (not table salt). Experiment with whole grains, flours, breads, and pastas like kamut, oat, quinoa, or spelt instead of wheat-based products. Buy raw nut butters instead of the no-stir kind, pure maple syrup instead of sugar, coconut oil instead of canola oil, and rolled oats instead of quick oats. Lastly, make sure your fridge is brimming full of fresh fruits and vegetables; that way you always have something to snack on and add to any meal.

We know it can be overwhelming, but just take small steps and soon you'll have a kitchen stocked with the best foods, and you'll feel inspired to prepare more foods at home. And don't forget that with your kitchen freshly made over, you just happen to be making over your health, too.

Stocking Your Plant-Based Kitchen

You don't need to buy everything at once. Buy fresh produce only in amounts that you need for the week. Stock up on pantry and freezer items as you can.

Fresh produce

This is what you're going to find yourself buying most frequently, as you're going to want it fresh — meaning you have to purchase it in small quantities. Depending on where you find it, you can get produce pretty inexpensively, although you may have to do some shopping around.

Keep this basic produce on hand as much as possible, because it's so nutritious and versatile:

>> Avocado

>> Broccoli

>> Cauliflower

>> Fresh fruit (in season), such as apples, bananas, berries, cherries, grapes, kiwi, melons, pears, and pineapple

>> Leafy green vegetables, such as bok choy, broccoli, cabbage, kale, lettuce, and spinach

>> Garlic

>> Lemons and limes

- » Mushrooms

- » Onions (red and white)

- » Sweet potatoes or squash

- » Tomatoes

Refrigerated items

The refrigerated section of the grocery store is where you'll find dairy alterna-tives, soy foods, and a few flavorful condiments, like sauerkraut and pickles.

You're likely to find chia seeds, flaxseeds, and hempseeds in the main aisles, but you should keep them in the fridge at home so they don't go rancid.

- » Chia seeds, flaxseeds, and hempseeds

- » Fresh ginger

- » Olives and pickles

- » Dijon mustard

- » Sauerkraut

- » Soy foods (miso paste, tempeh, and tofu)

- » Milks (almond, hempseed, oat, or organic soy)

- » Yogurt from coconut milk or coconut kefir

Frozen foods

Having some convenience foods and treats on hand is a great way to stay on track with your plant-based meals. This may mean all the difference between staying on and falling off the plant wagon — especially on those days when you're feeling a bit tired or unmotivated. Here's a list of frozen goods to get you started:

- » Frozen berries, peaches, and mangos

- » Frozen organic vegetables, including broccoli, edamame, green beans, mixed vegetables, peas, and spinach

- » Nondairy ice cream made from almond, coconut, or rice.

- » Sprouted-grain breads and wraps

- » Veggie burgers

Note: In some cases, frozen vegetables and fruits are more nutritious than fresh vegetables, especially if the frozen versions are organic. They're often picked at peak ripeness and flash-frozen soon afterward, thereby maintaining their nutrients. The nutrient content of fresh produce is affected by how much time passes between picking and eating, because nutrients degrade over time.

Pantry staples

Always keep these foundational items stocked in your pantry, cupboards, and the like. Some of these foods have a short shelf life, but you can keep others around for longer periods of time.

>> **Baking goods:** Arrowroot powder, baking powder, baking soda, and pure vanilla (and other) extracts.

>> **Dried beans:** Black beans, chickpeas, kidney beans, lentils, pinto beans, split peas, and white beans.

>> **Flavorings:** Cacao powder, carob, hot sauce or sriracha, and sea salt.

>> **Flours:** Almond flour, brown-rice flour, buckwheat flour, oat flour, or spelt flour.

>> **Herbs and spices:** Allspice, basil, bay leaves, chili powder, cinnamon, cloves, cumin, curry powder, five-spice powder, garlic powder, ground ginger, ground mustard, marjoram, onion powder, oregano, paprika, rosemary, sage, thyme, turmeric, whole black pepper, and whole nutmeg.

TIP

Store your herbs and spices away from heat and light sources. (In other words, don't store them over the oven or in the window, because the heat and light cause them to lose their flavor more quickly.) Replace herbs and spices that are older than one year. You can substitute 1 teaspoon of dried herbs for 1 tablespoon of chopped fresh herbs.

>> **Natural sweeteners:** Blackstrap molasses; coconut sugar; pure maple syrup or whole, unrefined cane sugar

>> **Naturally brewed soy sauce:** Liquid amino acids, shoyu, or tamari (wheat free)

>> **Nutritional yeast**

>> **Nuts and seeds:** Almonds, cashews, pecans, popcorn kernels, pumpkin seeds, sesame seeds, shelled sunflower seeds, and walnuts

>> **Nut and seed butters:** Almond, cashew, tahini, and walnut

>> **Oils:** Coconut, flaxseed, grapeseed, olive, and toasted sesame

- **Pasta and noodles (whole grain):** Brown-rice noodles, buckwheat soba noodles, and whole-grain pasta

- **Pseudo grains:** Amaranth, buckwheat, quinoa, and wild rice

- **Salsa**

- **Sea vegetables:** Arame, dulse, hijiki, kombu, nori, and wakame

- **Teas:** Green, herbal, and rooibos

- **Tomatoes (canned):** Crushed, diced, paste, sauce, or whole

- **Unsweetened dried fruit:** Apricots, cranberries, dates, figs, and raisins

- **Unsweetened fruit jams:** Blackberry, raspberry, strawberry, and so on

- **Unsweetened canned coconut milk**

- **Vinegars:** Balsamic, brown rice, coconut, red wine, and unpasteurized apple cider

- **Whole grains:** Barley, brown rice, millet, and spelt

- **Whole-grain products or sprouted grains:** Breads, cereals, pita breads, and wraps

Finding Alternatives to Common Ingredients

In Chapter 1, I mention that you can swap out plant-based ingredients for some of your favorite and most comforting ingredients. You may be at a loss and wonder how it's even possible to find a plant-based alternative to certain foods. The following sections cover some common ingredients and what the main go-tos are in the veggie world.

Milk

Luckily, you can find a plethora of nondairy milk alternatives, which are available at stores or easy enough to make at home. Some varieties include almond, Brazil nut, cashew, coconut, hempseed, and rice milk. You can easily substitute these (in equal measurements) into any recipe that calls for milk.

Choosing alternative milk doesn't mean you're missing out on calcium. Many nutritious plant-based foods, such as almonds, bok choy, and kale, are loaded with these nutrients. They're not just found in milk!

Eggs

People are often nervous about how to substitute an egg in baked goods. Well, you have more options than you likely think you do!

TIP

Try these; each makes the equivalent of one egg:

» 1 tablespoon of ground flaxseeds or ground chia seeds plus 3 tablespoons of water (soak for 5 to 10 minutes to allow the mixture to become gelatinous)

» ¼ cup mashed banana

» ¼ cup unsweetened applesauce

» 3 to 4 tablespoons *aquafaba* (the liquid from a can of chickpeas)

Meat

Meat is out on a plant-based diet. For a hearty, rich texture and something that fills you up, the main plant-based items to stock up on are beans, portobello mushrooms, tempeh, and tofu. Each of these items has a hearty, chewy texture, and you can marinate them in pretty much any sauce. You can also chop them up, grind them up, or use them any way you would use meat — as burgers, in stews and chili, or just baked on your plate.

For the sake of convenience, you can also keep a few store-bought packages of vegan burgers, sausages, or ground "beef" in the freezer for when you're short on time or feeling uninspired in the kitchen. Just remember that these should be consumed in moderation — your focus should always be on whole foods.

Cheese

This is usually one of the most difficult items for people to give up. Most people are addicted to cheese. The good news is that the plant world offers creamy, soft textures that are rich and decadent and can be used in place of cheese. Here are some of our favorites:

» Nutritional yeast

» Sliced avocado

>> Soaked and blended cashews

>> Sprouted soft organic tofu

All of these can be added to pizzas, quesadillas, sandwiches, tacos, and other dishes that need a cheesy flavor.

As for store-bought cheese, many vegan brands are available today. You may need to try a few to find the one you like best. Keep in mind that these vegan cheese options aren't health foods, so keep your consumption to a minimum.

Thickeners

Ever wonder what holds your meat gravy together? You probably don't want to know, so go for arrowroot powder, organic cornstarch, or tapioca. Each of these items makes your sauces and puddings gooey from natural sources.

You can find these items in most health-food stores or grocery stores in the baking section.

Getting the Must-Have Equipment

Having your kitchen set up correctly is just another way to make it easy and enjoyable to stay on track with your new plant-based habits. If everything you need is within arm's reach, it's easy not only to make delicious meals but also to choose healthy snacks.

You want to have a few essential things on hand when it comes time to make all this delicious food. If you don't have the right tools, it's that much more difficult to cook. In the following sections, we outline some of the basics. Check off the ones you have, go shopping for others, and put the rest on your wish list.

TIP

We highly recommend investing in good cookware and bakeware up front. It may be pricey, but it's a true investment that really makes a difference. Your food is only as good as what it comes in contact with. Choose good-quality stainless steel whenever and wherever possible.

Handy utensils

You may be surprised by how many of these you already have at home. Some you may use, and some may still be wrapped up in a box because you didn't know what to do with them! Here's a list of the basic utensils you should make sure you have:

TIP

» **Bakeware:** You'll need a variety — cookie sheets, rimmed baking sheets, muffin pans, square baking dishes, rectangular baking dishes, cake pans, and pie pans.

Rimmed baking sheets can be used to roast vegetables, bake tofu, roast nuts, make kale chips, and more! We suggest having at least two large ones. We often use them at the same time!

» **Colander:** This is similar to a strainer, but it has wider holes and a bigger base. It's good for washing vegetables and draining pasta.

» **Cutting boards (wooden):** You want at least one, maybe two, for cutting all your veggies. Aim for one that's at least 12 x 14 inches. You can get ones with rubber stoppers on the corners, or you can put a damp cloth beneath the board to prevent it from sliding.

» **Grater:** Use this for shredding vegetables.

» **Kitchen tongs:** Tongs are great for tossing stir-fries, mixing veggie salads, or picking up slices of tofu out of a pan. They're also good for plating food.

» **Knives:** Get yourself a set of good knives. If you're intimidated by the whole set, just start with these three: a chef's knife, a paring knife, and serrated knife.

» **Measuring cups:** Get a set of dry measuring cups for grains, flours, and seeds, and a set of wet measuring cups for milks, pure maple syrup, olive oil, and the like. Opt for the angled ones where you can see the measurements looking down.

» **Measuring spoons:** Get a set — preferably stainless steel — with measurements for 1 tablespoon, 1 teaspoon, ½ teaspoon, and ¼ teaspoon.

» **Microplane:** This type of grater is great for zesting lemons and oranges or grating ginger or garlic.

» **Mixing bowls:** Stainless steel bowls are lightweight and easy to clean. Glass bowls are also nice and clean up very well.

- **Pots and pans:** You want to have a range of sizes, including a small saucepan, a sauté pan, a skillet, and a soup pot.

- **Spatula:** This is essential for making perfect pancakes or flipping items in a pan.

- **Spoons (wooden and stainless steel):** You want a variety of spoons for mixing, stirring, and moving food around in a pan. Get a variety that feel and look nice and that clean up well.

- **Steaming basket or insert:** It's great to have a steamer on hand for quick veggie prep.

- **Strainer:** We suggest getting a set of two or three strainers in different sizes. They're handy tools for rinsing berries, grains, nuts, and seeds. You want the mesh to be fine enough that things like amaranth and quinoa don't seep through.

- **Vegetable peeler:** Be sure to get one with a good hand grip and a wide blade. You want a peeler that will do a variety of fruits and veggies, from apples to carrots to squashes.

- **Wire whisk:** This is great for combining liquids, such as a salad dressing, or mixing wet ingredients into dry ones. We suggest having at least one large and one small balloon whisk. We also find a flat whisk handy when cooking chunky sauces in a pan.

GLASS VERSUS PLASTIC STORAGE

When storing food, you should always use glass containers. Although cheaper and lighter, plastic is just downright harmful to your health because it leaches toxins into anything that is stored in it. This goes for solid foods and liquids, no matter whether you store things in a cupboard, in the fridge, or in the freezer.

You also most certainly do not want to put plastic in the microwave. In our opinion, you should just try to rid yourself of plastic altogether. Glass is cleaner and lasts longer; plus, it generally just looks better overall.

We encourage you to become conscious about the environment and your health all in one. You have a choice to make every day when it comes to food, including where you get it, how you take it home, and how you store it.

Helpful appliances

Here are some fun and helpful pieces of equipment that make your kitchen time and cooking experiences that much more efficient:

>> **Countertop blender:** You most definitely want one of these. This is essential for smoothies, cold soups, and even "ice cream." We suggest a high-speed blender for best results. They cost more but perform the best.

>> **Food processor:** This appliance is fabulous for quickly chopping, grating, and mixing. We use ours several times a week!

>> **Immersion blender:** This is a fabulous and handy tool for blending soups right in the pot. It's also good for sauces and dressings.

>> **Toaster oven:** This is a handy device so you don't have to turn on your regular oven when you just want to warm up something small.

Chapter **8**

Being a Savvy Shopper

When you embark on a new diet, it can be hard to figure out what's what and where to buy different items. Heck, even if you've been eating plant-based for a while, you may still be stumped when it comes to procuring the best stuff. Navigating farmers markets, health-food stores, and the organic section of your neighborhood grocery store can be enough to make you feel like you're running in circles.

Luckily, we have a few general rules that you can use to navigate toward the healthy foods and away from the traps. In this chapter, we go into these tips in detail: Shop the perimeter of the grocery store (where the fresh foods are stocked), avoid the center aisles (where junk food and sugary cereals lurk), choose real foods (such as 100 percent fruit juice or 100 percent whole grain), stay clear of foods with cartoons on the label, and avoid foods that contain more than five ingredients or artificial ingredients that you can't pronounce.

We also suggest other places to shop for plant-based foods, and we explain what the terms *organic* and *GMO* mean and why you should be familiar with them both.

Conquering the Grocery Store

You've got your list, and you know *what* to look for. Now let's get into the *where* of it all. Although you can use non-grocery-store resources (we talk about those in the next section), most people are probably most familiar with a standard grocery store, so that's where we want to start. This section is all about helping you figure out how to navigate the store so you can steer clear of the bad stuff and start filling your cart with the good stuff.

Picking up produce

When you first enter a grocery store, you more than likely find yourself right in the produce section, among all the colorful fruits and vegetables that you should fill your cart with. So, go ahead and start your shopping trip there by grabbing your usuals — whatever you're most comfortable with already (maybe things like bananas, broccoli, and carrots).

Next, we encourage you to explore new terrain. Perhaps that means venturing over to that corner that's filled with lots of green bunches of leaves (it's okay if you're a little intimidated). Just get to know them — many of them look similar, but they are, indeed, different. Check the labels above and below them and get used to noticing what arugula, collards, kale, and Swiss chard look like. Compare their colors, leaf shapes and sizes, and stems. Each of them holds different possibilities for you. These will become your new friends as you start to round out your plant-based diet.

TIP

If you're feeling a little lost, don't be afraid to ask an employee in the produce section for help. They know a lot about what each piece of produce is, what it does, and how to cook it.

When it comes to choosing organic versus local produce, just use your best judgment. To help you, the Environmental Working Group (EWG), an organization that provides information to protect public health and the environment, has done a fabulous job of outlining two lists, called the Dirty Dozen and the Clean Fifteen. They help consumers determine the best, safest produce to buy.

>> **Dirty Dozen** (www.ewg.org/foodnews/dirty-dozen.php**):** These types of produce are the biggest carriers of pesticides and chemical residues that can harm your health. When you buy these foods, you want to buy them in organic form and not in conventionally grown versions (as much as possible). If you do buy them conventionally once in a while, be sure to wash them well.

- Strawberries

- Spinach

- Kale, collard, and mustard greens

- Nectarines

- Apples

- Grapes

- Cherries

- Peaches

- Pears

- Bell peppers and hot peppers

- Celery

- Tomatoes

WARNING

Chemical residues and pesticides don't only reside on skins and peels; they're embedded within most parts of the fruit or vegetable.

>> **Clean Fifteen:** The Clean Fifteen is the produce that's okay to eat conventionally (that is, it doesn't have to be organic) in moderation, because it carries the least amount of pesticides and chemical residues:

- Avocados

- Sweet corn

- Pineapple

- Onions

- Papaya

- Sweet peas (frozen)

- Eggplant

- Asparagus

- Broccoli

- Cabbage

- Kiwi

- Cauliflower

- Mushrooms

- Honeydew melon

- Cantaloupe

REMEMBER

The EWG updates these lists every year. Keep up to date with the most current lists at www.ewg.org.

Dipping into the interior aisles

Most items in the interior aisles contain preservatives; cheap, poor–quality ingredients; excess sodium and sugar; and layers of packaging that can be damaging to the environment. Although most of the products on these shelves are garbage for your health, you can still find some relatively wholesome options with no or minimally added ingredients or preservatives. Some of the healthier items to look for in the aisles include the following:

>> Dry grains, such as brown-rice pasta, millet, quinoa, rice, and whole oats

>> Shelf-stable nondairy milks, such as almond milk or rice milk (***Remember:*** Refrigerate after opening.)

>> Whole-grain or brown-rice crackers made with wholesome ingredients

>> Raw and plain nuts and seeds

>> Dried organic legumes and beans (and even some canned organic beans)

>> Snack foods like brown-rice cakes, organic tortilla chips, and salsa

>> Liquids and sauces, such as apple-cider vinegar, olive oil, tahini, and tamari

>> 100 percent fruit juices made from apple, pear, or lemon

Seeing what's lurking in the freezer

The freezer section of the grocery store can also be a scary place if you're not aware of what's contained within those cases. Nothing is wrong with freezing per se — it keeps food in the state in which it was frozen. However, in many grocery stores, the freezer section acts just like the aisles, with row upon row of colorful packages filled with foods that have all kinds of unhealthy ingredients. Even many plant-based foods, such as frozen veggies, frozen pizzas, and veggie burgers, need to be considered very carefully — you want to make sure that they're made up of quality ingredients that you recognize, with no traces of dairy or other animal products, and that they're organic and not genetically modified (see more on that later in this chapter).

We like to keep frozen fruits and vegetables on hand. Not only are they convenient, but they're generally frozen at their peak ripeness, keeping all the nutrients intact. However, don't let these frozen items be a replacement for fresh produce. They may be great for soups, stews, and casseroles, but you can't make a salad with frozen vegetables; they carry lots of water and are often soggy.

TIP

Here are some of the healthier options you can find in your freezer section that are okay to take home:

» Fruits and berries

» Nondairy ice cream (in moderation for a treat)

» Organic veggie burgers made from beans, nuts, and seeds

» Sprouted-grain breads or wraps

» Tempeh

» Veggies like butternut squash, organic corn, peas, and spinach

Shopping Off the Beaten Path

When you're immersed in this world of plant-based eating for a bit of time, grocery-store shopping may begin to lose its appeal. You may find yourself wanting to set foot instead on alternative ground, which is actually now becoming more mainstream. Shopping at places like farmers markets and health-food stores or getting involved with a local community-supported agriculture (CSA) service will likely become your new terrain for shopping. Why? First, the diversity of products that fall within your new plant-based standards are boundless in these locations (although you still have to be a discerning consumer, because organic cheeses and the like still aren't healthy snacks). Also, at places like farmers markets, you get access to some of the freshest produce. Plus, when you shop at places like these, you support smaller businesses that typically have as much interest in your health as they do in making a sale. All around, you feel better about your choices. Here's why these places may be the next wave of your grocery-shopping experience.

Farmers markets

Farmers markets have popped up everywhere. They're a gathering of local vendors and farmers offering produce (and sometimes other fresh items) for direct sale to consumers. They usually happen weekly in a public place, such as a park or community center, and are typically busy. You won't find everything of a certain category in one place as you do at a grocery store — every vendor has something different to offer.

The main benefit of farmers markets, aside from all the food being extremely fresh, is that you get the chance to talk to the farmers about their products. They can tell you all about your new find, how to prepare it, and where exactly it came from. You can even ask about the growing methods, such as what pesticides were used (if any) and when it was harvested.

Some local farmers may still use mass suppliers. Get to know your local farmers' growing practices and legitimacy.

CSA programs

You can purchase an annual or seasonal share in farmers' land and receive fresh, seasonal produce from that farm in exchange for their monetary investment. In some cases, you prepay before the growing season. In other cases, you pay weekly for a delivery or pick up your share at a designated meeting place. These days, there's an evolution away from single-farm CSAs to multi-farm CSA services that give customers a wider variety of foods and more choices (which can sometimes be customized online). This is a nice way to get produce and sometimes other specialty goods without having to fight traffic in the parking lot (or aisles, for that matter).

CSAs are especially helpful to use when you're just starting out on a plant-based diet because the produce is sometimes selected for you (which can feel way less intimidating than trying to pick out your own stuff at the store). It's a great way to learn about different fruits and veggies and when they're at the height of their freshness. You can find CSAs in your area at www.localharvest.org or by searching the internet.

Health-food stores

Every major city — and most smaller ones — have at least a few health-food stores, and we're not just talking about Whole Foods. You can typically find a whole slew of smaller, privately or family-run businesses that are committed to stocking good-quality products, clean packaged products, and nutritional supplements.

Health-food stores are typically much smaller than supermarkets, so it's much easier to find what you're looking for, which makes them convenient and easy places to stock up. You may also get to know the owners well, making it likely that they'll order things in for you by request or make other special arrangements with you if needed. Either way, shopping at health-food stores is typically a lot smoother and more enjoyable than shopping at conventional grocery stores.

GROW YOUR OWN VEGGIES, CONTROL YOUR PRODUCT FROM SEED TO MOUTH

Growing your own garden has so many benefits and is an amazing way to get fresh, organic vegetables into your body! Consider these five benefits of growing your own veggies:

- **They're high in nutrition.** Homegrown produce is likely organic produce, which means you're not using any pesticides or other contaminants. This means that the food can have a higher vitamin and mineral content than store-bought foods.

- **They taste better.** Foods that are free of pesticides and harvested straight from the garden are fresher and taste better.

- **It's cost-effective.** Growing your own vegetables significantly reduces your food costs. It also saves you time at the grocery store, giving you more time in your garden!

- **It's environmentally friendly.** Home gardening lowers your carbon footprint by helping prevent soil erosion, improve water and air quality, save energy, and reduce transportation costs.

- **It's fun, educational, and beautiful.** Gardening can be a fun and satisfying experiment for individuals, families, and children. It also helps create a beautiful personal space.

To find out how to begin your garden, contact the farmers in your community, whether at farmers markets or through searches online, or contact a local cooperative extension office (just search the web for the name of your city and "cooperative extension"). They may be willing to give you a little lesson on how to make the best use of your backyard. You can also try gardening clubs, community gardens, and even gardening exchanges (where people who have yard space but don't know what to do with it partner with experienced gardeners who come in and garden, splitting the produce 50/50). Even if you live in an apartment, you can get your green thumb on with potted plants and vertical gardening techniques!

Organic and GMO: Figuring Out What It All Means to a Plant-Based Diet

Lots of people these days are talking about what it means to eat organic. This also brings to light the label *GMO* (short for *genetically modified organism*), which is becoming a hot topic of discussion because of the prevalence of GMO foods and the health dangers they present.

If you don't understand these labels, you're doing your body and your health a disservice — especially if you're a new plant-based eater making all kinds of transitions to better your overall well-being. This is just one more step in the right direction of good health.

Knowing what organic means

Eating organic is all about making a choice to eat foods that aren't treated with pesticides, herbicides, fungicides, and the like. It also likely supports agricultural practices that preserve and work toward bettering the condition of the soil. Organic soil has more nutrients, including minerals. This makes for foods that taste better and are better for you.

The standards for organic food come in several categories:

>> **100 percent organic:** Contains *only* organic ingredients and must be produced without synthetic fertilizers, pesticides, antibiotics, genetic engineering, irradiation, or growth hormones. A U.S. Department of Agriculture (USDA) or Canadian seal of certification may appear on the product.

>> **Organic:** Made with at least 95 percent organic ingredients. The remaining 5 percent must be approved by the USDA. No ionizing radiation is allowed. A USDA or Canadian seal may appear on the product.

>> **Made with organic ingredients:** Made with at least 70 percent organic ingredients. The remaining 30 percent may be agricultural products that aren't produced according to organic standards. It must be clear which ingredients are organic. These products can't display the USDA or Canadian organic seal.

REMEMBER

Many small organic farms can't afford the process of official certification, even though they adhere to all the organic practices the regulations require. You may encounter farms like this at your local farmers market, so feel free to ask the farmers directly about whether they follow sustainable farming practices.

It's not always possible to stick to organic eating 100 percent, but as with anything else in this book, just do the best you can. Refer to the Dirty Dozen and Clean Fifteen lists we mention in the "Picking up produce" section earlier in this chapter to help guide you when prioritizing your decisions about organic eating.

LOCAL VERSUS ORGANIC: CAN YOU HAVE IT ALL?

When it comes to local, organic, or local and organic, people get confused and want to know which is better. From our perspective, if you can get your hands on both, that's generally the way to go — but not always.

When you have to make the choice between local nonorganic or organic from across the world, it may be in your best interest to choose local. When food (even organic food) travels long distances, it loses its enzymes, nutrients, and life force, so you're left with an organic strawberry from South America that may have ripened on a truck, train, or plane. This means that unnatural gases and methods have been used to artificially stimulate the growth process.

Remember: In the end, you just need to use your best judgment.

Getting clear on GMOs

A genetically modified organism (GMO) is one that has been genetically modified in a lab to create combinations that do not occur naturally in nature. Most packaged foods that aren't labeled otherwise contain GMOs. Sounds crazy, right? GMOs can be found among crops such as canola, corn, soy, and sugar beets, all of which are found in abundance in packaged/processed foods. To avoid GMOs, avoid anything made with canola oil; eat whole plant-based foods; and choose organic varieties of corn, soy, and sugar.

Numerous scientific claims have created substantial debate about whether GMOs are beneficial or harmful. The initial theory was that GMOs could help prevent world hunger, give the world new varieties of foods, improve rural livelihoods, and help the environment. However, GMOs have proven to be unsustainable, because farmers have to purchase new seeds every year while destroying the land (because GMO crops can encourage herbicide-resistant weeds and insecticide-resistant pests that infest non-GMO crops). GMOs have also created numerous allergies (especially to soy) and health problems, all while contaminating large sources of the food supply.

TIP

You have a choice every time you buy food. Seek out resources like the Non-GMO Project (www.nongmoproject.org), which helps consumers find products that are free of GMOs. You need to know what you can do as a consumer and what you can do for your health.

3

Plant-Based Recipes for Success

Start your day with plant-based alternatives to eggs and bacon.

Check out salad, soup, and hand-held recipes that give you a midday plant-based boost.

Create incredible stir-fries, pasta dishes, and other entrees to nourish yourself at the end of the day.

Dress up any meal with simple plant-based sides.

Try your hand at making sensational snacks and appetizers.

Enhance your meals with tasty plant-based sauces and dressings.

Satisfy your sweet tooth with delicious plant-based desserts.

Chapter **9**

Brilliant Breakfasts

You've heard it before, and you know it's true: The key to a successful, highly energized day is eating a balanced breakfast. When you get the right plant-based foods into your body in the morning, you feel great — both mentally and physically. Knowing you have great options and feeling fantastic make you ready to tackle the day like a champion.

This chapter outlines several recipes for the most important meal of the day. From sweet to savory, there is something here for everyone. Start off right with these morning delights and see where the day takes you.

Wakey, Wakey, No Eggs and Bakey

You won't find any egg, sausage, or bacon recipes, or any other animal-based options, in this book. "So, then what do I eat for breakfast?" you may be asking. Just wait — this chapter is packed with powerful plant-based breakfast selections that fuel you up, give you energy, and don't weigh you down.

The standard, traditional breakfast of bacon and eggs — although it may be familiar and taste great — is heavy and high in salt and saturated fat. It can leave you feeling uncomfortable and doesn't provide the energy and vigor you need to thrive all day long. However, the good news is that there are many plant-based substitutes for your favorite breakfast items:

>> **Eggs:** A plant-based protein, such as sprouted tofu

>> **Sausage and bacon:** Marinated tempeh or baked tofu

>> **Yogurt:** Chia cereal, coconut yogurt, or mashed bananas.

>> **Milk:** Unsweetened almond milk, coconut milk, hempseed milk, or rice milk

REMEMBER

Whether you crave something sweet or savory in the morning, it's just a matter of finding the right foods to give you your fix for the day. If you don't get balanced ingredients in your body first thing in the morning, you can set yourself up for cravings, bloating, and an energy crash.

Easy to Make and Easy on the Go

If you want one meal to be easy and quick during the workweek, it's breakfast. Often, people neglect this meal because of limited time or poor planning. We often hear people complain that they don't eat a good breakfast because they don't have time or they think that making a decent breakfast is too complicated.

TIP

You can do a number of things to simplify breakfast preparation and make sure you start your day strongly:

>> Make some or all of your breakfast the night before, such as oatmeal, a smoothie, or soaked chia seeds.

>> Always have nut or seed milk ready to go in the fridge to use as a base for porridges and smoothies — or to add to coffee or tea.

>> Make a batch of muffins whenever you have time (perhaps on the weekend) and store them in the freezer. Then you can pull them out as needed for a simple breakfast.

>> If you like multiple-ingredient breakfasts, measure and portion out ingredients the night before. Store them in their own containers in the fridge or cupboard so they can be easily dumped into a bowl of oatmeal or a blender when you're half asleep.

>> Use glass or stainless-steel storage containers or glass water bottles for taking items on the go. These containers don't leak, and they keep your breakfast fresh.

>> Save the more involved recipes, such as pancakes and tofu scrambles, for the weekend when you have more time. Or make extra so you can warm up the leftovers the next day for a simple breakfast.

>> Throw caution to the wind and eat dinner leftovers for breakfast. Your first meal of the day doesn't have to be the typical breakfast fare you're used to. Sometimes we crave grains and veggies or a warm cup of soup to get going in the morning.

TIP

Try these super-simple ideas for a breakfast with no recipe required:

>> Two slices of sprouted-grain or whole-grain bread with nut or seed butter

>> A banana with a handful of nuts

>> Coconut yogurt topped with fruit

>> Apple slices with almond butter

>> Avocado spread on toast

Homemade Hempseed Milk

PREP TIME: ABOUT 5 MIN	COOK TIME: NONE	YIELD: 6 SERVINGS

INGREDIENTS

1 cup hempseeds

4 cups water

1 tablespoon coconut oil

2 tablespoons maple syrup or coconut nectar

1 teaspoon vanilla bean powder or ½ teaspoon vanilla extract

1 teaspoon cinnamon

DIRECTIONS

In a high–speed blender, place all the ingredients and blend for at least 1 minute.

PER SERVING: *Calories 263 (From Fat 189); Fat 21g (Saturated 26g); Cholesterol 0mg; Sodium 6mg; Carbohydrate 9g (Dietary Fiber 4 g); Protein 13g.*

TIP: You can substitute this homemade milk measure for measure in most recipes that call for dairy milk.

NOTE: This milk can be stored for up to 4 days and keeps best in the refrigerator in a glass jar.

VARY IT! Try swapping out the hempseeds for almonds, Brazil nuts, macadamia nuts, or sunflower seeds. If you swap out the hempseeds for a nut with skins, you'll need to strain the milk with a fine mesh colander, cheesecloth, or nut-milk bag to remove the skins from the liquid.

Liquid Nutrition Smoothie

PREP TIME: ABOUT 4 MIN	COOK TIME: NONE	YIELD: 2 SERVINGS

INGREDIENTS

2 cups almond milk, hempseed milk, or rice milk

2 to 4 tablespoons plant-based protein powder (such as Sunwarrior or Vega)

½ cup fresh or frozen blueberries or mixed berries

1 banana

½ cup fresh or frozen chopped mango, peach, or pear

½ cup ice

1 teaspoon coconut nectar or pure maple syrup

½ to 1 cup packed fresh spinach leaves

DIRECTIONS

1 In a blender, place all the ingredients and blend until the mixture is smooth and no lumps remain.

2 Pour into 2 glasses and enjoy.

PER SERVING: Calories 186 (From Fat 27); Fat 3g (Saturated 0g); Cholesterol 0mg; Sodium 283mg; Carbohydrate 31g (Dietary Fiber 4g); Protein 11g.

TIP: This smoothie will be creamier if your fruit is frozen, so opt for frozen fruit whenever possible (or just add more ice).

NOTE: The smoothie will keep for 8 hours in the refrigerator.

VARY IT! Try adding 1 tablespoon of any of these superfoods: acai berry powder, almond butter, cacao nibs, carob powder, chia seeds, coconut oil, flaxseed oil, goji berries, hempseeds, maca, or matcha green tea powder.

Superfood Berry Smoothie

PREP TIME: ABOUT 5 MIN	COOK TIME: NONE	YIELD: 2 SERVINGS

INGREDIENTS

1 avocado, peeled and pit removed

1 naval orange, peeled

1 cup chopped kale, tough stems removed

1 cup fresh or frozen spinach

1 cup frozen mixed berries

1 apple, cored

¼ cup raw walnuts

1 cup ice cubes

½ to 1 cup filtered water, as needed, to thin

DIRECTIONS

1 In a high-speed blender, place all the ingredients and blend until smooth.

2 Pour into 2 glasses and enjoy.

PER SERVING: *Calories 329 (From Fat 169); Fat 19g (Saturated 2g); Cholesterol 0mg; Sodium 35mg; Carbohydrate 42g (Dietary Fiber 12g); Protein 6g.*

Chocolate Nice Cream Breakfast Parfait

PREP TIME: ABOUT 5 MIN	COOK TIME: NONE	YIELD: 2 SERVINGS

INGREDIENTS

1 cup frozen banana slices

1 tablespoon creamy peanut butter

1 scoop plant-based protein powder or hemp powder (optional)

2 teaspoons unsweetened cocoa powder

1 teaspoon pure vanilla extract

1 to 2 tablespoons unsweetened nondairy milk, as needed, to thin

1 fresh banana, sliced

½ cup raw or toasted old-fashioned rolled oats

½ cup fresh blueberries

DIRECTIONS

1 In a food processor, place the frozen banana slices, peanut butter, protein powder or hemp powder (if using), cocoa powder, vanilla, and nondairy milk and process until smooth, stopping to scrape down the sides as necessary.

2 In individual glasses or bowls, layer the chocolate nice cream with fresh banana slices, rolled oats, and fresh blueberries.

PER SERVING: *Calories 271 (From Fat 57); Fat 6g (Saturated 1g); Cholesterol 0mg; Sodium 44mg; Carbohydrate 53g (Dietary Fiber 8g); Protein 7g.*

TIP: Toasting the oats will give them a sweet, nutty flavor. To toast rolled oats, heat a dry nonstick skillet over medium heat on the stove. Add the oats in a single layer and cook, stirring frequently to prevent burning, until they're golden brown and fragrant, about 5 to 7 minutes.

NOTE: Be patient — the frozen banana chunks sometimes take a few minutes to start breaking down. Resist the urge to add more milk unless absolutely necessary. The texture should be thick like ice cream, not pourable like a smoothie.

VARY IT! Try using sunflower seed butter instead of peanut butter for a nut-free version.

Blueberry Buckwheat Pancakes

PREP TIME: ABOUT 10 MIN	COOK TIME: 25 MIN	YIELD: 4–6 SERVINGS

INGREDIENTS

2 cups sifted buckwheat flour

½ teaspoon baking powder

½ teaspoon salt

1 teaspoon baking soda

2 teaspoons maple crystals or coconut sugar

3 tablespoons apple cider vinegar

2 cups rice milk

1 to 2 very ripe bananas, mashed

1 cup fresh or frozen blueberries

1 tablespoon coconut oil

DIRECTIONS

1 In a small bowl, combine the buckwheat flour, baking powder, salt, baking soda, and maple crystals or coconut sugar; set aside.

2 In a large bowl, combine the apple cider vinegar and rice milk. Let sit for 5 to 10 minutes; then add the mashed banana.

3 Add the dry ingredients to the wet ingredients, and beat only until blended. Then add the blueberries.

4 Place the coconut oil on a griddle and heat on medium. Using a 1-ounce ladle, pour the batter onto the greased griddle. Cook the pancakes until the bubbles in the batter break on the surface; flip and cook until browned. Repeat until you're out of batter.

5 Serve on a plate and top with cashew cream, cinnamon, coconut yogurt, fresh fruit, or maple syrup.

PER SERVING: *Calories 349 (From Fat 63); Fat 7g (Saturated 3g); Cholesterol 0mg; Sodium 701mg; Carbohydrate 65g (Dietary Fiber 10g); Protein 12g.*

VARY IT! Try these pancakes with different fruits, such as cranberries or strawberries, or make them even more decadent by adding some non-dairy chocolate chips. You can also substitute another gluten-free or whole-grain flour such as brown rice or oat flour for the buckwheat flour.

Fluffy Pumpkin Donuts

PREP TIME: ABOUT 10 MIN	COOK TIME: 10 MIN	YIELD: 6 SERVINGS

INGREDIENTS

1 cup oat flour

1¼ teaspoons baking powder

¼ teaspoon baking soda

1 tablespoon pumpkin pie spice

¼ teaspoon sea salt

1 tablespoon cornstarch

3 tablespoons water

⅓ cup 100 percent pure pumpkin puree

½ cup coconut sugar

¼ cup nondairy milk

1 teaspoon pure vanilla extract

1 teaspoon apple cider vinegar

DIRECTIONS

1 Preheat the oven to 350 degrees. Gently spritz a 6-cavity donut pan with cooking spray; set aside.

2 In a medium bowl, whisk together the oat flour, baking powder, baking soda, pumpkin pie spice, and salt; set aside.

3 In a small bowl, whisk together the cornstarch and water; set aside.

4 In another bowl, whisk together the pumpkin puree, coconut sugar, milk, vanilla, apple cider vinegar, and the cornstarch slurry from Step 3.

5 Stir the dry ingredients into the wet ingredients until just combined.

6 Fill the donut cavities using either a piping bag or a spoon.

7 Bake until set, about 8 to 10 minutes.

8 Let cool in the pan on a cooling rack for 5 minutes. Then turn the donuts out onto a cooling rack and let cool completely.

PER SERVING: *Calories 177 (From Fat 24); Fat 3g (Saturated 0g); Cholesterol 0mg; Sodium 137mg; Carbohydrate 19g (Dietary Fiber 2g); Protein 4g.*

TIP: Slather 1 tablespoon of raw creamy almond butter on the top of a donut for an added protein boost.

NOTE: Be sure to use certified gluten-free oat flour to ensure that these donuts are gluten-free, if needed.

Hearty Breakfast Cookies

PREP TIME: ABOUT 15 MIN | **COOK TIME: 12 MIN** | **YIELD: 14 SERVINGS**

INGREDIENTS

2 medium very ripe bananas, mashed well

½ cup raw creamy almond butter

¼ cup pure maple syrup

¼ cup unsweetened original almond milk, rice milk, or soy milk

1 teaspoon pure vanilla extract

1½ cups old-fashioned rolled oats

½ cup almond flour

¼ cup flax meal

¼ cup hempseeds

½ teaspoon baking soda

¼ teaspoon sea salt

½ cup dried fruit, like cranberries or raisins

DIRECTIONS

1 Preheat the oven to 350 degrees. Line a baking sheet with parchment paper; set aside.

2 In a medium bowl, place the mashed bananas, almond butter, maple syrup, milk, and vanilla and whisk until smooth; set aside.

3 In a small bowl, place the oats, almond flour, flax meal, hempseeds, baking soda, and salt and stir to combine.

4 Add the dry ingredients to the wet ingredients and stir until well incorporated.

5 Add the dried fruit and stir to distribute evenly.

6 Scoop up the mixture about ¼ cup at a time and form into round cookie shapes. Flatten the cookies as you place them on the prepared baking sheet. (They won't spread while baking.)

7 Bake until lightly browned on the bottoms and firm on the tops, about 11 to 13 minutes. The cookies will continue to firm up as they cool but will stay soft in texture.

PER SERVING: *Calories 245 (From Fat 141); Fat 16g (Saturated 2g); Cholesterol 0mg; Sodium 88mg; Carbohydrate 23g (Dietary Fiber 3g); Protein 6g.*

TIP: Make a double batch and stash them in the freezer for an easy grab-'n'-go breakfast or snack!

Apple Cinnamon Mini Muffins

PREP TIME: ABOUT 15 MIN	COOK TIME: 12 MIN	YIELD: 12–20 MINI MUFFINS

INGREDIENTS

1 cup kamut flour, oat flour, or spelt flour

½ cup rolled oats

1 teaspoon baking powder

½ teaspoon baking soda

¼ teaspoon cinnamon

¼ teaspoon sea salt

¼ cup coconut oil or grape-seed oil

¼ cup maple syrup

⅓ cup applesauce

½ cup rice milk

1 apple, seeded and cut into small cubes

½ cup raisins

DIRECTIONS

1 Preheat the oven to 350 degrees.

2 In a large bowl, combine the flour, oats, baking powder, baking soda, cinnamon, and salt; set aside.

3 In a medium bowl, combine the oil, maple syrup, applesauce, milk, and apple.

4 Pour the wet ingredients into the dry ingredients and mix well, making sure there are no lumps. Stir in the raisins.

5 Distribute the mixture evenly in a 24-cup mini-muffin pan. You can use coconut oil or grape-seed oil to grease the tin, or use paper liner cups.

6 Bake for 12 minutes.

7 Remove the pan from the oven and let sit for a few minutes; then remove the muffins and cool them on a cooling rack or tray.

PER SERVING: *Calories 140 (From Fat 45); Fat 5g (Saturated 4g); Cholesterol 0mg; Sodium 115mg; Carbohydrate 22g (Dietary Fiber 2g); Protein 2g.*

TIP: If you have empty muffin cups after filling the cups with batter, add water to the empty cups to prevent burning.

NOTE: Be sure to use unbleached parchment-paper cups. These are brown, not white. You don't want any residue leaching into your tasty muffins!

VARY IT! Use this recipe to make 8 to 12 full-size muffins — just be sure to extend the baking time to 20 minutes. You can also swap in a gluten-free flour, such as brown-rice flour.

Cherry Baked Oatmeal Muffins

PREP TIME: ABOUT 10 MIN	COOK TIME: 25 MIN	YIELD: 12 SERVINGS

INGREDIENTS

3 cups old-fashioned rolled oats

3 tablespoons raw shelled sunflower seeds

2 tablespoons flax meal

1½ teaspoons baking powder

1 teaspoon ground cinnamon

½ teaspoon sea salt

½ cup sunflower seed butter

½ cup pure maple syrup

½ cup unsweetened applesauce

½ cup unsweetened plain almond milk

1 teaspoon pure vanilla extract

1 cup dried cherries

DIRECTIONS

1 Preheat the oven to 350 degrees. Lightly spray a 12-cup muffin tin with cooking spray; set aside.

2 In a medium bowl, place the oats, sunflower seeds, flax meal, baking powder, cinnamon, and salt and stir together.

3 In a large bowl, place the sunflower seed butter and maple syrup and whisk until smooth. Then whisk in the applesauce, almond milk, and vanilla.

4 Stir the dry ingredients into the wet until thoroughly combined.

5 Stir in the dried cherries until dispersed well throughout.

6 Spoon the mixture into the muffin tin, filling each cavity to the top and pressing down to make sure it's compact.

7 Bake until the tops start to brown, about 22 to 25 minutes.

8 Let cool in the muffin tin on a wire rack for 10 to 15 minutes. Run a knife carefully along the edge of each muffin cup to loosen it from the sides. They should pop out easily after loosened. Eat them warm or continue cooling on the wire rack until completely cool.

PER SERVING: *Calories 227 (From Fat 74); Fat 8g (Saturated 1g); Cholesterol 0mg; Sodium 156mg; Carbohydrate 35g (Dietary Fiber 3g); Protein 6g.*

NOTE: This baked oatmeal can also be made in an 8-x-8-inch baking dish. Lightly spray the baking dish with cooking spray or line it with parchment paper. Bake until the top is firm and starting to brown, about 35 to 40 minutes.

VARY IT! Try chopped dates, dairy-free chocolate chips, dried cranberries, or raisins instead of dried cherries for a fun twist.

Morning Millet Granola

PREP TIME: ABOUT 8 MIN	COOK TIME: 25 MIN	YIELD: APPROXIMATELY 6 CUPS

INGREDIENTS

¾ cup pure maple syrup

1 tablespoon rice milk

¼ cup coconut oil

4 cups rolled oats

1½ cups puffed millet cereal or millet flakes

¾ cup sesame seeds

½ cup sunflower seeds

½ cup pumpkin seeds

1 cup unsweetened coconut flakes

¼ cup flaxseeds

1 cup chopped almonds

1 teaspoon sea salt

1½ cups apricots, cranberries, or raisins

DIRECTIONS

1 Preheat the oven to 300 degrees. Line 2 shallow pans or baking sheets with parchment paper; set aside.

2 In a large saucepan, place the maple syrup, rice milk, and coconut oil; set aside.

3 In a large bowl, mix the oats, millet, sesame seeds, sunflower seeds, pumpkin seeds, coconut flakes, flaxseeds, almonds, and salt. Toss well.

4 Add the syrup mixture to the large bowl and stir well.

5 Pour the mixture into the pans or baking sheets and bake for 15 minutes. Stir and bake for an additional 10 minutes.

6 Remove the granola from the oven and add the apricots, cranberries, or raisins.

7 Cool and store in an airtight container.

PER SERVING: *Calories 281 (From Fat 117); Fat 13g (Saturated 4.5g); Cholesterol 0mg; Sodium 73mg; Carbohydrate 41g (Dietary Fiber 5g); Protein 5g.*

TIP: Serve this granola with coconut yogurt and top it with fresh berries for a hearty breakfast delight.

NOTE: Don't add the raisins or other dried fruits too early — they get very hard if baked in the oven.

NOTE: Be sure that the dried fruit you buy is sulphite-free. Sulphites are preservatives that keep fruit "fresh" long after it has been harvested. Always check to make sure the dried fruit you buy is free of this additive.

VARY IT! Instead of millet, you can use amaranth flakes, oat bran, or quinoa.

Soaked Oats with Goji Berries

PREP TIME: ABOUT 10 MIN PLUS OVERNIGHT FOR SOAKING	COOK TIME: 2–10 MIN	YIELD: 1–2 SERVINGS

INGREDIENTS

½ cup whole rolled oats

½ cup water

1 tablespoon freshly squeezed lemon juice

½ cup almond milk or rice milk

1 tablespoon almond butter

1 banana, sliced

2 tablespoons goji berries

1 teaspoon cinnamon

¼ cup pumpkin seeds

1 tablespoon maple syrup

DIRECTIONS

1 In a bowl, combine the oats, water, and lemon juice. Cover with a plate and soak overnight at room temperature.

2 For cold oats, add the remaining ingredients to the bowl and enjoy. For warm oats, add all the ingredients to a pot with an additional splash of rice milk; warm for 5 minutes and serve.

PER SERVING: *Calories 433 (From Fat 144); Fat 16g (Saturated 2.5g); Cholesterol 0mg; Sodium 49mg; Carbohydrate 62g (Dietary Fiber 6g); Protein 15g.*

NOTE: If you like your pumpkin seeds or raisins soft, soak them overnight with the oats. If you want to make the warming process even easier, prepare this recipe in a slow cooker the night before and just turn on the heat for a few minutes in the morning to warm it up.

VARY IT! Try using some of these toppings instead for a different flavor: apple slices, cacao nibs, chia seeds, currants, hempseeds, pear slices, sunflower seeds, or walnuts.

Super Chia Banana Porridge

PREP TIME: ABOUT 10 MIN	COOK TIME: 15 MIN	YIELD: 1 SERVING

INGREDIENTS

¼ cup chia seeds

½ cup water or hempseed milk

½ to 1 ripe banana, mashed

1 teaspoon cinnamon

1 tablespoon softened coconut oil or nut butter

2 tablespoons fresh berries

Coconut flakes, for garnish

DIRECTIONS

1 Place the chia seeds and water or hempseed milk in a bowl and let soak for 10 minutes. Stir the soaked chia seeds until a gel-like consistency forms; add a bit more liquid if desired.

2 Add the mashed banana to the chia seeds. Combine until the mixture has a porridge-like consistency.

3 Stir in the cinnamon, coconut oil or nut butter, and berries.

4 Transfer to a bowl, garnish with coconut flakes for extra crunch, and enjoy.

PER SERVING: *Calories 382 (From Fat 243); Fat 27g (Saturated 13g); Cholesterol 0mg; Sodium 11mg; Carbohydrate 33g (Dietary Fiber 16g); Protein 8g.*

TIP: The ideal amount of time to soak chia is approximately 10 minutes for a thick consistency; for an even thicker consistency, soak it longer. If you want it thinner, add more liquid.

TIP: This breakfast is great on the go — you can prepare it the night before and have it ready to take with you in the morning.

VARY IT! Try sunflower seed butter or cashew butter instead of coconut oil for a variation. Also try adding a scoop of protein powder or topping the mixture with goji berries, hempseeds, or pumpkin seeds for an extra boost of protein.

Amaranth Porridge with Fruit Compote

PREP TIME: ABOUT 25 MIN, PLUS OVERNIGHT FOR SOAKING	COOK TIME: 20–30 MIN	YIELD: 4 SERVINGS

INGREDIENTS

1 cup dried amaranth

2 tablespoons freshly squeezed lemon juice

3 cups water

½ teaspoon sea salt

1 tablespoon freshly ground flaxseeds or other nuts or seeds

Fruit Compote (see the following recipe)

DIRECTIONS

1 Place the amaranth in a bowl and add enough water to cover the amaranth. Add the lemon juice and soak the grain overnight. In the morning, rinse and drain the amaranth and place in a pot with the water.

2 Bring to a boil over high heat, add the salt, reduce the heat to low, cover, and simmer for 20 to 30 minutes.

3 Remove from the heat, dish into bowls, sprinkle flaxseeds or nuts on top, and top with the Fruit Compote.

Fruit Compote

2 firm pears

1 teaspoon freshly squeezed lemon juice in 3 cups water

½ cup dried apricots

4 dried figs

2 cups apple juice

½ cup rice syrup

2 large pieces lemon peel

1 teaspoon coconut oil

Pinch of sea salt

1 cinnamon stick, 3 whole cloves, 1 teaspoon ground anise, and one 1-inch piece ginger in a tea bag (see below)

½ cup dried cranberries or raisins

1 Peel, core, and slice the pears into ¼-inch pieces. Place them in the lemon water; set aside. Slice the apricots and figs into ½-inch slices; set aside.

2 In a medium saucepan, place the apple juice, rice syrup, lemon peel, coconut oil, and salt and bring to a boil. Reduce the heat to low and simmer about 3 minutes.

3 Add the tea bag to the simmering liquid. Gently stir in the pears (discarding the liquid in which they were soaking), apricots, figs, and cranberries or raisins, and continue to simmer uncovered over medium heat for about 15 minutes.

4 Remove the tea bag. Strain the liquid into a small saucepan and set the fruit mixture aside in a bowl.

5 Boil the liquid until it's syrupy and reduced to about 1 cup. Remove from the heat. Serve chilled or warm.

PER SERVING: *Calories 512 (From Fat 54); Fat 6g (Saturated 1.5g); Cholesterol 0mg; Sodium 726mg; Carbohydrate 113g (Dietary Fiber 10g); Protein 9g.*

TIP: You can buy empty tea bags that you can fill yourself at home; be sure to buy ones without any bleach. Alternatively, you can use a tea infuser.

VARY IT! Instead of the compote, try serving the porridge with almond milk, coconut milk, coconut nectar, maple syrup, raw honey, or rice milk.

Breakfast Quinoa Bowl

PREP TIME: ABOUT 5 MIN	COOK TIME: 15–20 MIN	YIELD: 4 SERVINGS

INGREDIENTS

10 to 12 radishes, quartered

2 teaspoons olive oil

Sea salt to taste

Freshly ground black pepper to taste

1 small yellow onion, diced

2 tablespoons water

1 cup white quinoa, rinsed well under cold water

2 cups low-sodium vegetable broth

1 teaspoon turmeric

Juice of 1 lemon, divided

Dash of cayenne

1 tomato, seeded and diced

4 cups loosely packed arugula

DIRECTIONS

1 Preheat the oven to 425 degrees.

2 In a bowl, place the radishes, olive oil, salt, and pepper and toss to coat. On a rimmed baking sheet, spread out the radishes in an even layer.

3 Roast until tender and browned on the edges, about 15 to 20 minutes, shaking the pan halfway through the cooking time to redistribute the radishes.

4 Meanwhile, in a medium pot, add the onion and water and sauté over medium heat until soft and translucent, about 5 to 6 minutes.

5 To the saucepan, add the quinoa, broth, turmeric, juice of ½ lemon, cayenne, a pinch of salt, and a pinch of pepper. Bring to a boil, reduce the heat to medium-low, and simmer until the quinoa is tender, about 12 to 15 minutes.

6 Add the tomato and stir to combine.

7 In a medium bowl, toss the arugula with the juice from the other ½ lemon.

8 To serve, divide the arugula among 4 bowls, and top each bowl with ¼ of the quinoa mixture and ¼ of the radishes.

PER SERVING: *Calories 233 (From Fat 52); Fat 6g (Saturated 0g); Cholesterol 0mg; Sodium 54mg; Carbohydrate 37g (Dietary Fiber 4g); Protein 10g.*

TIP: This dish would make a great lunch or dinner, too. Serve it alongside cooked beans or the Orange Maple Marinated Tempeh (later in this chapter) for even more staying power.

NOTE: Raw radishes can be a bit spicy, but when they're roasted, they take on a mild, sweet, buttery flavor that is so delicious!

Turmeric Tofu Scramble

PREP TIME: ABOUT 5 MIN	COOK TIME: 20 MIN	YIELD: 6 SERVINGS

INGREDIENTS

1 tablespoon ground cumin

1 tablespoon ground turmeric

1 teaspoon coriander

½ teaspoon chili powder (optional)

½ teaspoon paprika

1 teaspoon dried thyme

Pinch cayenne pepper

¼ teaspoon sea salt

Freshly ground black pepper to taste

1 tablespoon grapeseed oil

1 onion, peeled and diced

1 green bell pepper, diced (optional)

Two 16-ounce packages firm tofu, drained

DIRECTIONS

1 In a small bowl, place the cumin, turmeric, coriander, chili powder (if using), paprika, thyme, cayenne, salt, and pepper and mix together; set aside.

2 In a sauté pan, add the grapeseed oil and warm over medium heat. Add the onion, bell pepper (if using), and spices from Step 1. Cook until the onion is softened, about 5 minutes.

3 With a fork, crumble the tofu into bite-size pieces and add it to the sauté pan. Stir to coat the tofu with the spice mixture. Sauté over medium to high heat until heated through, about 5 minutes.

PER SERVING: *Calories 185 (From Fat 90); Fat 10g (Saturated 1g); Cholesterol 0mg; Sodium 153mg; Carbohydrate 6g (Dietary Fiber 2.5g); Protein 15g.*

TIP: Serve the scramble with some sprouted-grain toast and steamed greens for a balanced breakfast.

Black Bean Breakfast Tacos

PREP TIME: ABOUT 5 MIN	COOK TIME: 5–7 MIN	YIELD: 3 SERVINGS

INGREDIENTS

1 tablespoon olive oil

½ teaspoon cumin

½ teaspoon smoked paprika

½ teaspoon chili powder

½ teaspoon oregano

¼ teaspoon garlic powder

¼ teaspoon salt

One 15-ounce can black beans, drained and rinsed

Juice of 1 lime

6 corn tortillas

1 avocado, peeled, pit removed, diced

1 tomato, diced

½ cup fresh cilantro, chopped

DIRECTIONS

1   In a skillet, warm the oil over medium heat. Add the cumin, paprika, chili powder, oregano, garlic powder, and salt and sauté until fragrant, about 1 to 2 minutes.

2   Add the black beans and sauté until heated through, about 3 to 4 minutes. Add the lime juice and stir to combine. Transfer to a bowl; set aside.

3   In the same skillet over medium heat, add 1 tortilla and cook until warmed, about 20 to 30 seconds. Carefully flip over and cook another 15 to 20 seconds on the other side. Repeat with the remaining tortillas.

4   To serve, add about ¼ cup of black beans to each tortilla. Top with diced avocado, diced tomato, and a sprinkle of chopped cilantro.

PER SERVING: *Calories 251 (From Fat 87); Fat 10g (Saturated 1g); Cholesterol 0mg; Sodium 312mg; Carbohydrate 35g (Dietary Fiber 11g); Protein 8g.*

TIP: Serve with roasted potatoes or hash browns and fresh fruit for a hearty, filling breakfast or brunch.

NOTE: Warming the tortillas makes them more pliable and less likely to tear, which corn tortillas are known for doing. If you'd like to keep the tortillas warm as you heat the rest, keep them covered on a plate or warmer.

VARY IT! This recipe is very versatile. Use chickpeas or pinto beans instead of black beans. Add a diced bell pepper or jalapeño pepper. Top with your favorite salsa instead of fresh tomato or guacamole instead of diced avocado.

Orange Maple Marinated Tempeh

PREP TIME: ABOUT 10 MIN, PLUS 1 HR FOR MARINATING	COOK TIME: 25 MIN	YIELD: 6 SERVINGS

INGREDIENTS

One 8.5-ounce package tempeh

¼ cup freshly squeezed orange juice

2 tablespoons tamari

3 tablespoons olive oil

1 tablespoon maple syrup

2 tablespoons minced white or red onion

1 clove garlic, minced

DIRECTIONS

1 Cut the tempeh lengthwise into 10 strips. (If it's frozen, thaw it slightly first.)

2 In a small bowl, add the orange juice, tamari, olive oil, maple syrup, onion, and garlic and mix to make the marinade.

3 In a casserole dish, place the tempeh and pour the marinade over it.

4 Marinate in the refrigerator for 1 to 6 hours.

5 Preheat the oven to 350 degrees.

6 Cover and bake for 20 minutes. Remove the cover and bake until the marinade is absorbed, about 10 minutes.

PER SERVING: *Calories 160 (From Fat 90); Fat 10g (Saturated 1.5g); Cholesterol 0mg; Sodium 340mg; Carbohydrate 10g (Dietary Fiber 4 g); Protein 9g.*

TIP: Use this recipe in place of bacon. Serve it alongside the Turmeric Tofu Scramble (see recipe earlier in this chapter) or with toast, avocado, and steamed spinach to make a delicious breakfast sandwich.

NOTE: You can prepare this dish ahead of time to allow the tempeh to absorb the flavors, or you can prepare it immediately after putting the marinade on it. Either way, it tastes delicious!

Chapter **10**

Soups and Salads

Soups and salads can be as light or as filling as you want them to be. They can be a starter to a heartier meal or satisfying enough to stand on their own. Whatever you're in the mood for, we've got a recipe for you here.

In this chapter, we give you some great ideas for throwing together soups and salads on the fly with what you have in your fridge, so you have endless options available.

Making a Meal of Salads and Soups

Many people think that salads and soups are only precursors to meals, but they can be the centerpieces of your meal, too. This section tells you how to make intricate and unique salads, along with hearty and filling soups that you can eat like a meal!

Making your fridge a salad bar

The best thing you can do to plan proper meals is to get some base ingredients and have them prepped and ready. When hunger strikes, you can just assemble them and go.

What to have ready:

>> **A cooked grain, such as brown rice, farro, or quinoa:** Be sure to cook your favorite grain ahead of time. Then seal it in a glass container so it's ready to go.

>> **Green leafy veggies, such as arugula, kale, leaf lettuce, or spinach:** These can be washed, stemmed, and chopped and then stored in a perforated bag or glass container.

WARNING

Don't leave them too long in the fridge after you've cut them or they'll start to turn brown.

>> **Veggies such as beets, bell peppers, cabbage, carrots, cucumber, seaweed (see Chapter 4), and tomatoes:** These can all be peeled, chopped, and prepared ahead of time and placed in glass containers for easy use and storage.

>> **Fruits such as apples, avocados, oranges, or strawberries.** Wash these ahead of time and cut them as you use them.

TIP

If you cut your fruit too early, it's more likely to oxidize and break down. When the flesh is exposed to air, apples and bananas turn brown, berries break down, and other items just get mushy. The best way to keep your fruit fresh is to cut it right before you use it.

>> **A hearty protein, such as black beans, chickpeas, kidney beans, lentils, tempeh, or tofu:** If you're cooking beans from scratch, be sure to rinse them after cooking and store them in a glass container. For tempeh and tofu, you can bake, grill, sauté, or marinate it; then they're ready to be used on demand.

>> **Herbs and spices, such as basil, mint, oregano, and parsley:** Be sure to stock both fresh and dried varieties of different herbs.

>> **Fun toppings, such as almond, dried cranberries, figs, hazelnuts, hempseeds, pumpkin seeds, raisins, sunflower seeds, or walnuts:** You can store these in glass jars or small containers and have them ready to go in your pantry.

KNOWING WHEN TO USE FRESH OR DRIED HERBS

Many recipes call for herbs. Sometimes they list fresh herbs in the ingredients list, and sometimes they list dried herbs. And sometimes they don't specify which type to use. So, when do you use fresh and when do you used dried?

- **Fresh herbs** are mostly used in dips, salads, and spreads. A recipe may call for them in a cooked dish; if that's the case, the herbs will be added toward the end so as not to destroy all their flavors by cooking.

- **Dried herbs** are best in soups, sauces, and marinades, where they have a chance to absorb liquid and transfer their flavor to the dish. Dried herbs are typically added at the beginning or midway through a recipe.

You can change up these items on a weekly basis, depending on what you have access to, giving yourself a healthy rotation for your own personal salad bar.

TIP

The best way to store any food, cooked or raw, is to seal it in a glass container. Glass is clean, nontoxic, and nonporous, and your food will stay fresher. Plastic containers leach chemicals into your food and stain easily; plus, food can spoil more quickly in them. Plastic can also break down over time, whereas glass has a much longer life. Yes, glass may travel a little heavier in your bag, but it's a much healthier and more sustainable choice.

KNOWING WHEN TO USE FRESH OR FROZEN VEGETABLES

Always opt for fresh vegetables and fruits in raw salads, where flavor and texture are key. For cooked dishes like soups, however, there is no hard and fast rule for using fresh versus frozen. Soups are a great vehicle for using up vegetables in the back of your fridge that may be on their last legs. But frozen vegetables work just as well, are extremely convenient, and require no chopping. Frozen mixed vegetables with carrots, corn, green beans, and peas are great for making vegetable soup.

Falling in love with soup as a meal

What could be better than having a full meal with all your main nutrients warmed up in a pot? Soup not only provides your body and brain with a balanced, veggie-happy meal but also nourishes you for the day.

Here are some general ideas for what to put in a satisfying soup:

» 4 to 8 cups of liquid base (veggie stock, water, miso paste, herbs, and spices)

» 1 to 3 cups of different veggies, such as broccoli, carrots, cauliflower, celery, kale, onions, peas, spinach, squash, or zucchini

» 1 to 2 cups of cooked beans, such as black beans, chickpeas, lentils, split peas, or white beans

» 1 to 2 cups of cooked whole grains: barley, brown rice, pasta, or quinoa

» 2 to 3 tablespoons of balsamic vinegar, fresh chopped herbs, fresh lemon juice, hot sauce, or tamari as a finisher

There aren't too many rules with soup, so here are some general steps for getting your soup on:

1. Sauté aromatics, like garlic and onion, in oil and stir in any dried spices to release their flavor.

2. Add veggies, which typically make up most of the soup.

3. Add a protein source, such as beans or whole grains.

4. Add the base, usually 4 to 8 cups of liquid, and simmer until the flavors meld and it's warm throughout.

5. Add the finishing touches (like freshly squeezed lemon, a splash of vinegar, or fresh herbs) just before serving.

TIP

Some soups require you to cook your grains and beans before you add them to the soup because they typically don't cook properly in the company of other ingredients. If so, cook them separately in another pot. Then you can add them along the way.

New Age Minestrone

INGREDIENTS

1 tablespoon olive oil

1 white onion, cut into large cubes

1 clove of garlic, minced

1 teaspoon sea salt

1 tablespoon dried oregano

1 tablespoon dried basil

4 cups water

1 bay leaf

1 butternut squash, peeled and cut into medium cubes

3 parsnips, peeled and cut into medium cubes

1 sweet potato, peeled and cut into large cubes

3 ribs celery, cut into medium pieces

1 large zucchini, cut into small chunks

4 to 5 cups of Swiss chard, cut into bite-size pieces

1 cup soaked and cooked kidney beans or one 14-ounce can kidney beans

½ cup cooked brown rice macaroni noodles

Salt to taste

Freshly ground black pepper to taste

DIRECTIONS

1 In a large pot, add the oil, onion, garlic, and sea salt, and sauté until the onion is soft and translucent, about 5 minutes.

2 Add the oregano and basil, and sauté for a few more minutes.

3 Add the water, bay leaf, squash, parsnips, and sweet potato to the pot. Bring everything to a boil and then reduce the heat to low. Simmer for 10 minutes.

4 Add the celery and zucchini. Turn up the heat again until the water boils. Then lower the heat, cover, and simmer for 40 to 45 minutes.

5 Stir until the squash falls apart, or press the squash against the side of the pot to break it down.

6 Add the chard, cover and simmer for 10 minutes.

7 Add the kidney beans and noodles. Season to taste with salt and pepper. Remove the bay leaf. Stir a few times and serve.

PER SERVING: *Calories 100 (From Fat 4.5); Fat 1.5g (Saturated 0g); Cholesterol 0mg; Sodium 421mg; Carbohydrate 20g (Dietary Fiber 5g); Protein 4g.*

TIP: Be sure to cook your macaroni noodles al dente in a separate pot so they don't get too hard or too soft. Then add them into the hot soup at the end.

Chunky Miso Soup

PREP TIME: ABOUT 10 MIN	COOK TIME: 40 MIN	YIELD: 8–10 SERVINGS

INGREDIENTS

8 cups water

One 1-inch piece kombu (sea vegetable)

5 dried or fresh shiitake mushrooms

1 small white onion, cut into small slices

2 large carrots, peeled and cut into small pieces

2 to 4 stalks of celery, cut into small pieces

1 block or 12 ounces firm tofu, cut into cubes

1 cup chopped bok choy

½ cup wakame (seaweed), soaked for 5 minutes and cut into bite-size pieces

One 16-ounce package brown rice vermicelli or soba noodles, cooked (optional)

⅔ cup miso paste, brown, white, or both

3 green onions, thinly chopped, for garnish

DIRECTIONS

1 In a large pot, bring the water to a boil. Add the kombu and mushrooms. (This adds extra nutrients to the soup broth.)

2 Add the onion, carrots, and celery. Reduce the heat to low and let the vegetables simmer for 30 minutes.

3 Add the tofu and simmer for another 10 minutes.

4 Add the bok choy and wakame, allowing it to wilt into the warm soup. Add the cooked noodles (if desired).

5 Remove 1 to 2 cups of the liquid to a bowl. Stir in the miso paste. When the miso paste is dissolved, pour the mixture back into the soup pot.

6 Ladle the soup into bowls and garnish with fresh green onions and serve.

PER SERVING: *Calories 149 (From Fat 27); Fat 3g (Saturated 0.5g); Cholesterol 0mg; Sodium 919mg; Carbohydrate 23g (Dietary Fiber 3g); Protein 10g.*

TIP: There are different varieties of miso. Brown miso is much richer and saltier; white miso is much lighter and sweeter. Try different varieties to see what tastes best to you.

NOTE: Always add miso paste at the end. Miso is very delicate and should never be boiled. Boiling destroys all its natural enzymes.

VARY IT! All seaweed is loaded with minerals, nutrients, and natural iodine. It's an excellent addition to your soup! If you can't get your hands on wakame, try arame, dulse, or nori.

Creamy Zucchini Soup

INGREDIENTS

2 tablespoons olive oil

1 small yellow onion, diced

2 cloves garlic, diced

½ teaspoon sea salt

1 large or 2 medium zucchini, chopped (about 3 cups)

One 15-ounce can white beans, drained and rinsed

4 cups low-sodium vegetable broth

2 cups fresh baby spinach

1 to 2 tablespoons chopped fresh parsley or dill (optional)

Juice of 1 lemon (optional)

DIRECTIONS

1 In a pot, warm the oil over medium heat. Add the onion and sauté until it's soft and translucent, about 5 to 6 minutes.

2 Add the garlic, salt, and zucchini and stir until fragrant, about 3 to 4 minutes.

3 Add the beans and broth. Increase the heat to bring to a boil. Then decrease the heat to medium–low, cover, and simmer for 15 minutes.

4 Turn off the heat, add the spinach, and stir to combine. Using an immersion blender, purée the soup until completely smooth.

5 Add the parsley or dill, if using, and a squeeze of fresh lemon, if desired, and serve.

PER SERVING: Calories 256 (From Fat 80); Fat 9g (Saturated 2g); Cholesterol 0mg; Sodium 219mg; Carbohydrate 33g (Dietary Fiber 7g); Protein 14g.

NOTE: This soup is heartier than it seems due to the white beans, but it's still light enough to serve as a starter. As a starter it, will serve about 6 people, as a light lunch, about 3 to 4.

TIP: If you don't have an immersion blender, you can carefully transfer the soup to a blender, blend until smooth, and transfer back to the pot. You may need to work in batches, though, because you should never fill the blender more than about halfway with hot liquid.

Butternut Squash Apple Soup

PREP TIME: ABOUT 15 MIN | COOK TIME: 38 MIN | YIELD: 4 SERVINGS

INGREDIENTS

1 tablespoon olive oil

1 sweet onion, peeled and diced

1 teaspoon sea salt

½ teaspoon ground cinnamon

¾ teaspoon yellow curry powder

½ teaspoon turmeric

¼ teaspoon freshly ground black pepper

1 small butternut squash, peeled, seeded, and chopped (about 4 cups)

1 apple, chopped

1¾ cups low- sodium vegetable broth, plus more as needed

¼ cup unsweetened nondairy milk, like almond, cashew, or soy

Roasted Pumpkin Seeds, for garnish (optional; see the following recipe)

DIRECTIONS

1 In a soup pot, warm the oil over medium heat. Add the onion and sauté until it's soft and translucent, about 5 to 6 minutes.

2 Add the salt, cinnamon, curry powder, turmeric, and pepper. Sauté until fragrant, about 1 to 2 minutes.

3 Add the squash, apple, and broth. Increase the heat to bring to a boil. Then decrease the heat to medium–low, cover, and simmer until the squash is fork tender, about 25 to 30 minutes.

4 Add the nondairy milk.

5 Using an immersion blender, purée until silky smooth.

6 Taste and adjust seasoning as necessary. Serve with a sprinkling of Roasted Pumpkin Seeds, if desired.

Roasted Pumpkin Seeds

½ cup raw shelled pumpkin seeds

¼ teaspoon olive oil

⅛ teaspoon sea salt

1 Preheat the oven to 325 degrees. Line a rimmed baking sheet with parchment paper.

2 Toss the pumpkin seeds with oil and salt and spread out in one single layer on the prepared baking sheet.

3 Roast 15 to 20 minutes, shaking the pan halfway through. Keep a close eye on them so they don't burn.

PER SERVING: *Calories 195 (From Fat 71); Fat 7g (Saturated 0g); Cholesterol 0mg; Sodium 541mg; Carbohydrate 30g (Dietary Fiber 5g); Protein 5g.*

TIP: If you don't have an immersion blender, you can carefully transfer the soup to a blender, blend until smooth, and transfer back to the pot. You may need to work in batches, though, because you should never fill the blender more than about halfway with hot liquid.

Mushroom Rice Soup

PREP TIME: ABOUT 10 MIN	COOK TIME: 55 MIN	YIELD: 6 SERVINGS

INGREDIENTS

2 tablespoons olive oil

1 small yellow onion, diced

1 tablespoon mellow white miso paste

2 teaspoons dried thyme

1 teaspoon dried rosemary

2 ribs celery, diced

2 carrots, peeled and diced

8 ounces baby bella or cremini mushrooms, sliced

½ cup wild rice blend

5 to 6 cups low-sodium vegetable broth

Sea salt to taste

Freshly ground black pepper to taste

DIRECTIONS

1 In a soup pot, warm the oil over medium heat. Add the onion and sauté until it's soft and translucent, about 5 to 6 minutes.

2 Add the miso paste and stir until relatively smooth.

3 Add the thyme, rosemary, celery, carrots, and mushrooms. Sauté until the mushrooms start to soften, about 5 minutes.

4 Add the wild rice blend and broth. Increase the heat to bring to a boil. Then decrease the heat to medium–low, cover, and simmer until the rice is tender, about 35 to 45 minutes.

5 Add the salt and pepper and serve.

PER SERVING: *Calories 161 (From Fat 56); Fat 6g (Saturated 1g); Cholesterol 0mg; Sodium 196mg; Carbohydrate 21g (Dietary Fiber 3g); Protein 8g.*

VARY IT! You can make this soup with any type of rice. Just adjust the cook time according to your rice package instructions.

Red Pepper Carrot Soup

PREP TIME: ABOUT 10 MIN	COOK TIME: 27 MIN	YIELD: 4 SERVINGS

INGREDIENTS

2 tablespoons olive oil

1 yellow onion, diced

2 cloves garlic, minced

3 carrots, peeled and chopped

2 red bell peppers, seeded and chopped

2½ cups low-sodium vegetable broth

¼ cup fresh parsley, chopped

Sea salt to taste

Freshly ground black pepper to taste

Splash of balsamic vinegar (optional)

DIRECTIONS

1   In a medium pot, warm the oil over medium heat. Add the onion and sauté until it's soft and translucent, about 5 to 6 minutes.

2   Add the garlic, carrots, and bell peppers and sauté until fragrant, about 2 to 3 minutes.

3   Add the broth and increase the heat to bring to a boil. Then decrease the heat to medium–low, cover, and simmer until the carrots are soft, about 20 minutes.

4   Add the parsley.

5   Using an immersion blender, purée the soup until smooth.

6   Add the salt and pepper.

7   Serve with a drizzle of balsamic vinegar over the top, if desired.

PER SERVING: *Calories 147 (From Fat 72); Fat 8g (Saturated 1g); Cholesterol 0mg; Sodium 86mg; Carbohydrate 16g (Dietary Fiber 3g); Protein 5g.*

TIP: If you don't have an immersion blender, you can carefully transfer the soup to a blender, blend until smooth, and transfer back to the pot. You may need to work in batches, though, because you should never fill the blender more than about halfway with hot liquid.

TIP: This soup is light and delicate and makes a great starter for a heavier meal. If you want to make it a meal on its own, serve it with roasted chickpeas on top and a hunk of crusty whole-grain bread. You can also blend a can of rinsed and drained chickpeas right into the soup (you may need to add more broth if you do this).

Velvety Green Vegetable Soup

PREP TIME: ABOUT 10 MIN	COOK TIME: 22 MIN	YIELD: 4 SERVINGS

INGREDIENTS

1 tablespoon olive oil

½ sweet onion, peeled and diced

4 cloves garlic, minced

2 ribs celery, chopped

1 teaspoon sea salt, or to taste

1 small head broccoli, chopped (about 2½ cups)

1 cup frozen green peas

3 green onions, sliced

2¾ cups low-sodium vegetable broth

4 cups baby spinach, baby kale, or baby chard (or a mix of all three)

One 15-ounce can cannellini beans, drained and rinsed

Juice of 1 lemon

2 tablespoons chopped fresh dill

5 fresh mint leaves

½ cup canned light coconut milk

DIRECTIONS

1 In a soup pot, warm the oil over medium heat. Add the onion and sauté until it's soft and translucent, about 5 minutes. Add the garlic, celery, and salt and sauté until fragrant, about 1 to 2 minutes.

2 Add the broccoli, peas, green onions, and broth. Increase the heat to bring to a boil. Then decrease the heat to medium-low, cover, and simmer until the vegetables are tender, about 10 to 15 minutes.

3 Carefully transfer the soup to a blender, add the baby greens, beans, lemon juice, dill, and mint. Blend until smooth, using the tamper to pack the greens down, if necessary.

4 Transfer the soup back to the soup pot, taste, and adjust seasonings to your liking. Add the coconut milk, if using; stir well to combine and serve.

PER SERVING: *Calories 264 (From Fat 75); Fat 8g (Saturated 2g); Cholesterol 0mg; Sodium 808mg; Carbohydrate 33g (Dietary Fiber 11g); Protein 14g.*

TIP: Light coconut milk is creamy without leaving a distinct coconut taste. We don't recommend using full-fat coconut milk. If you need to thin out the soup and don't want to use coconut milk, you can use unsweetened plain almond or soy milk, more vegetable broth, or water.

NOTE: If your blender is on the small side, you may need to work in batches to purée the soup.

VARY IT! Use any mix of leafy greens you like — arugula, chard, kale, red or green leaf lettuce, spinach, or watercress.

Coconut Curry Soup

INGREDIENTS

2 tablespoons olive oil

1 yellow onion, peeled and diced

3 cloves garlic, minced

1 tablespoon minced fresh ginger

1 red bell pepper, diced

1 large sweet potato, peeled and chopped into 1-inch cubes

2 tablespoons yellow curry powder

3 cups low-sodium vegetable broth

One 13.5-ounce can full-fat coconut milk

½ cup frozen green peas

Juice of ½ lime

¼ cup chopped fresh cilantro

DIRECTIONS

1 In a soup pot, warm the oil over medium heat. Add the onion and sauté until it's soft and translucent, about 5 to 6 minutes.

2 Add the garlic, ginger, bell pepper, sweet potato, and curry powder and sauté until fragrant, about 2 to 3 minutes.

3 Add the broth and increase the heat to bring to a boil; then decrease the heat to medium–low, and simmer until the sweet potato is tender, about 15 to 20 minutes.

4 Stir in the coconut milk, peas, lime juice, and cilantro. Stir to incorporate; simmer another 3 to 5 minutes to heat through and serve.

PER SERVING: *Calories 367 (From Fat 260); Fat 29g (Saturated 19g); Cholesterol 0mg; Sodium 112mg; Carbohydrate 24g (Dietary Fiber 4g); Protein 8g.*

NOTE: The potency of curry powder can differ by brand. Feel free to add a little more if yours isn't as strong in flavor.

VARY IT! Try swapping out the sweet potatoes for cubed butternut squash or pumpkin!

Lentil Rice Soup

INGREDIENTS

2 tablespoons olive oil

1 yellow onion, diced

2 cloves garlic, minced

1 teaspoon dried thyme

½ teaspoon freshly ground black pepper

2 ribs celery, diced

2 carrots, peeled and diced

1 cup dried green or brown lentils, picked over and rinsed

1 cup brown rice

One 15-ounce can diced tomatoes

1 tablespoon coconut aminos or tamari

8 cups low-sodium vegetable broth

1 teaspoon sea salt, or to taste

Juice of 1 lemon, or to taste

¼ cup fresh chopped parsley

DIRECTIONS

1 In a soup pot, warm the oil over medium heat. Add the onion and sauté until it's soft and translucent, about 5 to 6 minutes.

2 Add the garlic, thyme, and pepper, and sauté until fragrant, about 1 to 2 minutes. Add the celery and carrots and cook another 5 minutes so they start to soften.

3 Add the lentils, rice, tomatoes, coconut aminos or tamari, and broth and stir well. Increase the heat to bring to a boil. Then decrease the heat to medium–low, cover, and simmer until the lentils and rice are tender, but not mushy, about 30 to 40 minutes.

4 Add the salt, lemon juice, and parsley. Taste and adjust the seasoning as necessary and serve.

PER SERVING: *Calories 362 (From Fat 71); Fat 8g (Saturated 1g); Cholesterol 0mg; Sodium 354mg; Carbohydrate 57g (Dietary Fiber 13g); Protein 19g.*

Stuffed Pepper Soup

PREP TIME: ABOUT 10 MIN | COOK TIME: 40 MIN | YIELD: 6 SERVINGS

INGREDIENTS

2 tablespoons olive oil

1 yellow onion, peeled and diced

2 cloves garlic, minced

1 teaspoon dried basil

1 teaspoon dried oregano

2 tablespoons dried parsley

2 green bell peppers, seeded and diced

¾ cup long-grain brown rice, rinsed

½ cup dry brown lentils, picked over and rinsed

One 14-ounce can diced tomatoes

One 15-ounce can tomato sauce

6 cups low-sodium vegetable broth

1 tablespoon tamari

2 teaspoons liquid smoke (optional)

Salt to taste

Freshly ground black pepper to taste

DIRECTIONS

1 In a large soup pot, warm the oil over medium heat. Add the onion and sauté until it's soft and translucent, about 5 minutes. Add the garlic, basil, oregano, parsley, and bell peppers and sauté until fragrant, about 1 to 2 minutes.

2 Add the rice, lentils, tomatoes, tomato sauce, broth, tamari, and liquid smoke, if using. Increase the heat to bring to a boil. Then decrease the heat to medium-low, cover, and simmer until the rice and lentils are tender and cooked through, about 30 to 40 minutes.

3 Taste and adjust seasonings, adding salt and pepper, as needed; serve.

PER SERVING: *Calories 278 (From Fat 64); Fat 7g (Saturated 1g); Cholesterol 0mg; Sodium 714mg; Carbohydrate 43g (Dietary Fiber 9g); Protein 13g.*

NOTE: This soup will thicken up considerably as it sits. You may need to add more vegetable broth upon reheating any leftovers.

VARY IT! Use any color of bell pepper you like.

Roasted Cauliflower Soup

PREP TIME: ABOUT 10 MIN	COOK TIME: 30 MIN	YIELD: 4 SERVINGS

INGREDIENTS

2 medium heads cauliflower, chopped into small florets (about 8 cups), divided

2 tablespoons olive oil, divided

1½ teaspoons sea salt, divided

1 yellow onion, diced

3 cloves garlic, minced

2 teaspoons dried thyme

½ teaspoon freshly ground black pepper

¼ scant teaspoon ground nutmeg

2 cups low-sodium vegetable broth

1 to 2 cups unsweetened plain almond milk, divided

¼ cup nutritional yeast

Juice of 1 lemon

1 to 2 dashes of hot sauce (optional)

DIRECTIONS

1 Preheat the oven to 400 degrees.

2 In a large bowl, add the florets from one head of cauliflower. Drizzle with 1 tablespoon of the olive oil. Sprinkle with ½ teaspoon of the salt. Spread out into one even layer on a rimmed baking sheet. Bake 15 minutes, stir, and bake another 10 minutes until browned.

3 Meanwhile, in a soup pot, warm the remaining 1 tablespoon olive oil over medium heat. Add the onion and sauté until it's soft and translucent, about 5 to 6 minutes.

4 Add the garlic, thyme, the remaining 1 teaspoon of salt, pepper, nutmeg, and the florets from the remaining head of cauliflower. Stir until fragrant, about 2 to 3 minutes.

5 Add the broth and 1 cup of the milk. Increase the heat to bring to a boil; then decrease the heat and simmer until the cauliflower is soft, about 15 to 20 minutes.

6 Add the nutritional yeast, lemon juice, and hot sauce, if desired.

7 Using an immersion blender, puree the soup until silky smooth, adding an additional 1 cup of milk if you like a thinner soup.

8 Add the roasted cauliflower and serve.

PER SERVING: *Calories 218 (From Fat 83); Fat 9g (Saturated 1g); Cholesterol 0mg; Sodium 933mg; Carbohydrate 27g (Dietary Fiber 8g); Protein 12g.*

Vegetable Quinoa Soup

PREP TIME: ABOUT 10 MIN	COOK TIME: 26 MIN	YIELD: 4 SERVINGS

INGREDIENTS

6¼ cups low-sodium vegetable broth, divided

2 large carrots, peeled and diced

1 tablespoon balsamic vinegar, plus more for serving if desired

1 tablespoon tamari

One 28-ounce can diced tomatoes

½ cup dry quinoa, rinsed and drained

1 zucchini, diced

1 cup frozen green peas

1 teaspoon sea salt, or to taste

5 to 6 fresh basil leaves, chiffonade

2 tablespoons chopped fresh parsley

DIRECTIONS

1 In a soup pot, warm ¼ cup of the broth over medium heat. Add the carrots, vinegar, and tamari, and sauté until the liquid is absorbed, about 5 to 6 minutes.

2 Add the tomatoes, the remaining 6 cups of vegetable broth, and the quinoa. Increase the heat to bring to a boil; then reduce the heat to medium–low, cover, and simmer until the quinoa is tender, about 15 minutes.

3 Add the zucchini, peas, salt, basil, and parsley, and simmer until the peas are heated through, about 4 to 5 minutes.

4 Drizzle with balsamic vinegar, if desired, and serve.

PER SERVING: *Calories 231 (From Fat 38); Fat 4g (Saturated 1g); Cholesterol 0mg; Sodium 1,190mg; Carbohydrate 37g (Dietary Fiber 7g); Protein 15g.*

Vegan Chicken Noodle Soup

PREP TIME: ABOUT 15 MIN	COOK TIME: 23 MIN	YIELD: 4 SERVINGS

INGREDIENTS

2 tablespoons olive oil

1 yellow onion, diced

2 ribs celery, diced

2 carrots, peeled and diced

2 Yukon Gold potatoes, peeled and diced

2 teaspoons poultry seasoning

1 teaspoon sea salt

½ teaspoon freshly ground black pepper

2 ounces Butler Soy Curls (about 1½ cups)

8 to 10 cups low-sodium vegetable broth

8 ounces rotini noodles

2 tablespoons nutritional yeast

1 to 2 tablespoons fresh squeezed lemon juice

2 to 3 tablespoons chopped fresh parsley

DIRECTIONS

1 In a large soup pot, warm the oil over medium heat. Add the onion and sauté until soft and translucent, about 5 to 6 minutes.

2 Add the celery, carrots, potatoes, poultry seasoning, salt, and pepper and sauté until fragrant, about 1 to 2 minutes.

3 Add the soy curls, vegetable broth, and noodles. Increase the heat to bring to a boil; then reduce the heat to medium–low to simmer until the potatoes can be pierced easily with a fork, the soy curls are rehydrated and tender, and the noodles are cooked through, about for 10 to 15 minutes.

4 Remove from the heat, add the nutritional yeast, and stir well to incorporate.

5 Add the lemon juice and fresh parsley. Adjust the seasoning as necessary and serve.

PER SERVING: *Calories 495 (From Fat 96); Fat 11g (Saturated 1g); Cholesterol 0mg; Sodium 714mg; Carbohydrate 80g (Dietary Fiber 8g); Protein 21g.*

NOTE: If you can't find Butler Soy Curls at your grocery store, you can buy them directly from Butler Foods at `https://butlerfoods.com/soycurls.html` or order them through another online retailer like Amazon.

NOTE: This soup is quite thick, just the way we like it. If you prefer a thinner soup, add more broth or water and adjust seasoning as needed. Also note that the noodles and soy curls will continue to soak up liquid as it sits, so you'll likely need to add more broth or water if you're reheating leftovers.

TIP: If you don't have or can't find poultry seasoning, use 1 teaspoon each of dried sage and dried thyme.

VARY IT! You can substitute two 15-ounce cans of chickpeas, drained and rinsed, for the soy.

Arame Soba Noodle Salad

PREP TIME: ABOUT 15 MIN | COOK TIME: 15 MIN | YIELD: 4–6 SERVINGS

INGREDIENTS

6 cups water, divided

1 teaspoon dried basil

½ teaspoon dried rosemary

½ teaspoon sea salt

8 ounces buckwheat soba noodles

½ cup arame

2 cloves garlic, crushed

1 teaspoon fresh ginger, grated

¼ cup rice vinegar

¼ cup toasted sesame oil

3 tablespoons tamari

1 cup edamame, shelled and cooked (optional)

1 carrot, grated

1 cup chopped green onions

½ cup toasted pine nuts or black sesame seeds, for garnish

DIRECTIONS

1 In a large pot, bring 5 cups of the water to a boil. Add the basil, rosemary, salt, and noodles, and cook until the noodles are al dente, about 8 to 10 minutes; then rinse and drain the noodles.

2 In a separate dish, soak the arame in the remaining 1 cup of water for about 10 minutes; drain and set aside.

3 In a large bowl, whisk together the garlic, ginger, vinegar, sesame oil, and tamari. Add the warm noodles to the sauce and toss to coat. Let the noodles sit and absorb the sauce for 10 minutes to 1 hour. Then stir in the edamame, carrots, onions, and arame.

4 Divide among 4 to 6 small bowls and sprinkle with toasted pine nuts or sesame seeds before serving.

PER SERVING: *Calories 341 (From Fat 171); Fat 19g (Saturated 2g); Cholesterol 0mg; Sodium 735mg; Carbohydrate 36g (Dietary Fiber 4g); Protein 10g.*

NOTE: Enjoy this dish with a side of steamed greens. Add a dollop of tahini to make this salad extra creamy.

Quinoa Tabbouleh Salad

PREP TIME: ABOUT 10 MIN	COOK TIME: 25 MIN	YIELD: 8 SERVINGS

INGREDIENTS

1 cup quinoa

1½ cups water

1 pinch sea salt

1 clove of garlic, minced

1 teaspoon dry basil

2 tablespoons lemon juice

1 tablespoon apple cider vinegar

1 teaspoon honey or coconut nectar

2 teaspoons Dijon mustard

¼ cup olive oil

1 cup cooked chickpeas

½ cup chopped red onion

¼ cup chopped fresh parsley

¼ cup chopped fresh mint

2 cups fresh spinach, finely chopped

½ cucumber, diced

1 cup cherry tomatoes, quartered

DIRECTIONS

1 Rinse the quinoa and strain it through a fine mesh strainer. Add the rinsed quinoa to a pot and warm over medium-low heat until the moisture has evaporated and it smells kind of nutty, about 2 to 3 minutes.

2 Add the water and salt, bring to a boil, and cover. Reduce the heat to low and simmer the quinoa until all the water has been absorbed, about 12 to 15 minutes.

3 Meanwhile, make the dressing. In a bowl, combine the garlic, basil, lemon juice, apple cider vinegar, honey or coconut nectar, mustard, and olive oil until well mixed; set aside.

4 Turn off the heat and let the quinoa stand for 2 minutes. Then remove the quinoa and spread it out on a large plate or baking sheet to cool.

5 Place the quinoa in a bowl and combine with chickpeas, onion, parsley, mint, spinach, cucumber, and tomatoes.

6 Add the dressing to the quinoa mixture and gently stir from the bottom up. Serve.

PER SERVING: *Calories 192 (From Fat 81); Fat 9g (Saturated 1g); Cholesterol 0mg; Sodium 108mg; Carbohydrate 24g (Dietary Fiber 4g); Protein 6g.*

NOTE: Rinse the quinoa well in Step 1 to make it easier to cook and eat. Then dry-toast the quinoa to create a better consistency and prevent the quinoa from sticking while it's cooking in Step 2.

VARY IT! You can try using tahini instead of Dijon mustard in the dressing for a different tabbouleh experience. Also, if tomatoes aren't in season, swap them out for shredded or chopped carrots.

Kidney Bean Salad

PREP TIME: ABOUT 15 MIN	COOK TIME: NONE	YIELD: 6 SERVINGS

INGREDIENTS

¼ cup apple cider vinegar

1 teaspoon pure maple syrup

3 tablespoons extra-virgin olive oil

Two 15-ounce cans kidney beans, drained and rinsed, or 3 cups cooked kidney beans

1 English cucumber, diced

4 radishes, halved and thinly sliced

½ red onion, peeled and diced

½ cup fresh parsley, chopped

1 teaspoon sea salt, or to taste

¼ teaspoon freshly ground black pepper, or to taste

DIRECTIONS

1 In a medium bowl, whisk together the vinegar, maple syrup, and oil until smooth.

2 Add the kidney beans, cucumber, radishes, onion, parsley, salt, and pepper. Gently toss to combine, ensuring that all the salad ingredients are coated evenly with the dressing.

3 Serve immediately or cover and refrigerate until ready to serve.

PER SERVING: *Calories 186 (From Fat 62); Fat 7g (Saturated 1g); Cholesterol 0mg; Sodium 324mg; Carbohydrate 23g (Dietary Fiber 9g); Protein 9g.*

TIP: For an oil-free option, skip the dressing and use a squeeze of fresh lemon juice instead.

Kale and Cabbage Slaw Salad

PREP TIME: ABOUT 5 MIN PLUS 30 MIN FOR MARINATING	COOK TIME: NONE	YIELD: 10–12 SERVINGS

INGREDIENTS

1 head red cabbage

2 carrots

1 beet

1 head fennel

1 bunch kale (about 3 cups)

½ cup olive oil

¼ cup apple cider vinegar

Juice of 1 lemon

2 tablespoons raw honey or coconut nectar

2 tablespoons hempseeds

DIRECTIONS

1 Add the cabbage, carrots, beet, and fennel to a food processor and shred with a shredding blade.

2 Remove the stems from the kale, and then chop the kale into thin strips or bite-size pieces.

3 In a bowl, add the olive oil, apple cider vinegar, lemon juice, and raw honey or coconut nectar and mix together to make a vinaigrette.

4 Combine the vinaigrette with the shredded vegetables and toss until the cabbage and kale are well-coated.

5 Allow the salad to marinate in the fridge for 30 to 60 minutes.

6 Mix in the hempseeds just before serving.

PER SERVING: *Calories 178 (From Fat 117); Fat 13g (Saturated 3g); Cholesterol 0mg; Sodium 58mg; Carbohydrate 16g (Dietary Fiber 4g); Protein 4g.*

TIP: If you don't have a food processor, you can use a mandolin or hand-slice the cabbage, carrots, beet, and fennel into thin strips.

TIP: If you're using lacinato kale (dark kale), the stems are much softer and can be chopped into this salad. However, most other varieties, such as curly kale or red Russian, will need the stems removed.

NOTE: This salad can be consumed right after it's tossed together, but it will taste better and be easier to chew when it marinates longer. It also tastes great the next day!

VARY IT! Instead of olive oil, try chia seed oil, hempseed oil, or pumpkin seed oil for variety and a boost of omega-3 fatty acids. You can add sliced avocado on top of this salad to give it a nourishing boost.

Warm Festive Farro Salad

INGREDIENTS

1 cup farro (spelt), soaked overnight in enough water to cover it completely

½ butternut squash, peeled and cubed

¼ cup olive oil, plus 2 tablespoons, divided

1 clove garlic, minced

1 red onion, chopped

1 cup portobello mushrooms, chopped

⅓ cup currants or dried cranberries

1 cup thinly sliced rainbow chard or spinach

1 teaspoon sea salt

1 teaspoon oregano

1 dash herbes de Provence

3 tablespoons balsamic vinegar

¼ cup toasted walnuts or pine nuts

DIRECTIONS

1 Preheat the oven to 350 degrees.

2 Rinse the farro and place it in a pot with 1 cup of water. Bring to a boil, reduce the heat to medium-low, and simmer for 30 to 45 minutes. Set aside.

3 While the farro is cooking, place the butternut squash on a baking tray and toss with 1 tablespoon of the olive oil. Bake for 30 minutes.

4 In a skillet, warm 1 tablespoon of the olive oil with the garlic over medium heat. Add the onion, mushrooms, and currants or cranberries; sauté until softened, about 5 minutes.

5 Add the chard or spinach, salt, oregano, herbes de Provence, and balsamic vinegar. Let sit for a few minutes to let the flavors combine and the chard wilt.

6 In a large bowl, place the cooked farro and add 2 to 4 tablespoons of olive oil to taste. Add the butternut squash and the onion, mushroom, and chard mixture. Stir to combine. Top with walnuts or pine nuts and serve.

PER SERVING: *Calories 306 (From Fat 153); Fat 17g (Saturated 2g); Cholesterol 0mg; Sodium 251mg; Carbohydrate 31g (Dietary Fiber 4g); Protein 6g.*

VARY IT! For an extra dose of protein, add 1 cup of cooked white beans at the end of Step 6. This gives this dish a richer texture.

Coleslaw Pasta Salad

INGREDIENTS

One 16-ounce package macaroni noodles or other small to medium shaped pasta

1 cup frozen green peas

1½ cups vegan mayonnaise

3 tablespoons white vinegar

1 tablespoon yellow mustard

2 tablespoons cane sugar

¾ teaspoon sea salt, or to taste

¼ teaspoon freshly ground black pepper, or to taste

One 14-ounce package coleslaw mix

¼ cup chopped fresh parsley (optional)

DIRECTIONS

1 Cook the macaroni noodles in well-salted water according to package directions until al dente. Place the frozen peas in the bottom of a large colander and drain the cooked pasta over the top. Set aside to cool.

2 In a large bowl, whisk together the mayonnaise, vinegar, mustard, sugar, salt, and pepper until smooth.

3 Add the cooled pasta and peas to the bowl. Add the coleslaw mix. Mix well to incorporate all the ingredients and ensure that they're fully coated in the dressing.

4 Taste and adjust the seasoning as necessary. Stir in the fresh chopped parsley, if using.

5 Cover and refrigerate until ready to serve.

PER SERVING: *Calories 323 (From Fat 168); Fat 19g (Saturated 3g); Cholesterol 0mg; Sodium 278mg; Carbohydrate 33g (Dietary Fiber 3g); Protein 6g.*

TIP: This pasta salad can be made several days in advance.

Arugula Peach Salad with Lentils

INGREDIENTS

8 cups arugula

1½ cups cooked lentils (about ¾ cup dry lentils, cooked)

2 fresh peaches, pits removed, sliced

2 cups grape tomatoes, halved

½ cup sliced almonds

½ cup freshly squeezed orange juice

2 tablespoons red wine vinegar

1 tablespoon pure maple syrup

½ teaspoon sea salt

¼ cup extra-virgin olive oil

3 to 4 basil leaves, chiffonade

DIRECTIONS

1 In a large bowl, place the arugula, lentils, peaches, tomatoes, and almonds and toss to combine.

2 In a small bowl or jar, whisk together the orange juice, vinegar, maple syrup, and salt. Drizzle in the olive oil while whisking to combine. Stir in the basil.

3 Pour as much of the vinaigrette over the salad as you like, toss to coat, and serve.

PER SERVING: *Calories 405 (From Fat 191); Fat 21g (Saturated 3g); Cholesterol 0mg; Sodium 252mg; Carbohydrate 43g (Dietary Fiber 15g); Protein 15g.*

NOTE: Canned lentils, drained and rinsed, or packaged steamed lentils (found in the refrigerated section of some grocery stores) are perfect for this recipe. You can also use leftover cooked lentils that you have in your fridge.

VARY IT! If you don't have lentils, try it with chickpeas or white beans.

Massaged Kale Harvest Salad

PREP TIME: ABOUT 15 MIN | **COOK TIME: 12 MIN** | **YIELD: 6 SERVINGS**

INGREDIENTS

½ cup white quinoa, rinsed well with cold water

¾ cup water

1 bunch lacinato kale, tough stems and ribs removed, chopped

1 avocado pitted and peeled

1 pinch sea salt

1 cup shredded Brussels sprouts

2 carrots, shredded

1 or 2 tart apples or pears, cored and thinly sliced

½ cup toasted pecans or walnuts

¼ cup gold raisins or dried cranberries

¼ cup shelled pumpkin seeds

3 tablespoons apple cider vinegar

2 tablespoons Dijon mustard

1 tablespoon pure maple syrup

Salt to taste

Freshly ground black pepper to taste

DIRECTIONS

1 In a pot, add the quinoa and water and bring to a boil. Reduce the heat to low, cover, and simmer until the quinoa is cooked through and the water is absorbed, about 12 to 15 minutes. Remove from the heat, fluff with a fork, and let cool.

2 Meanwhile, in a large bowl, add the kale, avocado, and salt. With clean hands, "massage" the kale, making sure the avocado is completely mashed into the kale. Massage for several minutes to allow the kale to soften. Set aside.

3 When the quinoa is cool, add it to the kale along with the Brussels sprouts, carrots, apples or pears, pecans or walnuts, raisins or cranberries, and pumpkin seeds. Toss well with a spoon or two forks to combine.

4 In a small jar or bowl, whisk together the vinegar, mustard, maple syrup, and a sprinkle of salt and pepper, until smooth.

5 Drizzle the dressing over the salad, toss to coat, and serve.

PER SERVING: *Calories 241 (From Fat 113); Fat 13g (Saturated 2g); Cholesterol 0mg; Sodium 110mg; Carbohydrate 29g (Dietary Fiber 5g); Protein 7g.*

NOTE: To toast pecans or walnuts, heat a skillet over medium heat and add the nuts in a single layer. Cook, stirring frequently to prevent burning, until they're fragrant and starting to brown, about 3 to 4 minutes. Remove from the heat and let cool.

Orange Spinach Salad

INGREDIENTS

5 to 6 cups baby spinach

2 navel oranges, segmented

1 avocado, pitted, peeled, and diced

½ cup sliced almonds

⅓ cup unsweetened, plain vegan yogurt

¼ cup fresh orange juice

2 tablespoon fresh lime juice

1 to 2 tablespoons pure maple syrup (optional)

1 to 2 tablespoons water, if needed

Salt to taste

Freshly ground black pepper to taste

DIRECTIONS

1 In a serving bowl, combine the spinach, oranges, avocado, and almonds.

2 In a small bowl or jar, whisk together the yogurt, orange juice, lime juice, maple syrup, and water until smooth. Taste and add salt and pepper, if needed.

3 Drizzle as much or as little of the dressing as you like over the salad, toss to combine, and serve.

PER SERVING: *Calories 216 (From Fat 112); Fat 12g (Saturated 1g); Cholesterol 0mg; Sodium 38mg; Carbohydrate 24g (Dietary Fiber 6g); Protein 6g.*

VARY IT! Feel free to add more protein like chickpeas or white beans to this salad. Fresh berries like blackberries or sliced strawberries would be a great addition, too. Vegan feta (Violife makes a great one!) is delicious in this dish, too, and is worth the splurge.

Cucumber Chickpea Salad

PREP TIME: ABOUT 15 MIN	COOK TIME: NONE	YIELD: 6 SERVINGS

INGREDIENTS

1 English cucumber, chopped

1 pint grape tomatoes, halved or quartered

One 15-ounce can chickpeas, drained and rinsed

¼ red onion, diced

¼ cup fresh parsley, chopped

¼ cup tahini

3 tablespoons balsamic vinegar

Zest of 1 small lemon

Juice of ½ lemon, or more to taste

1 clove garlic, minced

¼ teaspoon sea salt, or to taste

¼ cup water, to thin, divided

Freshly ground black pepper to taste

DIRECTIONS

1 In a bowl, place the cucumber, tomatoes, chickpeas, onion, and parsley and toss well to combine. Set aside.

2 In a small bowl or glass jar, whisk the tahini, vinegar, lemon zest, lemon juice, garlic, and salt. Add the water 1 tablespoon at a time, whisking after each addition, until the desired consistency is reached. It should be pourable but not runny.

3 Pour the dressing (as little or as much as you like — you may not use it all) over the top of the salad and mix well to coat.

4 Finish the salad with freshly ground black pepper and an extra sprinkle of salt and squeeze of fresh lemon, if desired.

5 Serve immediately or chill until ready to serve.

PER SERVING: *Calories 148 (From Fat 56); Fat 6g (Saturated 1g); Cholesterol 0mg; Sodium 246mg; Carbohydrate 19g (Dietary Fiber 4g); Protein 5g.*

Hearts of Palm Salad

PREP TIME: ABOUT 10 MIN	COOK TIME: NONE	YIELD: 4 SERVINGS

INGREDIENTS

One 14-ounce jar hearts of palm, drained and thinly sliced

1 avocado, peeled, pitted, and cut into bite-size pieces

2 cups grape tomatoes, halved

1 English cucumber, chopped

1 recipe Lemon Vinaigrette (see the recipe in Chapter 15)

DIRECTIONS

1 In a bowl, add the hearts of palm, avocado, tomatoes, and cucumber. Toss gently to combine.

2 Drizzle as much or as little of the Lemon Vinaigrette over the salad as you like, toss to combine, and serve.

PER SERVING: *Calories 195 (From Fat 134); Fat 15g (Saturated 2g); Cholesterol 0mg; Sodium 693mg; Carbohydrate 15g (Dietary Fiber 6g); Protein 4g.*

Butter Lettuce Salad

PREP TIME: ABOUT 15 MIN	COOK TIME: NONE	YIELD: 4 SERVINGS

INGREDIENTS

8 cups chopped butter lettuce

1 apple, thinly sliced

4 radishes, thinly sliced

4 teaspoons nutritional yeast

2 green onions, sliced

2 tablespoons chopped fresh parsley

2 tablespoons chopped fresh dill

1 recipe Hempseed Ranch (see the recipe in Chapter 15)

Freshly cracked black pepper to taste (optional)

Juice of 1 lemon (optional)

DIRECTIONS

1 For each serving, place 2 cups of chopped butter lettuce in a salad bowl, followed by one-quarter of the apple slices, 1 sliced radish, 1 teaspoon nutritional yeast, one-fourth of the green onions, ½ tablespoon parsley, and ½ tablespoon dill.

2 Drizzle as much or as little of the Hempseed Ranch over the top as you like.

3 Finish with pepper and lemon juice, if you like, and serve.

PER SERVING: *Calories 178 (From Fat 92); Fat 10g (Saturated 1g); Cholesterol 0mg; Sodium 248mg; Carbohydrate 15g (Dietary Fiber 4g); Protein 9g.*

NOTE: If you don't plan on eating all 4 servings immediately, keep all the ingredients separate in airtight containers and plate just what you need. A squeeze of fresh lemon juice over the apple slices can help to preserve them.

Herb Roasted Potato Arugula Salad

PREP TIME: ABOUT 10 MIN | COOK TIME: 25 MIN | YIELD: 4 SERVINGS

INGREDIENTS

1 pound baby potatoes, halved

1 tablespoon olive oil

1 tablespoon chopped fresh parsley

1 tablespoon chopped fresh dill

1 teaspoon chopped fresh thyme

1 teaspoon chopped fresh rosemary

½ teaspoon sea salt

¼ teaspoon black pepper

2 cloves garlic, minced

3 cups arugula

Juice of 1 lemon

DIRECTIONS

1 Preheat the oven to 400 degrees.

2 In a bowl, toss the potatoes with the olive oil, parsley, dill, thyme, rosemary, salt, and pepper.

3 Spread the potatoes on a baking sheet in an even layer and bake for 15 minutes.

4 Sprinkle the potatoes with the garlic and toss, making sure to keep them in one even layer.

5 Return to the oven until the potatoes are brown and crispy on the edges, about 10 minutes.

6 When the potatoes are done, place them in a bowl with the arugula and toss to combine. Squeeze the lemon juice over everything, toss again, and serve.

PER SERVING: *Calories 141 (From Fat 33); Fat 4g (Saturated 1g); Cholesterol 0mg; Sodium 252mg; Carbohydrate 25g (Dietary Fiber 2g); Protein 3g.*

NOTE: Fresh herbs make all the difference in this dish! You can use dried herbs in a pinch, but you won't have the same bright flavor that fresh herbs provide.

Balsamic Roasted Beet Salad

PREP TIME: ABOUT 10 MIN	COOK TIME: 30 MIN	YIELD: 4 SERVINGS

INGREDIENTS

3 to 4 large beets, scrubbed really well and chopped into 1-inch cubes

1 tablespoon olive oil

¼ teaspoon sea salt

¼ teaspoon dried thyme

¼ teaspoon freshly ground black pepper

1 tablespoon balsamic vinegar

½ cup hazelnuts

5 to 6 cups baby chard, baby kale, or baby spinach

1 pear, thinly sliced

¼ cup fresh chopped parsley

Balsamic Maple Dressing (see the recipe in Chapter 15) or your favorite balsamic dressing

DIRECTIONS

1 Preheat the oven to 400 degrees. Line a rimmed baking sheet with parchment paper and set aside.

2 In a bowl, toss the beets with the oil, salt, thyme, and pepper. Spread out into one even layer on the prepared baking sheet. Roast, stirring every 10 minutes, until the beets are tender, about 30 to 40 minutes.

3 Add the balsamic vinegar to the beets and stir well to coat. Set aside to cool.

4 Meanwhile, in a small skillet, warm the hazelnuts in one even layer over medium heat. Cook, stirring frequently, until lightly browned and fragrant, about 5 to 10 minutes. Watch them closely — they burn easily.

5 In a serving bowl, add the baby greens, pear, parsley, roasted beets, and toasted hazelnuts. Toss to combine.

6 Drizzle with Balsamic Maple Dressing, as much or as little as you like, and serve.

PER SERVING: *Calories 472 (From Fat 369); Fat 41g (Saturated 5g); Cholesterol 0mg; Sodium 431mg; Carbohydrate 24g (Dietary Fiber 6g); Protein 5g.*

NOTE: Beet skins are edible, so you don't need to peel them. Just make sure to remove the greens and stems and scrub the beets really well.

NOTE: If you do peel the beets, keep in mind that they'll stain pretty much anything and everything, like wooden cutting boards, some countertops, fabric, and your hands! Peel them right over the sink under running water. You can wear gloves if you're really worried about it, but if you do it over the sink, you should be able to wash it off after a few tries.

Barbecue Ranch Chickpea Salad

PREP TIME: ABOUT 10 MIN	COOK TIME: 20 MIN	YIELD: 4 SERVINGS

INGREDIENTS

1 to 2 heads romaine lettuce, chopped (about 6 cups)

1 to 2 tomatoes, chopped

¼ cup diced red onion

One 15-ounce can black beans, drained and rinsed

1 cup fresh corn kernels (or frozen, thawed)

1 avocado, peeled, pitted, and diced

¼ cup chopped fresh cilantro

Roasted Chickpeas (see the following recipe), for garnish

¼ cup Hempseed Ranch (see Chapter 15) or your favorite vegan ranch dressing

¼ cup Smoky Barbecue Sauce (see Chapter 15) or your favorite vegan barbecue sauce

DIRECTIONS

1 In a large bowl, toss the lettuce, tomatoes, onion, black beans, corn, avocado, and cilantro.

2 Garnish with Roasted Chickpeas.

3 Drizzle with Hempseed Ranch and Smoky Barbecue Sauce and serve.

Roasted Chickpeas

One 15-ounce can chickpeas, drained and rinsed

1 teaspoon olive oil

¼ teaspoon sea salt

¼ teaspoon garlic powder

¼ teaspoon smoked paprika

⅛ teaspoon black pepper

(continued)

(continued)

1 Preheat the oven to 400 degrees. Line a rimmed baking sheet with parchment paper.

2 In a bowl, toss the chickpeas with the oil, salt, garlic powder, paprika, and pepper. Spread out in a single layer on the prepared baking sheet.

3 Roast, shaking the pan halfway through, until the chickpeas are slightly crunchy, about 20 to 30 minutes. The chickpeas will continue to crisp up as they cool.

PER SERVING: *Calories 337 (From Fat 137); Fat 15g (Saturated 2g); Cholesterol 0mg; Sodium 502mg; Carbohydrate 44g (Dietary Fiber 13g); Protein 11g.*

NOTE: The roasted chickpeas take the place of fried tortilla strips typically found in similar salads.

VARY IT! Add extra veggies if you want, like bell peppers, green onions, or zucchini.

Chapter **11**

Lovable Lunches

When it comes to lunch, you probably want to grab something quick and not spend too much time, if any, prepping it. However, you need to make sure it's balanced, varied, and filling enough to last you until snack time (see Chapter 14 for tips about snacks). Lunch recharges you after a busy morning and sets the tone for the rest of the day. You can make this meal easier on yourself with proper planning and organization.

The best way to tackle lunch as a beginning plant-based eater is to make a wonderfully wholesome wrap or sandwich or enjoy leftovers from the night before. All these options should contain plant-based protein, energizing carbohydrates, and healthy fats.

In this chapter, we give you some great ideas for making simple, quick lunches that you can pack and take with you for the workday or out on the town. If you're at home during the day, these are easy go-to meals that you can pull out and put together with very little effort.

Rethinking Handheld Lunches

Most people love a good, hearty sandwich. When meat is no longer in the picture, people often experience a sense of loss about what can go in between those slices of bread! Well, you have lots of options — more than you can even imagine.

But first, a note about bread: Pick a whole-grain or sprouted-grain bread made from barley, kamut, oats, or spelt. You can even opt for gluten-free breads and wraps made from brown rice, millet, or quinoa flour.

TIP

Food for Life, a brand available at most major grocery stores, has amazing sprouted-grain bread and tortillas, brown-rice wraps, and corn tortillas.

After you've chosen your bread, select your filling:

>> **Protein:** Go with hummus or another bean dip, grilled or baked tofu or tempeh, a veggie burger, falafel, or Spinach Almond Patties (see Chapter 13).

>> **Fat:** Try almond butter, avocado, cashew cheese, sunflower-seed butter, or tahini.

>> **Veggies:** Good options include beets, carrots, cucumbers, leafy greens, mushrooms, onions, radishes, sprouts, and tomatoes.

>> **Dressing:** Try a homemade salad dressing or other marinade, salsa, tomato sauce, Dijon mustard, pesto, or avocado spread. (Turn to Chapter 15 for lots of sauce and dressing recipes.)

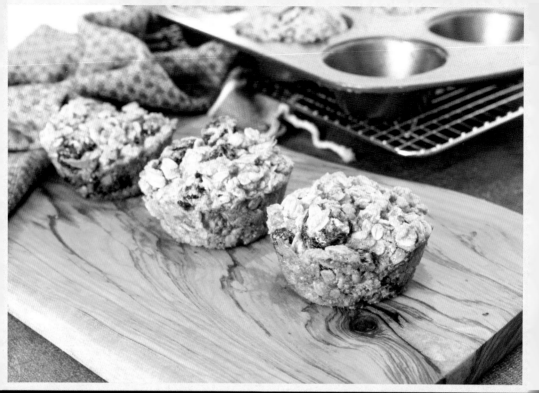

Cherry Baked Oatmeal Muffins (Chapter 9)

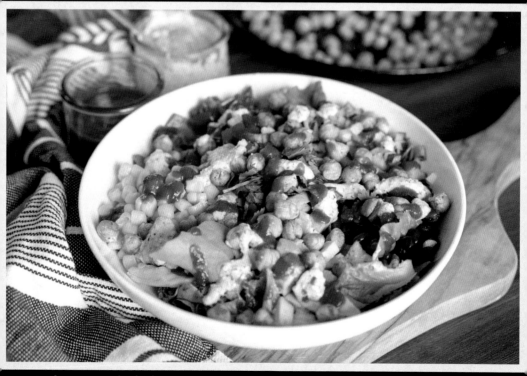

Barbecue Ranch Chickpea Salad (Chapter 10) with Hempseed Ranch (Chapter 15)

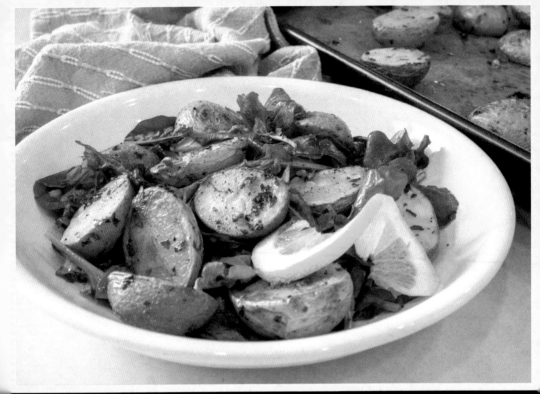

Herb Roasted Potato Arugula Salad (Chapter 10)

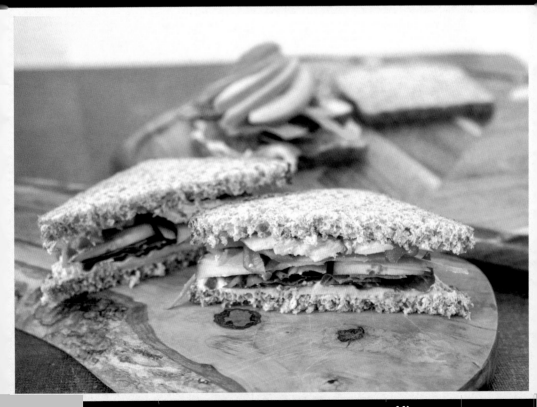

Humr								r 11)

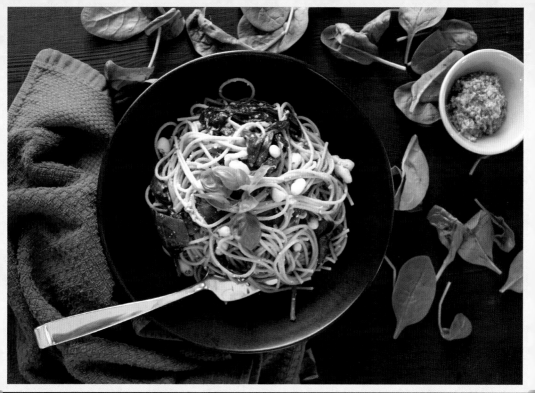

Zesty Pesto Pasta with White Beans (Chapter 12)

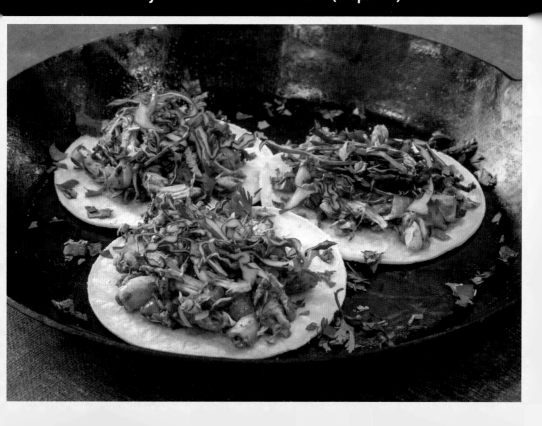

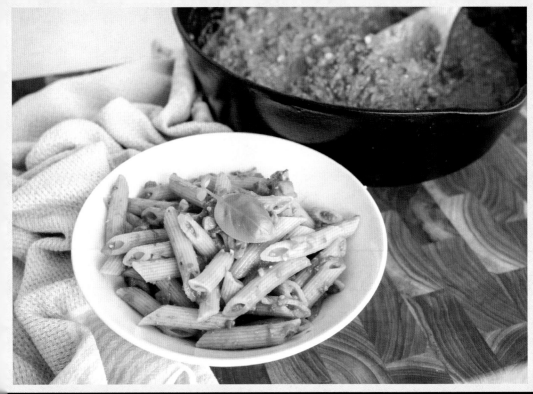

Chickpea Walnut Bolognese (Chapter 12)

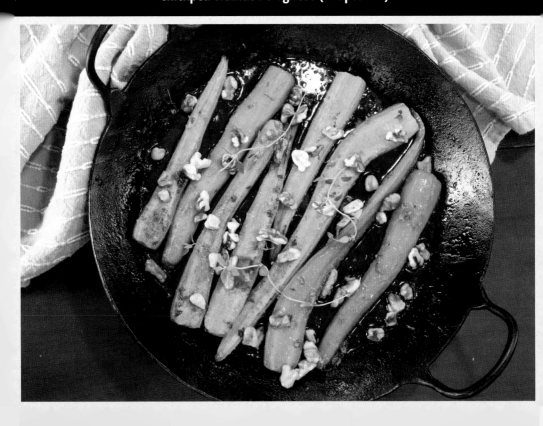

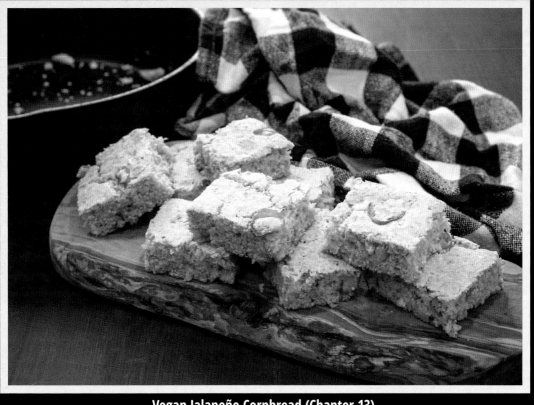

Vegan Jalapeño Cornbread (Chapter 13)

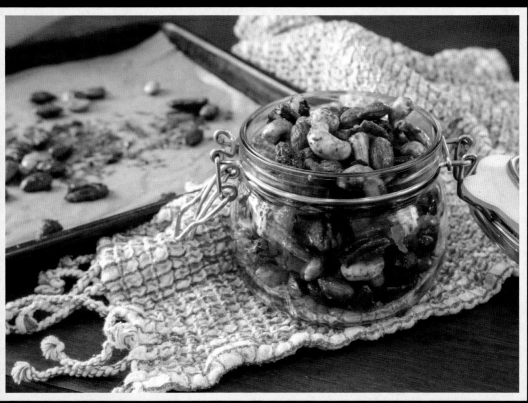

Spicy Herb Roasted Mixed Nuts (Chapter 14)

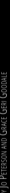

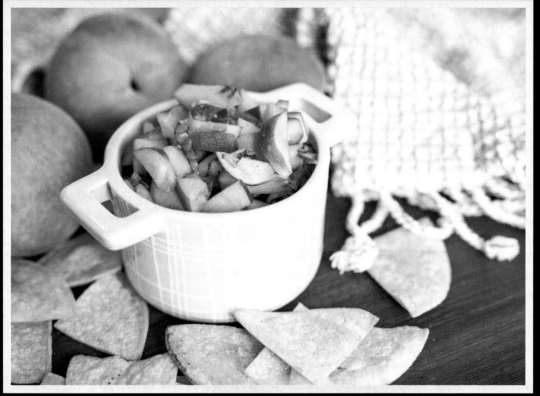

Fresh Peach Salsa with Homemade Tortilla Chips (Chapter 14)

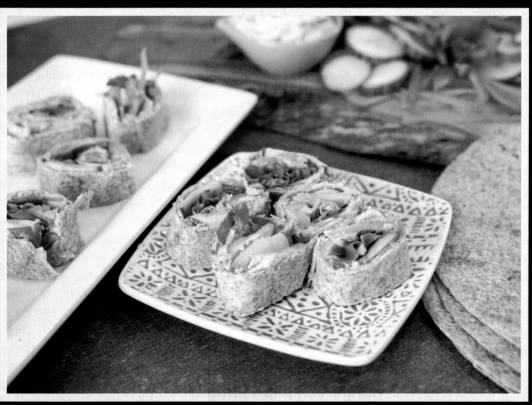

Hummus Tortilla Rollups (Chapter 14)

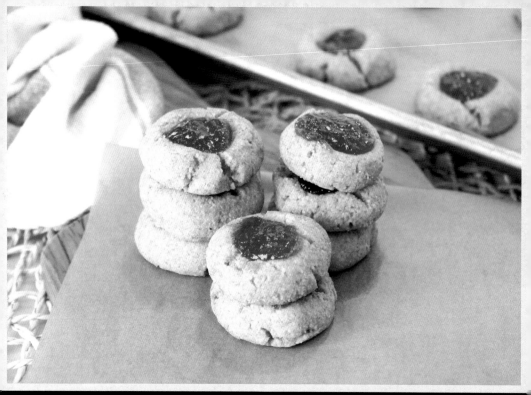

Jam Dot Cookies (Chapter 16)

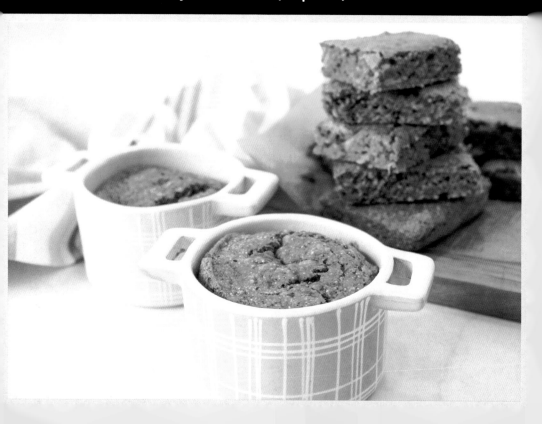

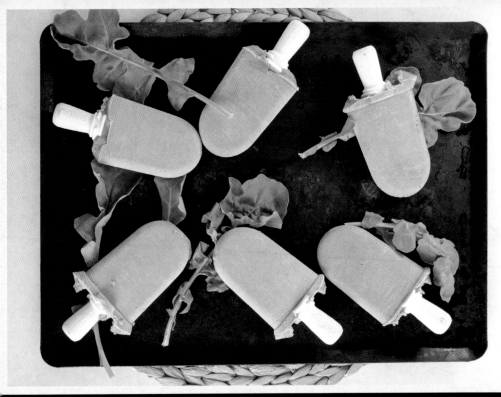

Smoothie Popsicles (Chapter 16)

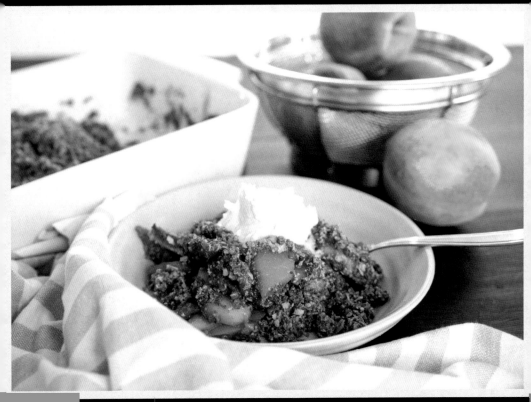

Warm Pe

MAKING A MEAL OUT OF SOUPS AND SALADS

Soups and salads aren't just for starters before a meal. Done right, they can *be* the meal. The key to a making a meal out of soup or salad isn't the portion size, but the balance of macronutrients.

Healthy plant proteins, like quinoa, beans, tofu, and lentils, are perfect in both soups and salads to fill you up. Add a variety of vegetables and a healthy fat, like avocado, nuts, or seeds, and you've got a nutritious meal that satisfies.

Texture is every bit as important as flavor when it comes to meal satisfaction. Include a variety of textures, like crispy (think bell peppers, cucumbers, or romaine lettuce), crunchy (think raw walnuts or roasted chickpeas), juicy (think cherry tomatoes, fresh peaches, or grapes), creamy (think avocado, cashew cream, or hummus), and chewy (think baked tofu, dried fruit, or farro) in your salads, and even as a garnish on your soups, for the most enjoyment.

Chapter 10 has great soup and salad recipes. Some worth trying for a standalone lunch are Vegan Chicken Noodle Soup, Vegetable Quinoa Soup, Arame Soba Noodle Salad, Kidney Bean Salad, and Quinoa Tabbouleh Salad.

Sunflower Seed Nori Rolls

PREP TIME: ABOUT 20 MIN	COOK TIME: 15 MIN	YIELD: 6 SERVINGS

INGREDIENTS

1 cup sunflower seeds, soaked for 10 to 12 hours

1 cup almonds, soaked for 10 to 12 hours

1 to 2 tablespoons fresh dill

1 tablespoon fresh oregano

1 teaspoon fresh sage, chopped

2 tablespoons lemon juice

1 tablespoon tamari

1 teaspoon fresh ginger

1 tablespoon dulse flakes

½ teaspoon sea salt

4 to 6 sheets raw nori

1 carrot, shredded

2 small beets, shredded

½ cucumber, sliced lengthwise

1 avocado, sliced lengthwise

Handful of sprouts (mung, sunflower, or pea shoots)

DIRECTIONS

1 In a food processor or high-speed blender, place sunflower seeds, almonds, dill, oregano, sage, lemon juice, tamari, ginger, dulse flakes, and salt and blend until uniform. For a smoother consistency, add a touch of water or blend longer.

2 Lay one nori sheet flat on a surface with the rough side facing up.

3 Spread about ¼ cup of seed spread on the nori sheet. (You can fill it to the edges if you want.)

4 Place the carrot, beets, cucumber, avocado, and sprouts in a relatively thin horizontal row toward the bottom of the sheet.

5 Roll by lifting the bottom edge closest to you and wrap it over all the veggies. Holding tight, continue to roll it all the way up. Seal it with some water or extra seed spread.

6 Repeat with the remaining nori sheet and remaining filling ingredients.

7 Cut the rolls, using a sharp, damp knife. Start in the center of the roll and keep cutting down the center of each half until you have 6 to 8 pieces.

PER SERVING: *Calories 494 (From Fat 351); Fat 39g (Saturated 4g); Cholesterol 0mg; Sodium 685mg; Carbohydrate 28g (Dietary Fiber 11g); Protein 18g.*

TIP: This recipe makes a great appetizer at a party and is extremely colorful. Make sure you load your nori rolls up with different veggies each time you make them.

NOTE: Be sure to use raw nori to make raw nori rolls. (It doesn't work if you buy the toasted kind.)

Tuna Salad Sandwiches

PREP TIME: ABOUT 10 MIN	COOK TIME: NONE	YIELD: 6 SERVINGS

INGREDIENTS

16 ounces extra-firm tofu

14 ounces canned artichoke hearts, drained and chopped small

3 tablespoons finely diced red onion

3 tablespoons finely diced dill pickles

1 rib celery, finely chopped

⅓ cup vegan mayonnaise, plus more for serving

1 tablespoon fresh lemon juice

1 teaspoon Dijon mustard

1 tablespoon dulse flakes (optional)

2 teaspoons Old Bay seasoning

½ teaspoon sea salt, or to taste

12 slices whole-grain or sprouted-grain bread, toasted

1 or 2 tomatoes, sliced

DIRECTIONS

1 Using clean hands, crumble the tofu into a big bowl until the pieces are fairly small.

2 Add the artichoke hearts, onion, pickles, celery, mayonnaise, lemon juice, mustard, dulse flakes, Old Bay seasoning, and salt. Mix well until fully combined. Taste and adjust the seasoning to your liking.

3 To serve, spread a thin layer of vegan mayonnaise on a slice of toasted bread, pile on the vegan tuna salad, add 1 or 2 slices of tomato, and top it off with another slice of toasted bread. Repeat to make the remaining 5 sandwiches.

PER SERVING: *Calories 291 (From Fat 116); Fat 13g (Saturated 2g); Cholesterol 0mg; Sodium 793mg; Carbohydrate 30g (Dietary Fiber 7g); Protein 16g.*

NOTE: If you use firm tofu, instead of extra-firm, be sure to press the tofu first. You can use a tofu press to do this, or simply wrap the block of tofu in a clean dish cloth or paper towels and place it between 2 plates, weighing down the top plate with bags of dry beans or canned goods, for about 20 minutes. Do not use soft or silken tofu.

VARY IT! Stuff the mixture into a pita pocket instead of between 2 slices of bread. Or skip the bread altogether and use whole-grain crackers to scoop up the tuna salad.

Curried Chickpea Salad Wraps

PREP TIME: 15 MIN	COOK TIME: NONE	YIELD: 4 SERVINGS

INGREDIENTS

Two 15-ounce cans chickpeas, drained and rinsed

1 rib celery, diced

1 sweet apple, cored and diced

2 green onions, sliced

1 tablespoon chopped fresh parsley

½ cup unsweetened dairy-free plain yogurt

2 tablespoons vegan mayonnaise

1 tablespoon Dijon mustard

1 tablespoon fresh lemon juice

1 tablespoon mild yellow curry powder

½ teaspoon sea salt, or to taste

¼ teaspoon freshly ground black pepper, or to taste

4 leaves romaine lettuce

Four 10-inch tortillas

DIRECTIONS

1   In a bowl, mash the chickpeas with a potato masher or a fork.

2   Add the celery, apple, onions, and parsley and mix well.

3   Add the yogurt, mayonnaise, mustard, lemon juice, curry powder, salt, and pepper. Mix well to combine.

4   Lay out 1 tortilla on a flat surface. Place 1 lettuce leaf on top of the tortilla. Spread ¼ of the chickpea mixture over the lettuce leaf. Fold in the sides of the tortilla about an inch, and then roll it up tightly from bottom to top. Cut in half for serving. Repeat to make the remaining 3 wraps.

PER SERVING: *Calories 448 (From Fat 107); Fat 12g (Saturated 2g); Cholesterol 0mg; Sodium 779mg; Carbohydrate 73g (Dietary Fiber 9g); Protein 13g.*

VARY IT! The filling for these wraps is also great served with whole-grain crackers instead of as a wrap.

Hummus Avocado Veggie Sandwiches

PREP TIME: ABOUT 10 MIN	COOK TIME: NONE	YIELD: 4 SERVINGS

INGREDIENTS

8 slices whole-grain, sprouted-grain, or gluten-free bread

1 cup Creamy Oil-Free Hummus (see Chapter **14**) or your favorite store-bought savory hummus variety, divided

2 cups arugula or fresh spinach, divided

2 carrots, peeled into ribbons or shredded, divided

½ English cucumber, thinly sliced, divided

1 red bell pepper, seeded and thinly sliced, divided

1 avocado, pitted, peeled, and thinly sliced, divided

DIRECTIONS

1 Toast the bread, if desired.

2 Spread 2 tablespoons of hummus on 1 slice of bread.

3 Top with ½ cup arugula or spinach, then a pile of carrot ribbons, 4 to 6 slices of cucumber, some bell pepper slices, and 3 to 4 avocado slices.

4 Spread another 2 tablespoons of hummus on a second slice of bread and place it on top of the sandwich, hummus side down.

5 Repeat with the remaining 3 sandwiches.

6 Cut the sandwiches in half before serving.

PER SERVING: *Calories 333 (From Fat 115); Fat 2g (Saturated 2g); Cholesterol 0mg; Sodium 399mg; Carbohydrate 45g (Dietary Fiber 11g); Protein 12g.*

NOTE: This recipe is extremely versatile. Try changing it by using sliced zucchini, radishes, tomatoes, pickled red onions, or sprouts.

Tofu Mushroom Collard Wraps

PREP TIME: ABOUT 15 MIN | COOK TIME: 16 MIN | YIELD: 4 SERVINGS

INGREDIENTS

5 to 6 large collard leaves

¼ cup coconut aminos or tamari

3 tablespoons tahini

1 tablespoon pure maple syrup

1 tablespoon rice vinegar

2 teaspoons sesame oil

Dash of hot sauce or sriracha, to taste

1 tablespoon grapeseed oil

2 ribs celery, diced

2 cloves garlic, minced

One 1-inch piece fresh ginger, peeled and minced

One 14- to 16-ounce package extra-firm tofu, drained and pressed

8 to 10 ounces shiitake mushrooms, chopped

2 green onions, sliced

¼ cup sliced almonds

DIRECTIONS

1 Bring a large pot of water to a boil. Turn the heat off. Wearing an oven mitt and using kitchen tongs, hold 1 collard leaf by the long stem and dip it into the boiling water. Make sure all of the leaf is covered for about 20 to 30 seconds. Drain off the excess water and transfer to a cutting board. Repeat with the remaining leaves.

2 Place 1 collard leaf on a cutting board and fold it half lengthwise. Using a sharp knife, carefully trim off the thick, woody stem. Don't cut the entire leaf in half — only cut up about halfway until the stem is thinner and more pliable. Set the leaves aside.

3 In a small bowl or jar, whisk the coconut aminos or tamari, tahini, maple syrup, vinegar, sesame oil, and hot sauce. Set aside.

4 In a large skillet, warm the grapeseed oil over medium heat. Add the celery, garlic, and ginger and sauté until fragrant, about 2 to 3 minutes.

5 Crumble the tofu into the pan and increase the heat to medium-high. Sauté until the tofu is starting to brown on the edges, about 4 to 6 minutes.

6 Add the mushrooms and sauté until they soften, about 5 minutes.

7 Add the prepared sauce from Step 3 and stir well to combine. Simmer for 1 to 2 minutes to heat through.

8 Add the onions and almonds and stir to incorporate. Remove from the heat.

9 Place 1 collard leaf flat on a cutting board or large plate. Overlap the split ends where you removed the stem so there are no gaps. Place about ¾ to 1 cup of filling (depending on the size of the leaf) on the overlapped part. Starting from that same end, fold up the bottom over the filling, fold in the sides, and then continue rolling from the bottom up as tightly as possible. Slice in half for serving. Repeat with the remaining collard leaves and filling.

PER SERVING: *Calories 209 (From Fat 134); Fat 15g (Saturated 1g); Cholesterol 0mg; Sodium 1,032mg; Carbohydrate 9g (Dietary Fiber 2g); Protein 13g.*

TIP: Start cooking the filling while the water is coming to a boil for the collard leaves to save yourself some time.

VARY IT! This filling is also delicious served over brown rice, cauliflower rice, or quinoa.

Mediterranean Pita Pockets

PREP TIME: ABOUT 15 MIN	COOK TIME: NONE	YIELD: 4 SERVINGS

INGREDIENTS

One 15-ounce can chickpeas, drained and rinsed

One 15-ounce can white beans, drained and rinsed

½ cup chopped cucumber

¼ cup chopped red onion

¼ cup sliced black olives

¼ cup chopped fresh parsley

¼ cup tahini

3 tablespoons red wine vinegar

1 tablespoon fresh lemon juice

1 clove garlic, minced

¼ teaspoon sea salt, or to taste

Water, as needed

4 pita pockets

2 cups fresh baby spinach

DIRECTIONS

1 In a bowl, combine the chickpeas, white beans, cucumber, onion, olives, and parsley. Toss to combine; set aside.

2 In a small jar or bowl, whisk together the tahini, vinegar, lemon juice, garlic, and salt. Whisk in water, 1 tablespoon at a time, until the mixture is a pourable dressing consistency.

3 Pour the dressing over the bean mixture and toss well to coat evenly.

4 Cut each pita pocket in half. Fill each half with ¼ cup spinach and about ½ cup of the bean mixture.

PER SERVING: *Calories 495 (From Fat 114); Fat 13g (Saturated 2g); Cholesterol 0mg; Sodium 785mg; Carbohydrate 82g (Dietary Fiber 15g); Protein 18g.*

TIP: I like the contrast of nutty chickpeas and creamy white beans, but you can use two cans of the same kind if that's what you have in your pantry.

NOTE: This Mediterranean salad is great on its own as a side dish.

Pickled Onion Pesto Grilled Cheese

PREP TIME: ABOUT 5 MIN, PLUS 30 MIN FOR PICKLING	COOK TIME: 7 MIN	YIELD: 4 SERVINGS

INGREDIENTS

1 red onion, peeled, halved, and sliced thin

½ cup red wine vinegar

½ cup water

1 tablespoon cane sugar

1 teaspoon sea salt

8 slices whole-grain, sprouted-grain, or gluten-free bread

2 to 3 tablespoons vegan butter or vegan mayonnaise

Basil Spinach Pesto (see Chapter 15)

8 slices vegan cheese

DIRECTIONS

1 In a bowl or jar, place the onions, vinegar, water, sugar, and salt and stir well to combine. Press the onions down into the liquid to ensure they're fully submerged. Let sit until the onions are softened and bright pink, at least 30 minutes.

2 When the pickled onions are ready, spread 1 to 2 teaspoons of vegan butter or vegan mayonnaise on 1 side of each slice of bread.

3 Heat a large skillet over medium heat and place 1 slice of bread, buttered side down, in the skillet. Spread 1 to 2 tablespoons of pesto over the nonbuttered side, top with 1 slice of cheese, pickled red onions, another slice of cheese, and a second slice of bread, buttered side up.

4 Cook until the first side is golden brown and crispy on the outside, about 3 to 4 minutes. Carefully flip the sandwich over and cook until the second side is golden brown and the cheese is melty, about 2 to 3 minutes.

5 Repeat with the remaining sandwiches. You can cook 2 sandwiches at once if your skillet is large enough, but don't overcrowd the pan.

PER SERVING: *Calories 418 (From Fat 241); Fat 27g (Saturated 10g); Cholesterol 0mg; Sodium 809mg; Carbohydrate 43g (Dietary Fiber 5g); Protein 9g.*

TIP: If the sandwich is browning faster than the cheese is melting, decrease the heat to medium-low or low.

NOTE: Be sure to shake or blot off any excess liquid from the pickled red onions before adding them to your sandwich; otherwise, your sandwich may get soggy. But don't get rid of the liquid in the jar — that's how you'll store the onions in the fridge. Any leftover pickled onions will keep in an airtight jar in the fridge for about 2 weeks.

Sweet Potato Black Bean Quesadillas

PREP TIME: ABOUT 10 MIN | **COOK TIME: 12 MIN** | **YIELD: 4 SERVINGS**

INGREDIENTS

2 medium sweet potatoes

1 tablespoon olive oil

1 teaspoon chili powder

1 teaspoon cumin

One 15-ounce can black beans, drained and rinsed

One 4-ounce can diced green chilies

½ cup frozen or fresh corn kernels

Juice of 1 lime, divided

½ teaspoon sea salt, or to taste

2 tablespoons nutritional yeast, optional

Four 10-inch sprouted-grain tortillas

Salsa, for serving, if desired

Guacamole, for serving, if desired

DIRECTIONS

1 Scrub the sweet potatoes well and pierce several holes in the skin on all sides using a fork. Place the sweet potatoes on a microwave-safe plate and microwave on high for 5 minutes. When done, the sweet potatoes should be tender and easily pierced with a fork. If they aren't quite cooked through yet, microwave in 1-minute increments until tender. Carefully remove from the microwave and set aside to cool.

2 Meanwhile, in a large skillet, warm the oil over medium heat. Add the chili powder and cumin and stir the spices around in the oil until fragrant, about 1 to 2 minutes.

3 Add the black beans, green chilies, corn, the juice of ½ lime, and salt, and stir to combine. Cook 4 to 5 minutes to heat through. Transfer to a bowl and wipe out the skillet with a paper towel or clean dish cloth.

4 When the sweet potato is cool enough to handle, cut it in half and scoop the flesh into a small bowl. Mash the sweet potato flesh with a fork. Add the nutritional yeast, if using, and a squeeze of the remaining ½ lime.

5 Lay 1 tortilla flat and spread ¼ of the sweet potato mixture over half of the tortilla. Top the sweet potato with about ⅓ cup of the bean mixture. Fold the other half of the tortilla over the top. Repeat with the remaining tortillas.

6 Spritz the skillet with cooking spray and heat it over medium-high heat. Place 2 of the quesadillas in the skillet side by side and cook until lightly browned and crispy on the bottom, about 2 to 3 minutes. Carefully flip the quesadillas over and cook until browned and crispy on the second side, about 2 to 3 minutes. Transfer the quesadillas to a cutting board and cut in half. Repeat with the remaining 2 quesadillas.

7 Serve warm with salsa and guacamole for dipping, if desired.

PER SERVING: *Calories 370 (From Fat 43); Fat 5g (Saturated 1g); Cholesterol 0mg; Sodium 762mg; Carbohydrate 71g (Dietary Fiber 14g); Protein 14g.*

VARY IT! To save a few minutes, you can use canned 100 percent pure pumpkin instead of the sweet potato. You'll need about 1 cup.

Discovering the Joy of One-Pot Dishes

Soups and stews are the most common one-pot dishes everyone thinks of, but there are plenty more out there to try. Beans, grains, pastas, and stir-fries all can be made easily in one pot, and many of them come together in 30 minutes or less, making them perfect for an easy lunch.

Make your life easier by keeping your pantry stocked with quick-cooking ingredients, like jasmine rice or quick-cook brown rice, quinoa, BPA-free canned beans, red lentils, and whole-grain pasta.

MAXIMIZING YOUR LEFTOVERS

An easy way to enjoy lunch without doing any extra work during the day is to make more dinner than you need the night before. Pack up the leftovers, and they're ready to go for the next day's lunch! This method may require some planning so you can get more ingredients. Items such as pasta, quinoa salads, and noodle dishes keep well in a glass container overnight for lunch the next day.

Another way to maximize your leftovers is to have one meal item that can be used in different ways. For instance, if you make a bean dip, veggie patty, or guacamole, you can find different ways to enjoy them — in a wrap, on a salad, on top of whole grains, or in pasta. You'll find many ways to use the same ingredient more than once while still getting variety.

One-Pot Hummus Pasta

PREP TIME: ABOUT 10 MIN | **COOK TIME: 10 MIN** | **YIELD: 6 SERVINGS**

INGREDIENTS

16 ounces whole-grain penne pasta or other medium shaped pasta

½ to 1 cup pasta cooking water

1 cup Creamy Oil-Free Hummus (see Chapter 14) or your favorite savory hummus variety

1 pint (2 cups) grape tomatoes, halved

2 cups fresh spinach leaves, chopped

Juice of 1 lemon

½ teaspoon kosher salt, or to taste

¼ teaspoon freshly ground black pepper, or to taste

DIRECTIONS

1 In a large pot on the stove, cook the pasta according to package directions in well-salted water. Before draining, reserve 1 cup of the pasta cooking water and set aside.

2 Transfer the cooked noodles back to the pot. Add the hummus, tomatoes, spinach, lemon juice, salt, and pepper. Stir to combine.

3 Add ½ cup of the reserved pasta cooking water and stir well until the sauce is creamy and smooth. Add more pasta cooking water, if needed, to reach the desired consistency.

4 Taste and adjust the seasoning, as needed. Add more salt, pepper, lemon juice, or even more hummus, as desired.

PER SERVING: *Calories 364 (From Fat 43); Fat 5g (Saturated 1g); Cholesterol 0mg; Sodium 308mg; Carbohydrate 67g (Dietary Fiber 5g); Protein 13g.*

TIP: This recipe is easily made gluten free by choosing gluten-free pasta noodles.

NOTE: If you forget to reserve the pasta water, you can use vegetable broth, unsweetened almond milk, or even just plain water. Start with ¼ cup because these options are thinner and not as viscous as pasta cooking water. Add more as needed. Be sure to taste and adjust the seasonings as necessary before serving.

Quinoa and Chickpeas with Spinach

PREP TIME: ABOUT 15 MIN	COOK TIME: 25 MIN	YIELD: 6 SERVINGS

INGREDIENTS

1 tablespoon extra-virgin olive oil

1 medium onion, chopped

3 cloves garlic, minced

1 cup water

¾ cup freshly squeezed orange juice

½ teaspoon sea salt

Zest from 1 orange, approximately ½ tablespoon

1 cup quinoa, rinsed and drained

½ cup raisins

1 cup cooked chickpeas or canned chickpeas

1 to 2 cups spinach leaves, trimmed, washed, drained, and dried

Sea salt to taste

½ teaspoon ground cinnamon

¼ cup toasted pine nuts or almonds

1 orange, cut into wedges

DIRECTIONS

1 In a large pot, warm the oil over medium heat. Add the onion and sauté until it has softened and begun to brown, about 5 minutes. Add the garlic and sauté until golden, about 1 to 2 minutes.

2 Add the water and orange juice and bring to a boil. Add the salt, orange zest, and quinoa and return to a boil. Reduce the heat, cover, and simmer for 12 minutes, or until all the liquid is absorbed.

3 Remove the quinoa from the heat, keep it covered, and let sit for 3 minutes.

4 Add the raisins, chickpeas, and spinach and stir to combine. Cover and let sit just until the spinach has wilted a bit, about 3 to 4 minutes.

5 Stir in the cinnamon and another squeeze of fresh orange juice. Garnish with toasted pine nuts or almonds and orange wedges.

PER SERVING: *Calories 198 (From Fat 63); Fat 7g (Saturated 0.5g); Cholesterol 0mg; Sodium 173mg; Carbohydrate 31g (Dietary Fiber 4g); Protein 6g.*

Chapter **12**

Super Suppers

We know, dinner can seem daunting. It's the pinnacle of the day's meals. It's what everyone looks forward to after a hard day of work or school. It's the heartiest and most filling of all meals. But don't panic! Supper in the plant-based world is manageable (and fun!) because you have so many different ways to prepare the same food. It's all about simple creativity!

If you're just starting out on a plant-based diet or you simply don't have time to spend all day cooking dinner, consider cooking more food than you need for one meal and then building your next dinner around the leftovers. The good news is that most plant-based foods last longer in the fridge than meat does because they don't have the same bacteria issues. Plus, some items can even be frozen. That way, on busy weeknights, you can just pull out a soup or stew from the freezer, make a fresh salad, or steam greens or grains as an easy side component, and — voilà! — a full, super supper is served!

WARNING

Don't leave items in the freezer too long — they'll not only lose their nutrients but also get freezer burn and have to be thrown out. On average, consider a freezer time of no more than three months.

Rethinking What Your Dinner Plate Should Look Like

When it comes to dinnertime — whether you're cooking for one, three, or five — it's important to think about versatility and variety. Make sure that everyone in the family is satisfied. A typical plate that many people are accustomed to is broken up in three ways: a piece of meat, some kind of starch (typically, white potatoes or rice), and an overcooked veggie. This "pie plate" concept goes out the window on a plant-based diet. Instead, think of your plate or bowl as having so much variety, texture, and color that exact portions or amounts don't really matter.

When thinking of dinner from now on, don't think of foods as their own sections of the plate; they may be layered together in a pot or casserole dish instead. Or maybe you have just two things on your plate, such as a quinoa salad and a homemade veggie burger, which can be combined and eaten together. Or a plate may be made up of mostly carbohydrates that together make a perfect plant protein. Also, many lunch items can be served for dinner, and vice versa.

In time, you'll discover so much more variety when you make the switch to plants. Your dinners become colorful and dazzling sensations that you'll love.

TIP

If you have kids or (ahem) picky adults in the family, try these tips for keeping their minds and tummies happy:

>> Get them involved in the process to add their own flair to pasta or pick what veggies go into the stir-fry.

>> Let them help with age-appropriate prep work.

>> Always have their favorite veggies and grains available at dinner — either as a stand-alone dish or as an ingredient in new dishes to encourage them to try new things.

>> Introduce new items slowly. Don't unleash a seven-course meal of dishes they've never had. Make sure a new addition is just one part of a dinner that's full of familiar foods.

Black Bean Cumin Burgers

PREP TIME: ABOUT 15 MIN	COOK TIME: 40 MIN	YIELD: 8 TO 12 SERVINGS

INGREDIENTS

1 cup dried black beans, soaked overnight and rinsed, or 2 cans black beans, drained and rinsed

1 cup grated sweet potatoes

½ cup almond butter

½ cup diced red onion

¼ cup brown-rice flour

2 tablespoons tamari

3 cloves garlic, minced

1 tablespoon cumin

DIRECTIONS

1 Preheat the oven to 350 degrees and line a baking sheet with parchment paper.

2 Place the soaked beans in a pot with water (cover the beans by 1 to 2 inches). Bring the water and beans to a boil. Lower the heat and simmer for 1½ hours. Remove from the heat and drain.

3 Place the beans in a bowl and mash. Stir in the remaining ingredients.

4 Scoop ⅓ cup of the batter to form a burger patty and place on the baking sheet. Continue until all the batter is used.

5 Bake until golden brown, about 30 minutes. Serve.

PER SERVING: *Calories 217 (From Fat 81); Fat 9g (Saturated 1g); Cholesterol 0mg; Sodium 405mg; Carbohydrate 26g (Dietary Fiber 7g); Protein 9g.*

TIP: Enjoy this burger on a sprouted-grain bun or wrap, with brown rice or quinoa, or on a salad for a complete dinner. You may want to add some salsa or avocado for a tasty topping.

VARY IT! For a nut-free option, use sunflower-seed butter instead of almond butter.

Vegan Burgers with Apricot Jalapeño Jam

PREP TIME: ABOUT 5 MIN | COOK TIME: 15 MIN | YIELD: 4 SERVINGS

INGREDIENTS

4 vegan burgers

1 cup arugula

4 burger buns

Apricot Jalapeño Jam (see the following recipe)

Drizzle of Smoky Barbecue Sauce (see Chapter 15) or your favorite store-bought brand

¼ cup thinly sliced red onion

DIRECTIONS

1 Cook the burgers according to package directions.

2 Place a small handful of arugula on a bottom bun, top with 1 burger, a dollop or two of jam, a drizzle of barbecue sauce, and a few onion slices. Finish with the top bun. Repeat for the remaining burgers. Serve.

Apricot Jalapeño Jam

¾ cup dried apricots

3 to 4 jalapeño peppers, ribs and seeds removed if you like a milder heat, diced

1 teaspoon fresh lemon juice

2 tablespoons cane sugar, or to taste

2 tablespoons white vinegar

¾ to 1 cup water, divided

1 In a small pot, place all the ingredients (start with ¾ cup water). Bring to a boil. Decrease the heat to medium–low and simmer for 15 minutes.

2 Using an immersion blender, or transferring to a blender, blend the mixture until pureed. Add the remaining ¼ cup water, if needed, to thin. A few chunks in the jam is fine — it doesn't need to be perfectly smooth.

PER SERVING: *Calories 246 (From Fat 32); Fat 3g (Saturated 1g); Cholesterol 0mg; Sodium 430mg; Carbohydrate 45g (Dietary Fiber 7g); Protein 13g.*

NOTE: The recipe for Apricot Jalapeño Jam makes about 1 cup. You likely won't use it all for 4 burgers. Store leftovers in an airtight container in the fridge for 4 to 5 days.

Mushroom and Chickpea Loaf

PREP TIME: ABOUT 20 MIN	COOK TIME: 55 MIN	YIELD: 6–8 SERVINGS

INGREDIENTS

2 tablespoons grapeseed oil

2 teaspoons minced garlic

1 cup chopped onions

2 medium carrots, chopped

½ cup chopped zucchini

1 cup chopped mushrooms

1½ cups chickpeas (soaked overnight and cooked), or one 14-ounce can chickpeas

1½ cups cooked white beans

⅓ cup dried wheat-free bread crumbs

¼ cup tomato sauce

2 tablespoons nutritional yeast

1 tablespoon arrowroot powder

1 tablespoon Dijon mustard

½ cup whole rolled oats

¼ teaspoon ground pepper

1 teaspoon dried basil

¼ teaspoon cumin

1 teaspoon oregano

1 tablespoon tamari

DIRECTIONS

1 Preheat the oven to 350 degrees.

2 In a large sauté pan, warm the oil over medium-high heat.

3 Add the garlic, onions, and carrots and cook until the onions are soft and translucent, about 4 to 5 minutes.

4 Stir in the zucchini and mushrooms and sauté until softened, about 8 minutes.

5 In a food processor, combine the zucchini mixture and the remaining ingredients. Pulse on and off until the mixture is finely chopped and well combined. Press into a loaf pan greased with grapeseed oil.

6 Bake uncovered for 40 minutes.

7 Allow the loaf to set for approximately 20 minutes to cool. Remove from the pan and slice into 8 to 10 slices.

8 Serve with the Hearty Vegetable Cacciatore (see the recipe in this chapter), Tahini Miso Gravy (see Chapter 15), or extra tomato sauce.

PER SERVING: *Calories 174 (From Fat 54); Fat 6g (Saturated 0.5g); Cholesterol 0mg; Sodium 414mg; Carbohydrate 25g (Dietary Fiber 6g); Protein 7g.*

NOTE: Dried chickpeas need to cook for 1½ to 2 hours, and dried white beans need to cook for 45 to 60 minutes.

Hearty Vegetable Cacciatore

PREP TIME: ABOUT 15 MIN	COOK TIME: 30 MIN	YIELD: 6 SERVINGS

INGREDIENTS

2 tablespoons olive oil

2 cloves garlic, minced

1 cup diced leeks or diced onions

1 cup diced carrots

1 cup diced celery

3 cups sliced mushrooms

½ cup finely chopped fresh basil or 1 teaspoon dried basil

2 tablespoons fresh oregano or 1 teaspoon dried oregano

3 bay leaves

2 cups tomato sauce

1 teaspoon sea salt

½ cup finely chopped parsley

1 to 2 cups cubed firm tofu

DIRECTIONS

1 In a large saucepan, warm the oil over medium heat. Add the garlic and leeks or onions and cook until soft, about 5 minutes.

2 Add the remaining ingredients and cook until the moisture has evaporated and the dish is reduced and thickened, about 15 to 30 minutes. Remove the bay leaves.

3 Serve with whole-grain or gluten-free pasta, brown rice, or quinoa, or enjoy on its own.

PER SERVING: *Calories 147 (From Fat 72); Fat 8g (Saturated 1.5g); Cholesterol 0mg; Sodium 858mg; Carbohydrate 12g (Dietary Fiber 4g); Protein 9g.*

VARY IT! Instead of tofu, opt for white beans, chickpeas, or fava beans for a hearty vegetarian source of protein. Or use this as a sauce to top the Mushroom and Chickpea Loaf (see the recipe in this chapter).

COOKING WITH OILS: WHAT TO USE AND WHEN

The world of oil is a mysterious, liquidy place. Understanding it isn't as hard as it seems, though, and understanding which ones should be used greatly enhances recipes and cooking techniques. Here's a quick rundown of which oils to use in which circumstances:

- On low to medium heat, try olive (regular, not extra-virgin), safflower oil, sesame oil, or sunflower oil.

- If a recipe calls for high heat, go with coconut oil or grapeseed oil.

- When no heat is required (as in raw recipes), extra-virgin olive oil, flaxseed oil, chia seed oil, or hempseed oil is the best. ***Note:*** These oils should *never* be used with heat.

When certain oils are heated beyond their smoke point (which means they start smoking in the pan), they're no longer stable and they become toxic to the body. Be mindful of which oil you're using at which temperature.

Want to skip the oils altogether? In most cases, you can sauté or roast with vegetable broth or water instead.

Sweet Potato Shepherd's Pie

PREP TIME: ABOUT 30 MIN	COOK TIME: 45 MIN	YIELD: 10 SERVINGS

INGREDIENTS

Grapeseed oil, for greasing baking dishes

2¼ cups water, divided

2 teaspoons olive oil

1 clove garlic, peeled and crushed

1 onion, peeled and sliced

1 teaspoon sea salt

2 ribs celery, washed and chopped

1 bay leaf

1 to 2 cups butternut squash, peeled, halved, deseeded, and cut into small pieces

2 cups cooked kidney beans or 1 can or kidney beans

½ head cauliflower, cut into slices of chopped

2 medium zucchini, sliced

½ head broccoli, finely chopped

3 medium carrots, sliced

2 tablespoons finely chopped fresh parsley

1 teaspoon arrowroot

4 sweet potatoes, steamed for 15 minutes until soft, and mashed (reserve a small amount of cooking water)

Dash of tamari

DIRECTIONS

1 Preheat the oven to 350 degrees. Grease 1 large baking dish or 2 small baking dishes with grapeseed oil.

2 In a large saucepan, heat ¼ cup of the water and the olive oil. Add the garlic, onion, salt, celery, and bay leaf and simmer for 3 minutes.

3 Add the squash and heat for another 3 minutes, stirring. Pour in the remaining 2 cups of water and bring to a boil over medium heat. Simmer gently for 10 minutes, stirring occasionally.

4 Add the kidney beans, cauliflower, zucchini, broccoli, and carrots. Simmer until the squash is just tender, about 5 minutes. Stir in the parsley and arrowroot.

5 Transfer to 1 large baking dish or 2 small baking dishes.

6 In a small bowl, mix the sweet potato mash with a little of the steamed cooking water. Add the tamari.

7 Using a fork or the back of a spoon, spread the sweet potato mixture over the vegetable mixture. Bake until the pie is set, about for 15 to 20 minutes.

8 To serve, scoop out a large square of the pie and serve with a side of cooked millet, brown rice, or quinoa and some steamed leafy green vegetables like kale.

PER SERVING: *Calories 152 (From Fat 12); Fat 1.5g (Saturated 0g); Cholesterol 0mg; Sodium 238mg; Carbohydrate 31g (Dietary Fiber 7g); Protein 6g.*

TIP: To give this dish more flavor, add a few spoonsful of Tahini Miso Gravy (see Chapter 15).

Tangy Tempeh Teriyaki Stir-Fry

PREP TIME: ABOUT 15 MIN	COOK TIME: 15 MIN	YIELD: 8 SERVINGS

INGREDIENTS

2 tablespoons toasted sesame oil

¼ cup tamari

1 to 2 cloves garlic, minced

1 tablespoon minced ginger

Juice of 1 orange

1 to 2 tablespoons brown-rice vinegar

1 tablespoon brown-rice syrup

One 10.5-ounce package of tempeh or tofu, cut into small cubes

1 onion, chopped

1 cup chopped carrots

1 cup chopped celery

1 head (about 2 cups) broccoli or cauliflower, cut into florets

1 head (about 2 cups) bok choy, chopped

¼ cup sesame seeds

DIRECTIONS

1 In a bowl, make the marinade by combining the sesame oil, tamari, garlic, ginger, orange juice, vinegar, and brown-rice syrup; set aside.

2 In a medium saucepan or wok, combine the tempeh or tofu with ¾ of the marinade. Add the onions, carrots, and celery. Cover and simmer over medium heat for 5 to 10 minutes.

3 Place the broccoli or cauliflower in the saucepan or wok and cook until just tender.

4 Combine the bok choy with the tempeh or tofu and stir with the remaining marinade until the bok choy softens a bit.

5 Make sure everything is well coated. Top with sesame seeds and serve with brown rice, soba noodles, or quinoa.

PER SERVING: Calories 129 (From Fat 63); Fat 7g (Saturated 1g); Cholesterol 0mg; Sodium 551mg; Carbohydrate 11g (Dietary Fiber 3g); Protein 6g.

TIP: For extra flavor, marinate the tempeh or tofu cubes in half of the marinade for up to 1 hour before making this dish to allow the flavors to absorb.

NOTE: Be sure not to overcook your green veggies — you want them to remain green. The goal is to keep them crisp and tender. Add them at the end and let them cook down with the warmth of the stir-fry.

VARY IT! Try this stir-fry with different veggies that are in season. Peppers, asparagus, and Japanese eggplant can all be swapped in to make different variations.

Eggplant Green Curry with Tofu

PREP TIME: ABOUT 10 MIN	COOK TIME: 32 MIN	YIELD: 6 SERVINGS

INGREDIENTS

2 tablespoons tamari

One 14.5-ounce block extra-firm tofu, drained and cut into 1-inch cubes

½ teaspoon sea salt

¼ teaspoon freshly ground black pepper

2 tablespoons grapeseed oil, divided

1 medium eggplant, cut into cubes

½ yellow onion, diced

3 cloves garlic, minced

3 to 4 tablespoons green curry paste

One 13.5-ounce can full-fat coconut milk

1 red bell pepper, sliced into thin strips

4 to 5 Thai basil leaves or regular basil leaves

Squeeze of fresh lime juice

3 cups cooked rice, for serving

DIRECTIONS

1 Heat a large nonstick skillet over medium–high heat. Add the tamari and tofu in 1 even layer. Cook for 8 to 10 minutes, stirring occasionally, until all sides are browned. Sprinkle with the salt and pepper, transfer to a bowl or plate, and set aside.

2 In the same skillet, heat 1 tablespoon of the oil over medium–high heat. Add the eggplant and sauté until seared on all sides, about 4 to 5 minutes. Transfer to the same bowl or plate with the tofu.

3 In the same skillet, heat the remaining 1 tablespoon of oil over medium heat. Add the onion and sauté until soft and translucent, about 4 to 5 minutes.

4 Add the garlic and green curry paste and sauté until fragrant, about 1 to 2 minutes. Add the coconut milk and whisk to combine until the curry paste is completely mixed in and smooth.

5 Add the red bell pepper and simmer until hot and bubbly, about 10 minutes.

6 Add the basil leaves and lime juice. Add the tofu and eggplant back to the skillet and stir to combine.

7 Serve hot over the cooked rice.

PER SERVING: *Calories 396 (From Fat 203); Fat 23g (Saturated 13g); Cholesterol 0mg; Sodium 685mg; Carbohydrate 40g (Dietary Fiber 4g); Protein 12g.*

NOTE: Different brands of curry paste have varying levels of spicy heat. We like Thai Kitchen Green Curry Paste, which is fairly mild. If yours is spicier, you may want to start with just 2 tablespoons and add more as needed.

TIP: The skin of eggplant is edible. You can peel it if you like, but it's really just personal preference. We usually leave it on.

Zesty Pesto Pasta with White Beans

PREP TIME: ABOUT 5 MIN	COOK TIME: 20 MIN	YIELD: 6 SERVINGS

INGREDIENTS

1 tablespoon sea salt

One 16-ounce package whole-grain or gluten-free pasta

Pesto Sauce (see the following recipe)

1 cup cooked white beans

2 cups spinach or Swiss chard

DIRECTIONS

1 Boil a large pot of water, add sea salt, and cook the pasta until al dente or tender, about 7 to 10 minutes. Drain, but keep the pasta in the pot.

2 On low to medium heat, add the Pesto Sauce, beans, and spinach or Swiss chard to the cooked pasta. Stir until well combined and the spinach has wilted.

3 Place a few ladles of the pasta into a bowl and serve alongside a salad or a bowl of minestrone soup.

Pesto Sauce

¼ cup pine nuts or walnuts, toasted

2 cups fresh basil

¼ cup olive oil

1 to 2 cloves garlic

2 tablespoons fresh lemon juice

1 teaspoon white miso

Salt to taste

Freshly ground black pepper to taste

1 Grind the nuts in a food processor until you get a paste.

2 Add the remaining ingredients and process for a few minutes until well combined.

PER SERVING: *Calories 279 (From Fat 90); Fat 10g (Saturated 1g); Cholesterol 0mg; Sodium 28mg; Carbohydrate 40g (Dietary Fiber 6g); Protein 8g.*

NOTE: Gluten-free pasta, like brown-rice pasta, often takes about 15 minutes to cook.

Chickpea Walnut Bolognese

INGREDIENTS

16 ounces medium shaped pasta, like penne, rotini, or farfalle

1 cup raw shelled walnuts

One 15-ounce can chickpeas, drained and rinsed

1 tablespoon olive oil

1 yellow onion, diced

2 cloves garlic, minced

2 tablespoons tomato paste

1 tablespoon tamari or coconut aminos

1 tablespoon balsamic vinegar

2 teaspoon dried oregano

2 teaspoons dried basil

One 28-ounce can crushed tomatoes

1½ cups low-sodium vegetable broth

1½ teaspoons sea salt

½ teaspoon freshly ground black pepper

¼ to ½ teaspoon crushed red pepper flakes (optional)

DIRECTIONS

1 Fill a large pot with water, salt well, add the pasta, and cook according to package directions until al dente.

2 Meanwhile, add the walnuts to the bowl of a food processor and pulse several times to chop into small pieces. Add the chickpeas and pulse a few more times to break them up. Don't overprocess them — you want the mixture chunky like the texture of ground meat. Set aside.

3 In a large, deep skillet, warm the oil over medium heat. Add the onion and sauté until soft and translucent, about 5 to 6 minutes.

4 Add the garlic, tomato paste, tamari or coconut aminos, vinegar, oregano, and basil. Stir to combine until the tomato paste is fully incorporated.

5 Add the tomatoes, broth, salt, pepper, and red pepper flakes, if using. Stir to combine and simmer 15 to 20 minutes.

6 Serve the sauce over the pasta.

PER SERVING: *Calories 513 (From Fat 138); Fat 15g (Saturated 2g); Cholesterol 0mg; Sodium 893mg; Carbohydrate 79g (Dietary Fiber 7g); Protein 18g.*

TIP: Sprinkle individual servings with nutritional yeast for an extra protein boost and a cheesy-like topping.

Autumn Risotto

PREP TIME: ABOUT 15 MIN	COOK TIME: 40 MIN	YIELD: 6 SERVINGS

INGREDIENTS

1 small butternut squash, peeled and cubed (about 4 cups)

3 tablespoons olive oil, divided

1 teaspoon dried thyme

1 teaspoon dried sage

4 to 6 cups low-sodium vegetable broth

1 yellow onion, diced

1½ cups Arborio rice

½ cup dry white wine

¼ cup nutritional yeast

Sea salt to taste

Freshly ground black pepper to taste

¼ cup shelled pumpkin seeds, for garnish

Sprinkle of fresh thyme, for garnish (optional)

¼ cup vegan Parmesan cheese, for garnish (optional)

DIRECTIONS

1 Preheat the oven to 400 degrees. Line a rimmed baking sheet with parchment paper and set aside.

2 Toss the butternut squash with 1 tablespoon of the oil and the thyme and sage. Spread into one even layer on the prepared baking sheet and roast until tender, about 25 to 35 minutes, stirring once halfway through cooking.

3 Meanwhile, in a pot, bring the broth to a simmer and keep warm.

4 In a large, deep skillet, warm the remaining 2 tablespoons of oil over medium heat. Add the onion and sauté until soft and translucent, about 5 to 6 minutes.

5 Add the rice and stir to combine. Cook for 2 to 3 minutes to toast the rice, stirring occasionally.

6 Add the wine and stir until absorbed, about 4 to 5 minutes.

7 Add ½ cup of warm broth and stir until absorbed. Continue adding broth ½ to 1 cup at a time until it's absorbed, stirring constantly, until the rice is creamy and tender yet still al dente. This whole process could take anywhere from 20 to 30 minutes. You may not use the full 6 cups of broth, but it's better to have too much than too little. Any leftover broth can be stored in an airtight container in the fridge.

8 When the rice is tender, add the nutritional yeast and stir to combine. Taste and add salt and pepper, as needed. Stir in the roasted butternut squash.

9 Garnish with pumpkin seeds, fresh thyme (if using), and vegan Parmesan cheese (if using).

PER SERVING: *Calories 385 (From Fat 96); Fat 11g (Saturated 2g); Cholesterol 0mg; Sodium 65mg; Carbohydrate 60g (Dietary Fiber 5g); Protein 11g.*

Cheesy Chili Mac

PREP TIME: ABOUT 15 MIN | **COOK TIME: 30 MIN** | **YIELD: 6 SERVINGS**

INGREDIENTS

16 ounces macaroni noodles

1 tablespoon olive oil

1 yellow onion, diced

1 green bell pepper, seeded and diced

1 jalapeño pepper, ribs and seeds removed, diced

1 teaspoon chili powder

1 teaspoon cumin

½ teaspoon dried oregano

Pinch of cayenne (optional)

One 28-ounce can diced tomatoes

One 15-ounce can red kidney beans, rinsed and drained

¼ cup raw unsalted cashews, soaked in hot water for 15 to 20 minutes

1 roasted red pepper from a jar

½ cup nutritional yeast, or more to taste

1 tablespoon mellow white miso paste

1 teaspoon onion powder

½ teaspoon garlic powder

¼ to ½ cup water, to thin

Salt to taste

Freshly ground black pepper to taste

Diced avocado, for topping (optional)

Chopped cilantro, for topping (optional)

Squeeze of fresh lime juice, for topping (optional)

DIRECTIONS

1 Fill a large pot with water, salt well, add the macaroni, and cook according to package directions until al dente, about 8 to 10 minutes.

2 Meanwhile, in a large skillet, warm the oil over medium heat. Add the onion and sauté until soft and translucent, about 5 to 6 minutes.

3 Add the bell pepper, jalapeño pepper, chili powder, cumin, oregano, and cayenne, if using. Stir until fragrant, about 1 to 2 minutes.

4 Add the tomatoes and kidney beans. Reduce the heat to medium–low, cover, and simmer for 15 minutes.

5 While the tomato sauce is simmering, add the cashews, red pepper, nutritional yeast, miso paste, onion powder, garlic powder, and water to a high-speed blender and blend until completely smooth.

6 Add the cooked noodles to the tomato sauce. Pour in the cheese sauce and stir to combine.

7 Taste and salt and pepper, as necessary. Top with avocado, cilantro, and/or lime juice (if desired) before serving.

PER SERVING: *Calories 499 (From Fat 88); Fat 10g (Saturated 2g); Cholesterol 0mg; Sodium 729mg; Carbohydrate 85g (Dietary Fiber 9g); Protein 20g.*

VARY IT! Use black beans instead of kidney beans if you prefer. Add 1 cup of corn kernels or diced zucchini for more veggies.

Spinach Artichoke Pasta Bake

PREP TIME: ABOUT 10 MIN	COOK TIME: 29 MIN	YIELD: 6 SERVINGS

INGREDIENTS

16 ounces medium-shaped pasta, like rotini, penne, or medium shells

1 cup raw cashews, soaked for 20 minutes in hot water

⅓ cup nutritional yeast

2 tablespoons tamari

1 tablespoon fresh lemon juice

1½ cups unsweetened, plain nondairy milk, like almond milk, oat milk, or soy milk

1½ teaspoons sea salt

¼ teaspoon freshly ground black pepper

2 tablespoons olive oil

1 yellow onion, diced

3 cloves garlic, minced

2 tablespoons all-purpose flour

One 14.5-ounce can artichoke hearts, chopped

5 ounces baby spinach, chopped

¼ cup fresh parsley, chopped

1 cup panko breadcrumbs

2 tablespoons melted vegan butter or olive oil

DIRECTIONS

1 Preheat the oven to 350 degrees.

2 Fill a large pot with water, salt well, add the pasta, and cook according to package directions until al dente.

3 Meanwhile, in a high-speed blender, add the cashews, nutritional yeast, tamari, lemon juice, milk, salt, and pepper. Blend until smooth. Set aside.

4 In a large skillet, warm the oil over medium heat. Add the onion and sauté until soft and translucent, about 5 to 6 minutes. Add the garlic and flour and whisk until no white flour remains.

5 Add the artichokes and spinach and stir to combine.

6 Pour in the cashew sauce from Step 3 and cook to heat through, about 2 to 3 minutes.

7 Add the cooked pasta and fresh parsley and stir to combine. Pour into a 7-x-11 baking dish or similar.

8 In a small bowl, combine the breadcrumbs with the butter or oil and mix until well moistened. Sprinkle evenly over the top of the pasta.

9 Bake until bubbly and heated through, about 15 to 20 minutes. Serve.

PER SERVING: *Calories 680 (From Fat 210); Fat 23g (Saturated 4g); Cholesterol 0mg; Sodium 987mg; Carbohydrate 96g (Dietary Fiber 10g); Protein 24g.*

VARY IT! This creamy dish is delicious straight from the stove top if you don't feel like baking it. Just skip the breadcrumb topping.

Vegan Sloppy Joes

INGREDIENTS

16 ounces vegan ground beef

2 tablespoons olive oil

½ yellow onion, peeled and diced

1 green bell pepper, seeded and diced

2 small carrots, finely diced or shredded

2 cloves garlic, minced

One 15-ounce can tomato sauce

¼ cup ketchup

¼ cup brown sugar

2 tablespoons vegan Worcestershire sauce

1 to 2 teaspoons liquid smoke

1 teaspoon yellow mustard

1 teaspoon dried oregano

½ teaspoon salt, or to taste

¼ teaspoon freshly ground black pepper, or to taste

6 burger buns

Pickles, for topping (optional)

Tomato slices, for topping (optional)

Avocado, for topping (optional)

Red onion slices, for topping (optional)

DIRECTIONS

1 Heat a large nonstick skillet over medium–high heat. Add the vegan ground beef and sauté until hot and cooked through, about 5 to 7 minutes, breaking it up with the back of a wooden spoon and stirring frequently. Transfer to a bowl or plate and set aside.

2 In the same skillet, heat the oil over medium heat. Add the onion, green bell pepper, and carrots and sauté until the onion is soft and translucent, about 5 to 6 minutes. Add the garlic and sauté 1 minute.

3 Add the tomato sauce, ketchup, brown sugar, Worcestershire sauce, liquid smoke, mustard, and oregano. Bring the mixture to a boil, decrease the heat to low, and simmer uncovered for 20 minutes, until thick and bubbly.

4 Add the cooked vegan ground beef and stir until evenly coated. Simmer until heated through, about 5 to 10 minutes.

5 Serve on buns with pickles, tomato, avocado, and/or onion, if desired.

PER SERVING: *Calories 362 (From Fat 108); Fat 12g (Saturated 2g); Cholesterol 0mg; Sodium 996mg; Carbohydrate 49g (Dietary Fiber 7g); Protein 17g.*

NOTE: If you can't find vegan Worcestershire sauce, use equal amounts of balsamic vinegar and molasses (regular, not blackstrap) for a similar flavor profile.

TIP: Toast the buns before serving for a nice texture contrast.

VARY IT! You can use 2½ cups of cooked lentils in place of the vegan ground beef, if you prefer.

Black Bean Quinoa Chili

PREP TIME: ABOUT 10 MIN | **COOK TIME: 23 MIN** | **YIELD: 6 SERVINGS**

INGREDIENTS

2 tablespoons olive oil

1 yellow onion, diced

1 green bell pepper, seeded and diced

2 carrots, peeled and shredded

2 tablespoons unsweetened cocoa powder

1 tablespoon chili powder

2 teaspoons cumin

1 teaspoon smoked paprika

1 teaspoon dried oregano

1 teaspoon allspice

1 teaspoon sea salt, or to taste

1 teaspoon liquid smoke (optional)

Three 15-ounce cans black beans, drained and rinsed

One 28-ounce can diced tomatoes

1 cup dry white quinoa

2 cups low-sodium vegetable broth

1 cup fresh or frozen corn kernels

Squeeze of fresh lime, for topping (optional)

Avocado or guacamole, for topping (optional)

Vegan sour cream, for topping (optional)

Hot sauce, for topping (optional)

Chopped fresh cilantro, for topping (optional)

Sliced green onions, for topping (optional)

Crushed tortilla chips, for topping (optional)

DIRECTIONS

1 In a soup pot, warm the oil over medium heat. Add the yellow onion and sauté until soft and translucent, about 5 to 6 minutes. Add the green bell pepper, carrots, cocoa powder, chili powder, cumin, paprika, oregano, allspice, salt, and liquid smoke, if using. Mix well and sauté until the spices are fragrant, 1 to 2 minutes.

2 Add the black beans, tomatoes, quinoa, and broth and stir. Be sure the liquid is completely covering the quinoa; add a bit more broth or water, if needed. Increase the heat to bring to a boil, cover, reduce the heat to medium-low, and simmer until the quinoa is tender, about 15 to 20 minutes.

3 Add the corn and mix well. Taste and adjust the seasonings as necessary.

4 Serve with lime juice, avocado or guacamole, sour cream, hot sauce, cilantro, green onions, and tortilla chips, if you like.

PER SERVING: *Calories 310 (From Fat 57); Fat 6g (Saturated 1g); Cholesterol 0mg; Sodium 753mg; Carbohydrate 50g (Dietary Fiber 16g); Protein 17g.*

TIP: Be sure to use *unsweetened* cocoa powder. If you prefer, you can use a shot of espresso, 1 cup of strong black coffee, or 2 squares of dairy-free dark chocolate instead. If you're using squares of dark chocolate, add it when you add the tomatoes and broth and let it melt slowly. Don't use milk chocolate or any other sweet chocolate.

NOTE: This chili recipe will thicken up considerably as the quinoa cooks. If you find it a bit too thick for your liking, add an extra cup or so of broth or water and stir well to incorporate.

Vegan Sausage and Roasted Vegetables Sheet-Pan Meal

PREP TIME: ABOUT 15 MIN	COOK TIME: 30 MIN	YIELD: 6 SERVINGS

INGREDIENTS

2 sweet potatoes, peeled and chopped into 1-inch cubes

1 pound Brussels sprouts, trimmed and halved

2 bell peppers, any color, seeded and sliced

1 to 2 red onions, halved and sliced

1 tablespoon olive oil

1 tablespoon dried oregano

1 teaspoon garlic powder

½ teaspoon sea salt

¼ teaspoon freshly ground black pepper

4 vegan sausages (large, thick links, not breakfast-style), sliced

½ cup tahini

3 to 4 tablespoons hot sauce, or to taste

2 tablespoons pure maple syrup

2 tablespoons tamari or coconut aminos

¼ cup water, to thin, or more as needed

1 bunch kale, tough stems and ribs removed, chopped

DIRECTIONS

1 Preheat the oven to 400 degrees. Line 2 rimmed baking sheets with parchment paper and set aside.

2 In a large bowl, toss the sweet potatoes, Brussels sprouts, peppers, and onions with the olive oil, oregano, garlic powder, salt, and pepper. Spread out into 1 even layer on the prepared baking sheets. Roast for 15 minutes.

3 Add the sausages to the pans, again spreading out into 1 even layer. Roast until the vegetables are tender and the sausage is browned, about 10 to 15 minutes.

4 Meanwhile, in a small bowl or jar, add the tahini, hot sauce, maple syrup, tamari or coconut aminos, and water. Whisk together until completely smooth.

5 Add the chopped kale to a bowl and drizzle with 1 tablespoon of the sauce. Using clean hands, massage the kale with the sauce for 1 or 2 minutes to soften.

6 To serve, add a serving of kale to each plate, top with a serving of roasted sausages and vegetables. Drizzle with more sauce, as desired.

PER SERVING: *Calories 418 (From Fat 222); Fat 25g (Saturated 4g); Cholesterol 0mg; Sodium 1,031mg; Carbohydrate 37g (Dietary Fiber 9g); Protein 20g.*

NOTE: The sauce recipe makes about 1¼ cups, which is about 2 to 3 tablespoons per serving. If you have leftovers, serve it with tofu or tempeh, over baked potatoes, on grain bowls, or drizzled over tacos.

TIP: Serve up a side of brown rice or quinoa if you want to stretch this meal even further.

NOTE: If you don't want to use store-bought vegan sausages, feel free to toss the roasted vegetables with some cooked beans or lentils or baked tempeh or tofu instead.

VARY IT! Don't like the tahini sauce in this recipe? Try this dish with Basil Spinach Pesto, Smoky Barbecue Sauce, or Tahini Miso Gravy instead. The recipes for all three are in Chapter 15.

Red Lentil White Bean Stew

PREP TIME: ABOUT 10 MIN | **COOK TIME: 27 MIN** | **YIELD: 6 SERVINGS**

INGREDIENTS

2 tablespoons olive oil

1 large yellow onion, diced

2 carrots, peeled and diced

3 cloves garlic, minced

2 teaspoons smoked paprika

1 teaspoon dried thyme

½ teaspoon cumin

¼ teaspoon freshly ground black pepper, or to taste

1 cup dried red split lentils, picked over and rinsed

Two 15-ounce cans white beans, rinsed and drained

4 cups low-sodium vegetable broth

One 28-ounce can diced tomatoes

1 teaspoon sea salt, or to taste

¼ cup chopped fresh parsley

DIRECTIONS

1 In a soup pot, warm the oil over medium heat. Add the onion and sauté until soft and translucent, about 5 to 6 minutes.

2 Add the carrots, garlic, paprika, thyme, cumin, and pepper and sauté until fragrant, about 1 minute.

3 Add the lentils, beans, broth, and tomatoes. Increase the heat to bring to a boil, cover, decrease the heat to medium–low, and simmer until the lentils are tender, about 15 to 20 minutes.

4 Add the salt and chopped parsley. Stir to combine. Serve.

PER SERVING: *Calories 305 (From Fat 49); Fat 5g (Saturated 1g); Cholesterol 0mg; Sodium 671mg; Carbohydrate 49g (Dietary Fiber 14g); Protein 18g.*

TIP: A side of crusty bread is the perfect texture contrast for this stew.

NOTE: Red split lentils get very soft when cooked, and they don't retain their shape. They do, however, add a protein-packed punch to this dish and contribute to the thickness of the stew. Most red lentils sold in grocery stores are actually red split lentils. Check the package if you're unsure.

VARY IT! Use chickpeas instead of white beans.

Barbecue Jackfruit Tacos

PREP TIME: ABOUT 10 MIN	COOK TIME: 20 MIN	YIELD: 6 SERVINGS

INGREDIENTS

One 20-ounce can green jackfruit in brine, drained, rinsed, and patted dry

2 tablespoons olive oil

1 yellow onion, peeled and diced

1 jalapeño pepper, seeded and finely diced

1 teaspoon tamari

2 teaspoons chili powder

1 teaspoon cumin

1 teaspoon dried oregano

½ teaspoon salt, or to taste

½ cup Smoky Barbecue Sauce (see Chapter 15) or your favorite store-bought barbecue sauce

Twelve 6-inch corn tortillas

Shredded red or green cabbage or a combo of both, for garnish

Sliced avocado, for garnish

Chopped fresh cilantro, for garnish

Fresh squeeze lime juice, for garnish

DIRECTIONS

1 In a large bowl, place the dried jackfruit. Using 2 forks, pull the pieces of jackfruit apart until they resemble shreds. Set aside.

2 In a large skillet, warm the oil over medium heat. Add the onion and jalapeño pepper and sauté until the onion is soft and translucent, about 5 to 6 minutes.

3 Add the shredded jackfruit and cook, stirring occasionally, until the edges are browned and crispy, about 8 to 10 minutes.

4 Add the tamari, chili powder, cumin, oregano, and salt. Stir and cook until fragrant, about 1 minute.

5 Add the Smoky Barbecue Sauce, stir to combine, and cook until heated through, about 2 to 3 minutes.

6 Wrap the tortillas in slightly damp paper towels and heat in the microwave in 30-second increments until warm.

7 To serve, place 2 to 3 tablespoons of the jackfruit mixture on each tortilla and garnish with the toppings of your choice.

PER SERVING: *Calories 274 (From Fat 56); Fat 6g (Saturated 1g); Cholesterol 0mg; Sodium 445mg; Carbohydrate 54g (Dietary Fiber 5g); Protein 5g.*

TIP: Corn tortillas can be a bit finicky and tend to fall apart, especially if the filling ingredients are wet. To combat this problem, try doubling up the tortillas before adding the filling. The tortilla closest to the filing will soak up the juices, keeping the outside tortilla intact. You can use flour tortillas, if you prefer.

NOTE: Be sure to use young green jackfruit in brine! Ripe jackfruit is sweet and not the flavor you want for this recipe.

Chapter **13**

Simple Sides

Sides dishes are important for balancing out a meal. They're the perfect way to boost the amount of fruits and vegetables in your diet. They're useful in bringing additional nutrients, textures, and flavors to complete the dining experience. They can be simple or fancy, light or filling, raw or cooked. Almost anything can pose as a side dish, but in this chapter, we give you some delicious ideas that you'll turn to time and time again.

Adding Variety with Sumptuous Sides

It's all about the sides. If you have nothing to put on your plate besides your main course, the plate looks very empty. It's your sides that make a meal whole. They're also the perfect platform to make your meal special.

Whether your side is greens and mushrooms or roasted potatoes, make sure you have enough variety, color, texture, and balance to make your lunch or dinner that much more exciting. Of course, you can also pair your sides with other sides or some of the snack options we mention in Chapter 14 for a tapas-style meal!

Consider this: If your entree remains the same for a few meals, but you change up your sides, it'll still feel like you're eating from different menus. It's a perfect approach for those hectic weekday dinners.

These ideas for sides will get your creative wheels turning:

>> Sautéed leafy, green veggies, such as chard, collards, kale, or spinach, with a small amount of garlic and olive oil

>> Steamed asparagus, broccoli, and green beans topped with Tahini Miso Gravy (see Chapter 15)

>> Roasted vegetables like broccoli, Brussels sprouts, carrots, cauliflower, sweet potatoes, or a combination of several, with a drizzle of olive oil and a sprinkle of salt and pepper

>> Baked sweet potato, roasted squash, or spaghetti squash

>> Cooked whole-grain noodles or grains served with one of the sauce recipes in Chapter 15

To keep meals hearty and interesting, opt for two different kinds of veggies — one green and one root (for example, sautéed greens and yam fries) — or try serving several sides to make a complete meal.

Garlic Oregano Yam Fries

PREP TIME: ABOUT 15 MIN	COOK TIME: 45 MIN	YIELD: 4 SERVINGS

INGREDIENTS

2 tablespoons coconut oil, plus extra for greasing

2 cloves garlic, minced

1 tablespoon coarsely chopped pumpkin seeds

1 tablespoon dried oregano

1 teaspoon dried basil

Sea salt to taste

4 medium yams or sweet potatoes, cut into wedges or chunks

DIRECTIONS

1 Preheat the oven to 300 degrees. Lightly grease a baking sheet with coconut oil and set aside.

2 In a bowl, combine the garlic, pumpkin seeds, oregano, basil, coconut oil, and sea salt.

3 Add the yams, stirring with your hands to make sure all the pieces are covered with the mixture.

4 Spread the yams on the baking sheet and bake for about 45 minutes. If you prefer them crispier, leave them in the oven for an extra 10 to 20 minutes.

PER SERVING: *Calories 254 (From Fat 81); Fat 9g (Saturated 6g); Cholesterol 0mg; Sodium 235mg; Carbohydrate 40g (Dietary Fiber 6g); Protein 4.5g.*

NOTE: Don't be tempted to increase the temperature to cook the fries quicker because the garlic may burn.

Rosemary Cauliflower Mashed Potatoes

PREP TIME: ABOUT 5 MIN	COOK TIME: 55 MIN	YIELD: 8 SERVINGS

INGREDIENTS

3 cups water

1 cup millet, rinsed

1 head cauliflower, chopped into florets

1 clove garlic

2 tablespoons olive oil

¼ cup chopped fresh rosemary

½ teaspoon sea salt

DIRECTIONS

1 In a large pot, bring the water to a boil.

2 Place the rinsed millet in the boiling water, reduce the heat to low, and simmer for 25 minutes.

3 Add the cauliflower and garlic and continue to simmer until the cauliflower is soft when pierced with a fork, about 20 minutes.

4 Turn off the heat and let the pot stand for another 10 minutes.

5 Using a potato masher, mash the cauliflower until you get a thick, creamy texture.

6 Stir in the olive oil, rosemary, and salt.

PER SERVING: *Calories 133 (From Fat 45); Fat 5g (Saturated 0.5g); Cholesterol 0mg; Sodium 139mg; Carbohydrate 20g (Dietary Fiber 2.5g); Protein 3g.*

TIP: For a really creamy texture with a unique flavor, try roasting the cauliflower and garlic in an oven at 300 degrees for 30 minutes instead of simmering it. Then combine the cauliflower, garlic, and cooked millet and mash them together.

NOTE: Serve this dish with Tahini Miso Gravy (see Chapter 15) for a perfect side dish to a hearty plant-based meal.

VARY IT! Try using turnips, parsnips, squash, carrots, or beets instead of cauliflower for a different color and flavor.

Spinach Almond Patties

PREP TIME: ABOUT 20 MIN	COOK TIME: 30 MIN	YIELD: 10 SERVINGS

INGREDIENTS

4 cups fresh spinach, washed, dried, and stems removed

1 medium onion, chopped

1¼ cups wheat-free bread-crumbs

1½ cups ground almonds or ground almond meal, divided

2 tablespoons olive oil

2 tablespoons tamari

½ cup brown-rice flour

1 teaspoon dried dill

DIRECTIONS

1 Preheat the oven to 350 degrees. Lightly oil a cookie sheet and set aside.

2 In a food processor, place the spinach and onion and blend on high until they're wet and blended.

3 Add the breadcrumbs, ¾ cup of the almonds or almond meal, olive oil, tamari, rice flour, and dill and blend until all the ingredients are combined to form a paste.

4 Fill a small bowl with water for wetting your hands while flat-tening the mixture into patties.

5 Place the remaining ¾ cup ground almonds or almond meal on a large plate. Flatten the spinach mixture into 10 patties about 2 inches wide and 1 inch thick. Press them into the ground almonds or almond meal, coating the outside of each patty.

6 Place the finished patties on the cookie sheet and cook for 30 minutes.

7 Allow the patties to cool on the cookie sheet and then place them in a bowl or on a platter.

8 Serve the patties in wraps or on sprouted-grain buns, along with a fresh salad, steamed greens, brown rice, or quinoa.

PER SERVING: *Calories 214 (From Fat 117); Fat 13g (Saturated 1g); Cholesterol 0mg; Sodium 317mg; Carbohydrate 21g (Dietary Fiber 5 g); Protein 5g.*

NOTE: These patties should be approximately the size of a small burger or slider.

VARY IT! Instead of making flat patties, you can roll the mixture into balls about the size of a ping-pong ball.

Collards with Portobello Mushrooms

PREP TIME: ABOUT 5 MIN	COOK TIME: 25 MIN	YIELD: 10 SERVINGS

INGREDIENTS

¾ pound collard greens

1 cup water

2 tablespoons olive oil

2 teaspoons minced garlic

⅓ cup thinly sliced scallions

2 to 3 portobello mushrooms, cut into thin slices

Pinch of salt

DIRECTIONS

1 Wash the collard greens, remove the stalks, and stack 4 to 5 leaves. Roll the leaves like a cigar and slice into thin ribbons.

2 To steam the collards, place the water in the bottom of a pot with a lid and bring the water to a boil. Add the collards to a steaming basket and place the basket in the pot. Cover and steam over medium heat for 5 minutes, stirring occasionally. Remove the collards from the pot and set aside.

3 In a skillet, warm the oil over medium heat. Add the garlic and scallions and sauté until fragrant, about 30 seconds to 1 minute. Increase the heat to medium–high and add the mushrooms and a pinch of salt to draw out some liquid. Cook, stirring constantly, until the mushrooms are tender, about 5 to 6 minutes.

4 Reduce the heat to low, stir in the cooked collards, cover, and cook until warm, about 5 minutes. Serve.

PER SERVING: Calories 39 (From Fat 27); Fat 3g (Saturated 0g); Cholesterol 0mg; Sodium 161mg; Carbohydrate 2g (Dietary Fiber 1 g); Protein 1g.

NOTE: Collards are one of the toughest greens to break down, so they require a bit of steaming at the beginning to start the cooking process. You can skip Step 2 and simply sauté the collards in the pan with the mushrooms, but the cooking time will be closer to 10 minutes.

Citrus Wild Rice and Broccoli

PREP TIME: ABOUT 10 MIN	COOK TIME: 45 MIN	YIELD: 8 SERVINGS

INGREDIENTS

1 cup wild rice, soaked overnight in 2 cups of water

2 cups water

½ teaspoon sea salt

2 tablespoons orange zest or the zest of 1 orange

¼ cup fresh-squeezed orange juice

2 tablespoons lemon juice

2 teaspoons balsamic vinegar

¼ teaspoon ground cinnamon

½ teaspoon sea salt

¼ cup olive oil

1 head broccoli

½ cup sliced or supremed orange segments

⅓ cup cranberries

½ cup hazelnuts or pecans

DIRECTIONS

1 Drain the soaked rice and place it in a medium saucepan. Add the water and salt and bring to a boil. Lower the heat, cover, and simmer until the grains have burst open and are tender but still chewy, about 35 to 45 minutes. Drain and set aside in a medium bowl.

2 While the rice is cooking, make the vinaigrette: In a large mason jar, place the orange zest, orange juice, lemon juice, vinegar, cinnamon, salt, and olive oil. Tightly seal the lid on the jar and shake to mix the ingredients together. Set aside.

3 Cut the broccoli into small florets and place in a steamer basket over boiling water until they're dark green and tender, about 3 minutes. Run the broccoli under cool water to halt the cooking.

4 Pour the vinaigrette over the rice. Add the broccoli, cranberries, orange segments, and nuts to the rice, mix, and serve.

PER SERVING: *Calories 200 (From Fat 108); Fat 12g (Saturated 1g); Cholesterol 0mg; Sodium 268mg; Carbohydrate 21g (Dietary Fiber 3g); Protein 5g.*

NOTE: If you can't get your hands on wild rice, use a long-grain brown rice or wild-rice blend. The salad will taste just as delicious! This salad tastes great both warm and cold out of the fridge. Also, be sure not to over-steam your broccoli. You want to make sure it's green — not brown — when you place it in your salad.

VARY IT! Instead of broccoli, try green beans, snap peas, or snow peas for a unique variation.

Roasted Asparagus with Lemon Dill Sauce

| PREP TIME: ABOUT 5 MIN | COOK TIME: 15 MIN | YIELD: 4 SERVINGS |

INGREDIENTS

1 to 2 bunches asparagus, tough woody ends snapped off

1 to 2 tablespoons olive oil, for drizzling

Pinch of sea salt

Lemon Dill Sauce (see the following recipe)

DIRECTIONS

1 Preheat the oven to 425 degrees. Line a rimmed baking sheet with parchment paper.

2 Drizzle the asparagus with olive oil and sprinkle with a pinch of salt. Toss to coat.

3 Spread the asparagus spears out into one even layer on the prepared baking sheet. Roast until tender and browned, about 12 to 15 minutes.

4 Serve with Lemon Dill Sauce.

Lemon Dill Sauce

½ cup plain, unsweetened, nondairy yogurt

1 to 2 tablespoons freshly squeezed lemon juice

½ teaspoon garlic powder

½ teaspoon onion powder

¼ teaspoon sea salt, or to taste

1 to 2 tablespoons fresh chopped dill

In a small bowl, whisk together all the ingredients until fully combined. Chill until ready to serve.

PER SERVING: *Calories 75 (From Fat 36); Fat 4g (Saturated 1g); Cholesterol 0mg; Sodium 182mg; Carbohydrate 8g (Dietary Fiber 3g); Protein 3g.*

NOTE: Thinner asparagus spears will be done in a shorter amount of time than thicker spears. Adjust your roasting time as necessary.

VARY IT! Don't care for dill? Try a simple squeeze of lemon or Balsamic Maple Dressing (see Chapter 15).

Oven-Roasted Carrots

PREP TIME: ABOUT 5 MIN	COOK TIME: 25 MIN	YIELD: 6 SERVINGS

INGREDIENTS

2 pounds carrots, peeled, thicker ones halved lengthwise

2 tablespoons olive oil or grapeseed oil

1½ teaspoons chopped fresh thyme, plus extra for garnish

¾ teaspoon ground cumin

½ teaspoon sea salt

¼ teaspoon freshly ground black pepper

Juice of ½ orange

3 tablespoons pure maple syrup

½ cup raw walnuts, chopped

DIRECTIONS

1 Preheat the oven to 425 degrees. Line a rimmed baking sheet with parchment paper.

2 Place the carrots on the baking sheet. Drizzle with oil and sprinkle the thyme, cumin, salt, and pepper over the top. Toss the carrots until they're evenly coated. Spread them out into 1 single layer. Roast for 15 minutes.

3 Meanwhile, in a small bowl, whisk together the orange juice and maple syrup.

4 Pour the orange maple mixture over the roasted carrots, toss well, and spread back out evenly in 1 single layer. Roast until the carrots start to brown and caramelize and are tender when pierced with a fork, about 5 to 10 minutes.

5 While the carrots are roasting the final time, heat a dry skillet over medium-high heat. Add the walnuts and toast them, stirring frequently to prevent burning, until they're fragrant and starting to darken, about 3 to 5 minutes. Watch them closely so they don't burn. After the walnuts are toasted, pour them out onto a plate in 1 even layer to cool down. They'll continue to get crunchier as they sit.

6 Place the carrots on a plate or platter and sprinkle with the toasted walnuts and extra thyme, if desired. Serve.

PER SERVING: *Calories 186 (From Fat 93); Fat 10g (Saturated 1g); Cholesterol 0mg; Sodium 262mg; Carbohydrate 23g (Dietary Fiber 5g); Protein 3g.*

TIP: Make these oil-free by using a splash of vegetable broth instead of oil to help the spices stick to the carrots.

NOTE: Be sure not to add the maple syrup and orange juice mixture until the last 5 to 10 minutes of roasting. The high sugar content of these ingredients can burn easily if you add them too soon.

VARY IT! Fresh oregano, rosemary, or marjoram can all be used instead of thyme.

Vegan Jalapeño Cornbread

PREP TIME: ABOUT 10 MIN	COOK TIME: 30 MIN	YIELD: 8 SERVINGS

INGREDIENTS

1½ cups medium-ground cornmeal

½ cup spelt flour

1 tablespoon baking powder

¼ teaspoon baking soda

¾ teaspoon sea salt

1 cup unsweetened, plain almond milk

1 tablespoon apple cider vinegar

¼ cup aquafaba, the liquid from a can of chickpeas

¼ cup pure maple syrup

½ cup fresh or frozen corn kernels

1 jalapeño pepper, ribs and seeds removed, diced

1 jalapeño pepper, sliced

DIRECTIONS

1 Preheat the oven to 400 degrees. Line a 9-inch round cake pan with parchment paper or gently spray with cooking spray.

2 In a bowl, add the cornmeal, flour, baking powder, baking soda, and salt and whisk together.

3 In a separate bowl, add the milk, vinegar, aquafaba, and maple syrup and whisk together.

4 Mix the dry ingredients into the wet ingredients until combined.

5 Add the corn and diced jalapeño and stir to combine.

6 Pour into the prepared pan, top with jalapeño slices, and bake until a toothpick inserted into the center comes out clean, about 25 to 30 minutes.

7 Let cool in the pan on a cooling rack before cutting into slices.

PER SERVING: *Calories 177 (From Fat 9); Fat 1g (Saturated 0g); Cholesterol 0mg; Sodium 179mg; Carbohydrate 39g (Dietary Fiber 2g); Protein 3g.*

TIP: Serve with soups, stews, chilis, saucy beans, or seasoned lentils — or simply grab a slice as a snack!

Green Bean Broccoli Sauté

INGREDIENTS

1 tablespoon olive oil

½ red onion, sliced

1 pound fresh green beans

1 average head broccoli, chopped into florets

2 cloves garlic, minced

1 teaspoon minced fresh ginger

2 tablespoons coconut aminos or tamari

Juice of ½ lime, plus more to taste

1 tablespoon sesame seeds

DIRECTIONS

1 In a large skillet, warm the oil over medium heat. Add the onion and sauté until softened, about 3 to 4 minutes.

2 Add the green beans and broccoli and stir. Cover the skillet with a lid and cook 7 to 8 minutes.

3 Add the garlic, ginger, and coconut aminos or tamari and sauté another 2 minutes, uncovered.

4 Add the lime juice and sesame seeds just before serving.

PER SERVING: *Calories 150 (From Fat 48); Fat 5g (Saturated 1g); Cholesterol 0mg; Sodium 564mg; Carbohydrate 23g (Dietary Fiber 8g); Protein 8g.*

TIP: Serve over brown rice or soba noodles with baked tofu for a complete meal.

Baked Veggie Potato Fritters

PREP TIME: ABOUT 15 MIN	COOK TIME: 35 MIN	YIELD: 5 SERVINGS

INGREDIENTS

3 cups coarsely shredded russet potatoes (about 2 medium potatoes)

1 cup coarsely shredded zucchini

1 cup finely shredded carrots

1 teaspoon dried parsley

¾ teaspoon sea salt

½ teaspoon garlic powder

¼ teaspoon paprika

¼ teaspoon turmeric

¼ cup chickpea flour

DIRECTIONS

1 Preheat the oven to 400 degrees. Line a baking sheet with parchment paper and set aside.

2 Wrap the potatoes, zucchini, and carrots in a clean kitchen cloth, very sturdy paper towels, or cheese cloth, and squeeze out as much liquid as possible. Just when you think you've squeezed out all the liquid, squeeze a little more. This is the key to crispy fritters — don't skip this step!

3 Add the potatoes, zucchini, and carrots to a bowl along with the parsley, salt, garlic powder, paprika, turmeric, and flour. Mix well to combine.

4 Take about ¼ to ⅓ cup of the mixture and form it into a thin patty. Place it on the prepared baking sheet and press down slightly to flatten it. The thinner you can make the patties, the better. Repeat to make the remaining 4 patties.

5 Bake for 20 minutes, gently flip the fritters over, and bake another 10 to 15 minutes until golden brown on both sides and crispy on the edges.

PER SERVING: *Calories 98 (From Fat 5); Fat 1g (Saturated 0g); Cholesterol 0mg; Sodium 305mg; Carbohydrate 21g (Dietary Fiber 2g); Protein 3g.*

TIP: Serve with Smoky Barbecue Sauce, Tahini Miso Gravy, or Creamy Avocado Dill Sauce (all in Chapter 15).

Roasted Potato and Pepper Hash

PREP TIME: ABOUT 10 MIN	COOK TIME: 35 MIN	YIELD: 4 SERVINGS

INGREDIENTS

1½ pounds red potatoes, scrubbed clean and chopped into 1-inch pieces

2 bell peppers, any color, seeded and chopped

1 red onion, peeled and chopped

1 tablespoon olive oil

1 teaspoon paprika

1 teaspoon dried oregano

½ teaspoon garlic powder

¼ teaspoon sea salt, or to taste

¼ teaspoon freshly ground black pepper, or to taste

DIRECTIONS

1 Preheat the oven to 400 degrees.

2 In a large bowl, place the potatoes, bell peppers, and onion. Drizzle with olive oil and toss to coat.

3 Add the paprika, oregano, garlic powder, salt, and pepper. Toss to coat evenly.

4 Spread out evenly onto a rimmed baking sheet in one even layer.

5 Roast for 20 minutes, stir, and roast another 10 to 15 minutes until the vegetables are tender and browned.

PER SERVING: *Calories 226 (From Fat 35); Fat 4g (Saturated 1g); Cholesterol 0mg; Sodium 146mg; Carbohydrate 43g (Dietary Fiber 5g); Protein 5g.*

TIP: Chop the peppers and onions the same size and slightly larger than the potatoes so they're all done at the same time.

NOTE: This dish is delicious for breakfast next to the Turmeric Tofu Scramble (see Chapter 9).

VARY IT! Use beets, butternut squash, or sweet potato instead of the potatoes for a twist.

Sautéed Garden Vegetables

PREP TIME: ABOUT 10 MIN	COOK TIME: 8 MIN	YIELD: 4 SERVINGS

INGREDIENTS

2 tablespoons olive oil

1 red onion, thinly sliced

1 medium zucchini, cut in half lengthwise and thinly sliced

2 cloves garlic, minced

½ teaspoon sea salt, or to taste

¼ teaspoon freshly ground black pepper, or to taste

1 cup frozen green peas

3 to 4 large Swiss chard leaves, stems removed, chopped

2 tablespoons Dijon mustard

1 tablespoon pure maple syrup

1 tablespoon balsamic vinegar

DIRECTIONS

1 In a skillet, warm the oil over medium heat. Add the onion and sauté until it starts to soften, about 4 to 5 minutes.

2 Add the zucchini, garlic, salt, and pepper and sauté 2 minutes.

3 Add the green peas, Swiss chard, mustard, maple syrup, and vinegar. Stir to coat the vegetables in the sauce evenly. Sauté until heated through, about 2 to 3 minutes. Serve immediately.

PER SERVING: *Calories 151 (From Fat 67); Fat 7g (Saturated 1g); Cholesterol 0mg; Sodium 444mg; Carbohydrate 19g (Dietary Fiber 4g); Protein 4g.*

TIP: Pair with cooked quinoa for an easy light lunch.

Orzo with Cherry Tomatoes and Basil

PREP TIME: ABOUT 5 MIN	COOK TIME: 12 MIN	YIELD: 4 SERVINGS

INGREDIENTS

1 cup dry orzo

1 tablespoon olive oil

16 ounces cherry or grape tomatoes, halved

½ teaspoon sea salt, or to taste

¼ teaspoon freshly ground black pepper, or to taste

Zest of 1 lemon

Juice of ½ lemon, or to taste

10 to 15 basil leaves, chiffonade

DIRECTIONS

1 Fill a pot with water, salt well, add the orzo, and cook according to package directions until al dente, about 8 to 10 minutes. When the orzo is done, drain, and set aside.

2 In the same pot, add the oil and warm over medium-high heat. Add the tomatoes, salt, pepper, and lemon zest and stir to combine. Sauté until the tomatoes start to soften and give off their juices, about 3 to 4 minutes. Remove from heat.

3 Add the cooked orzo back to the pot and add the lemon juice and basil. Stir to combine. Taste and adjust the seasoning as necessary. Serve warm or room temperature.

PER SERVING: *Calories 126 (From Fat 36); Fat 4g (Saturated 0g); Cholesterol 0mg; Sodium 240mg; Carbohydrate 20g (Dietary Fiber 3g); Protein 4g.*

TIP: Add a drizzle of balsamic vinegar or crumbled vegan feta cheese right before serving for extra indulgence.

NOTE: Serve this dish alongside pan-fried tofu or tempeh, cauliflower steaks, grilled portobello mushrooms, vegan meatballs or sausages, sautéed white beans and a dollop of pesto, or seasoned steamed lentils.

VARY IT! Instead of orzo, try this dish with brown rice or quinoa, cooked according to package directions.

Raw Corn and Radish Salad

PREP TIME: ABOUT 10 MIN	COOK TIME: NONE	YIELD: 6 SERVINGS

INGREDIENTS

Kernels cut from 4 large ears of fresh sweet corn (about 4 cups)

1 cup thinly sliced radishes

¼ cup fresh cilantro, chopped

Juice of 1 to 2 limes, to taste

1½ teaspoons smoked paprika

½ teaspoon cumin

Salt to taste

Freshly ground black pepper to taste

DIRECTIONS

1 In a large bowl, place all the ingredients and toss well to mix. Taste and adjust seasoning as needed.

2 Serve immediately or chill in the fridge up to 2 days until ready to serve.

PER SERVING: *Calories 85 (From Fat 7); Fat 1g (Saturated 0g); Cholesterol 0mg; Sodium 10mg; Carbohydrate 20g (Dietary Fiber 2g); Protein 3g.*

TIP: Get your hands on the freshest sweet corn you can for this recipe!

Chapter **14**

Appetizers and Snacks

Snacking is an important part of a healthy diet. Between-meal eats can help keep overall hunger at bay and prevent overeating at mealtimes. It's also a great way to increase the essential nutrients your body needs in a day. Plus — let's be honest — we all love to snack!

The goal for successful snacking is to reach for nutritious foods that make you feel energized, not junk foods that make you feel sluggish. The good news is, you have plenty of friendly plant-based options from which to choose.

In this chapter, we explain how snacking is beneficial to your health and how to balance the flavors your body craves. Then we provide all sorts of recipes that will satisfy your hunger when you just want a quick bite.

TIP

Plan out your snacks just as you would your meals so you're not caught in the position of being ravenous and reaching for the first bite you can find, which may not be the healthiest.

Boosting Your Metabolism with Healthy Snacking

An old adage says that the more often you eat, the faster your metabolism functions. Although a lot of metabolism is genetics, you can influence it by how frequently you eat. When you wait a long time between meals, your metabolism actually slows down to conserve your body's remaining fuel and energy. When you eat more often throughout the day, it stays in high gear. Why does this matter? Well, having a faster (or higher) metabolism means you can turn your food into energy and burn your energy efficiently and quickly. When your metabolism slows down, the calories are slower to burn away and ultimately can turn into extra weight. Snacks keep the furnace burning.

To boost your metabolism, you need to have regular snacks in addition to your three meals. So, you may eat upwards of five times a day, depending on your metabolism, appetite, and activity levels.

When you think of the average snack, chances are, you envision one favorite item — a bag of pretzels or perhaps a cookie, or maybe you're one of the good ones and reach for an apple! But your snack probably isn't as powerful as it could be, even if you do reach for the apple. The key is to make the snack a little more complex, especially on a plant-based diet.

REMEMBER

Snacks should be balanced, meaning they have a good ratio of plant protein, complex carbohydrates, and healthy fat so you're left feeling satisfied and satiated.

To get started, try the plant-based (and much healthier) replacements for some common snacks we all know and love in Table 14-1.

TABLE 14-1   Healthy Snack Options

Instead of . . .	Try . . .
Potato chips	Kale chips or tortilla chips with salsa or hummus
Soda pop	Natural, 100 percent fruit juice; coconut water; or kombucha (see the nearby sidebar)
Candy bar	Homemade balanced energy bar (see the Brown-Rice Crispy Bars recipe, later in this chapter)
French fries	Baked sweet potato fries dipped in hummus
Latte, hot chocolate, or chocolate milk	Homemade chocolate smoothie (see the Chocolate Banana Super Smoothie recipe, later in this chapter)
Donuts	Homemade muffins topped with Almond Butter and Cinnamon Dip (see the recipe later in this chapter)

Choosing Sweet or Savory Snacking

Snacks generally fall into one of two taste categories: sweet or savory (think: salty). If you don't crave one, you often crave the other — or sometimes even both at the same time. If you're hungry but you don't know what you're craving, eat something that contrasts with your last meal. That way, you'll not only help balance your blood-sugar levels but also feel satisfied all day long.

TIP

Eating something savory after eating something sweet can help slow down the rate at which glucose is released into your blood, so be mindful of the last meal you ate. Did you last eat a fruit salad or a fruit smoothie? If so, for your next meal or snack, you may want to consider something savory like nuts, seeds, dried seaweed, or guacamole with corn chips. You may not realize it, but you'll feel better with this contrast.

Sometimes it's best to have both sweet *and* savory flavors in the same snack. Try adding a pinch of sea salt to your apple or into your muffin batter. This little bit of salt makes the sweetness taste sweeter while helping to balance your cravings. It may sound a little strange, but it works! *Note:* You can technically do the reverse (add a bit of sweetener to something savory), but it doesn't often work as well.

Here are some ideas for savory munchies and add-ins:

>> Brown rice cakes

>> Dulse flakes

>> Gluten-free or whole-grain crackers

>> Non-GMO corn chips

>> Nuts and seeds with a pinch of sea salt or a splash of *tamari* (natural soy sauce)

>> Sprouted-grain tortillas

>> Toasted nori or other seaweeds

And here's a list to appeal to your sweet tooth:

>> Almond butter

>> Apple butter

>> Cacao nibs or dairy-free dark chocolate chips

>> Coconut butter or flakes

>> Dried fruit, such as cranberries, goji berries, goldenberries, and raisins

>> Fresh fruit

Edamame Hummus

INGREDIENTS

2 cups cooked, shelled edamame beans

¼ cup tahini

¼ cup freshly squeezed lemon juice

2 cloves garlic, minced

1 teaspoon chopped or minced ginger or ½ teaspoon ground dry ginger

1 teaspoon tamari

1 teaspoon toasted sesame oil, plus extra for serving

2 tablespoons olive oil

¼ cup water

½ teaspoon sea salt

Black sesame seeds (optional)

DIRECTIONS

1 In a food processor, place the edamame, tahini, lemon juice, garlic, ginger, tamari, sesame oil, and olive oil and blend until smooth.

2 With the motor still running, slowly add the water and sea salt until the desired consistency is reached.

3 Transfer the dip to a bowl and sprinkle with the sesame seeds (if desired) and a few drops of sesame oil. Serve with brown-rice crackers.

PER SERVING: *Calories 102 (From Fat 72); Fat 8g (Saturated 1g); Cholesterol 0mg; Sodium 141mg; Carbohydrate 5g (Dietary Fiber 1g); Protein 4g.*

Sweet Pea Guacamole

PREP TIME: ABOUT 15 MIN	COOK TIME: NONE	YIELD: 10 SERVINGS

INGREDIENTS

1 cup frozen green peas or fresh when in season, blanched

4 green onions, cut into 2-inch slices

3 to 5 tablespoons freshly squeezed lemon or lime juice

1 teaspoon ground cumin

½ teaspoon ground coriander

¼ teaspoon garlic powder or 1 clove fresh garlic, peeled

8 sprigs parsley

1 jalapeño pepper, finely chopped, or ¼ teaspoon hot sauce (optional)

¼ teaspoon sea salt

2 large ripe avocados

¾ cup chopped tomatoes

DIRECTIONS

1 In a food processor, place the peas, onions, lemon or lime juice, cumin, coriander, garlic, parsley, jalapeño or hot sauce (if desired), and salt and process until well blended and smooth.

2 Cut the avocados in half, remove the pits, and scoop out the flesh into a medium bowl (see Figure 14-1). Mash the avocados and mix in the ingredients from the food processor.

3 Stir in the tomatoes and adjust the seasoning to taste.

4 Serve with corn tortilla chips, slices of jicama, or whole-grain crackers.

PER SERVING: *Calories 66 (From Fat 36); Fat 4g (Saturated 0.5g); Cholesterol 0mg; Sodium 68mg; Carbohydrate 7g (Dietary Fiber 3g); Protein 2g.*

TIP: For a flavor boost, top off this dip with an extra squirt of lime juice and a dash of sea salt.

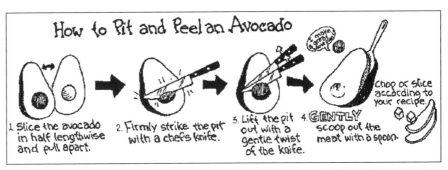

FIGURE 14-1: Pitting and extracting the meat from an avocado.

Illustration by Elizabeth Kurtzman

Fresh Peach Salsa with Homemade Tortilla Chips

INGREDIENTS

4 ripe peaches, pits removed, chopped (about 2 cups)

¼ red onion, finely diced

1 jalapeño pepper, ribs and seeds removed, finely diced

6 to 8 basil leaves, chiffonade

Juice of 1 naval orange

Sea salt to taste

Twelve 4-inch corn tortillas

DIRECTIONS

1 In a bowl, place the peaches, onion, jalapeño pepper, basil, orange juice, and a pinch of salt and mix well. Set aside while the chips bake.

2 Meanwhile, preheat the oven to 350 degrees.

3 Cut each tortilla into 6 triangles and lay them out in 1 even layer on a rimmed baking sheet. Bake for 5 to 6 minutes. Turn over each chip with tongs and bake another 6 to 8 minutes until they start to brown. Watch them closely as all ovens vary and the chips can burn easily.

4 Remove from the oven and immediately sprinkle with salt. The chips will continue to crisp up as they cool.

5 Serve the chips with the salsa.

PER SERVING: *Calories 97 (From Fat 8); Fat 1g (Saturated 0g); Cholesterol 0mg; Sodium 11mg; Carbohydrate 22g (Dietary Fiber 3g); Protein 2g.*

TIP: If you like your salsa spicy, leave the ribs and seeds in the jalapeño.

NOTE: The salsa can be made 1 to 2 days ahead. Place in an airtight container in the fridge until ready to serve.

VARY IT! Try this recipe with freshly diced pineapple or strawberries instead of peaches.

White Bean Dip with Dill

PREP TIME: ABOUT 5 MIN	COOK TIME: 45 MIN	YIELD: 8–10 SERVINGS

INGREDIENTS

Two 14-ounce cans navy beans, rinsed and drained, or 1 cup dry beans, soaked overnight

½-inch piece of kombu, if using dry beans

2 cloves garlic

¼ cup freshly squeezed lemon juice

2 to 4 tablespoons tahini

1 tablespoon olive oil

Salt to taste

Freshly ground black pepper to taste

1 bunch fresh dill or basil, finely chopped

DIRECTIONS

1 If using dry beans, place the beans, kombu, and 4 cups of water in a large pot, and cook for 45 to 60 minutes. If using canned beans, proceed to the next step.

2 In a food processor or blender, place the garlic, lemon juice, and half of the beans and blend well.

3 Add the remaining beans, tahini, olive oil, salt, and pepper and blend until smooth. (Add water if a thinner consistency is desired.)

4 Transfer the spread to a bowl and stir in the dill.

5 Serve with a side of whole-grain or gluten-free crackers and veggies, or scoop 2 tablespoons of dip onto a wrap or sprouted-grain bread for a sandwich.

PER SERVING: *Calories 125 (From Fat 36); Fat 4g (Saturated 0.5g); Cholesterol 0mg; Sodium 70mg; Carbohydrate 17g (Dietary Fiber 7g); Protein 6g.*

TIP: If you want the beans to be nice and soft for pureeing, cook them for at least 1 hour.

VARY IT! Try this dip with different beans, such as black beans, chickpeas, kidney beans, or lentils.

Almond Butter and Cinnamon Dip

PREP TIME: ABOUT 3 MIN	COOK TIME: NONE	YIELD: 2 SERVINGS

INGREDIENTS

¼ cup almond butter

1 teaspoon cinnamon

1 tablespoon raw honey or pure maple syrup

DIRECTIONS

1 In a bowl, place all the ingredients and stir with a fork or spoon to combine.

2 Enjoy this dip with sliced apples, bananas, or pears for a nourishing and balanced snack. You can also spread it onto whole-grain toast, crackers, or rice cakes.

PER SERVING: *Calories 231 (From Fat 162); Fat 18g (Saturated 2g); Cholesterol 0mg; Sodium 73mg; Carbohydrate 16g (Dietary Fiber 4g); Protein 7g.*

TIP: This dip is great to eat as an energizing snack before a workout.

VARY IT! If you're allergic to nuts, use hempseed butter, sunflower seed butter, or tahini as an alternative and it'll taste just as delicious!

Buffalo Cauliflower Dip

PREP TIME: ABOUT 10 MIN | **COOK TIME: 45 MIN** | **YIELD: 8 SERVINGS**

INGREDIENTS

1 small head cauliflower, diced into small bite-size florets

1½ cups raw cashews, soaked in hot water for 20 to 30 minutes

1 cup unsweetened, plain dairy-free yogurt

¼ cup nutritional yeast

2 tablespoons fresh lemon juice

½ teaspoon sea salt

¾ cup buffalo sauce

¾ cup unsweetened, plain almond milk

1 tablespoon olive oil

1 yellow onion, diced

2 cloves garlic, minced

1 tablespoon poultry seasoning

2 green onions, diced

DIRECTIONS

1   Preheat the oven to 425 degrees. Line a rimmed baking sheet with parchment paper.

2   Spread the chopped cauliflower out into one even layer on the baking sheet. Roast until the cauliflower is tender and browned on the edges, about 20 to 25 minutes.

3   While the cauliflower is roasting, drain and rinse the cashews and place them in a high-speed blender along with the yogurt, nutritional yeast, lemon juice, salt, buffalo sauce, and milk. Blend until smooth and creamy. Set aside.

4   When the cauliflower is almost done roasting, warm the oil in a large skillet over medium heat. Add the onion and sauté until soft and translucent, about 5 to 6 minutes. Add the garlic and poultry seasoning, stir, and sauté for 1 minute.

5   Add the roasted cauliflower and sauce from the blender into the skillet. Stir well to combine.

6   Pour the mixture into an 8-x-8-inch baking dish and bake until hot throughout, about 20 minutes.

7   Sprinkle the green onions over the top.

8   Serve hot with whole-grain baguette slices, tortilla chips, or celery sticks.

PER SERVING: *Calories 253 (From Fat 161); Fat 18g (Saturated 3g); Cholesterol 0mg; Sodium 759mg; Carbohydrate 19g (Dietary Fiber 3g); Protein 8g.*

TIP: If you don't have or can't find poultry seasoning, use 2 teaspoons of dried sage and 1 teaspoon of dried thyme instead.

NOTE: Not all buffalo sauce is vegan and even some that are contain questionable ingredients. Try Tabasco brand buffalo sauce for a clean store-bought version.

Creamy Oil-Free Hummus

PREP TIME: ABOUT 15 MIN	COOK TIME: NONE	YIELD: 8 SERVINGS

INGREDIENTS

One 15-ounce can no-salt-added chickpeas

⅓ cup tahini

3 to 4 tablespoons freshly squeezed lemon juice

3 tablespoons aquafaba, the liquid from the can of chickpeas

2 cloves garlic

1 teaspoon cumin

½ teaspoon sea salt, or to taste

2 to 4 tablespoons cold water, if needed, to thin

DIRECTIONS

1 Drain the can of chickpeas over a measuring cup or bowl. Set aside the liquid for later.

2 Rinse the drained chickpeas under cold water and then transfer to a plate or bowl lined with paper towels or a clean dish cloth and rub the chickpeas dry.

3 Remove the skins from the chickpeas. The skins should already by starting to come off from rubbing them, but if not, simply squeeze a chickpea between your fingers and it should slide right out of its skin.

4 In a food processor, place the skinned chickpeas, tahini, lemon juice, aquafaba, garlic, cumin, and salt and puree until smooth and creamy, stopping to scrape down the sides as necessary to ensure that all the ingredients are fully incorporated.

5 If you want to thin out the hummus a bit, add water 2 tablespoons at a time through the top feed tube while the food processor is running, until the desired consistency is reached.

6 Serve with crudités or pita chips.

PER SERVING: *Calories 102 (From Fat 51); Fat 6g (Saturated 1g); Cholesterol 0mg; Sodium 183mg; Carbohydrate 10g (Dietary Fiber 2g); Protein 4g.*

VARY IT! Optional add-ins: 1 jarred roasted red pepper, 1 chipotle pepper in adobo, a few sun-dried tomatoes, or a handful of cilantro and squeeze of lime juice.

NOTE: Aquafaba is the leftover liquid from cooked chickpeas. The most consistent aquafaba comes from canned chickpeas, but you can make your own by cooking dry garbanzo beans. Although there is no real nutrient value in this starchy liquid, it's naturally gluten-free and low in calories and has the ability to mimic the consistency of eggs, dairy, and oil in certain recipes. Always choose no-salt-added beans in BPA-free cans to avoid unnecessary sodium and chemicals.

Roasted Carrot Bean Dip

PREP TIME: ABOUT 10 MIN	COOK TIME: 25 MIN	YIELD: 12 SERVINGS

INGREDIENTS

2 cups peeled and chopped carrots (about 4 to 5 medium carrots)

1 sweet onion, peeled and roughly chopped

1 tablespoon olive oil, plus more as needed for consistency

Salt to taste

Freshly ground black pepper to taste

½ cup raw walnuts

One 15-ounce can navy beans, drained and rinsed well under cold water

1 roasted red pepper (jarred)

1 tablespoon balsamic vinegar

1 teaspoon tarmari or coconut aminos

4 cloves garlic, peeled

1 teaspoon dried basil

2 teaspoons smoked paprika

DIRECTIONS

1 Preheat the oven to 400 degrees. Line a rimmed baking sheet with parchment paper.

2 Place the carrots and onions on the baking sheet, drizzle with olive oil, and toss to coat. Sprinkle with salt and pepper and spread out the vegetables into one even layer.

3 Roast the vegetables for 15 minutes, add the walnuts to the baking sheet with the vegetables in an even layer, and roast until the vegetables are tender, the edges are browned, and the walnuts have turned a shade darker, about 10 minutes.

4 In a food processor, place the roasted vegetables and walnuts, along with the navy beans, red pepper, vinegar, tamari or coconut aminos, garlic, basil, and paprika. Pulse until smooth. Add more olive oil, 1 tablespoon at a time, if needed to achieve a smoother consistency, if desired.

5 Serve with whole-grain crackers, raw vegetables, or crusty whole-grain bread.

PER SERVING: *Calories 91 (From Fat 37); Fat 4g (Saturated 0g); Cholesterol 0mg; Sodium 145mg; Carbohydrate 12g (Dietary Fiber 4g); Protein 3g.*

TIP: Try this dip as a spread for sandwiches and wraps or dollop it on grain bowls for more flavor.

NOTE: This dip can be served warm, room temperature, or cold.

VARY IT! For a nut-free option, use shelled pumpkin seeds instead of walnuts.

Super Brazil and Goldenberry Trail Mix

INGREDIENTS

1 cup Brazil nuts, chopped

1 cup unsweetened coconut flakes

½ cup goldenberries

¼ cup goji berries

½ cup pumpkin seeds

Pinch of sea salt (optional)

DIRECTIONS

Place all the ingredients in a large glass jar or container and shake.

PER SERVING: *Calories 158 (From Fat 133); Fat 15g (Saturated 5g); Cholesterol 0mg; Sodium 3mg; Carbohydrate 5g (Dietary Fiber 2g); Protein 4g.*

TIP: To make this snack nut-free, choose sunflower seeds instead of Brazil nuts.

NOTE: Goldenberries and goji berries are different from your typical apricot or raisin (which can also be used). They're more tart and tangy than sweet. Both are superfood fruits with protein, antioxidants, and fiber. You can find them at health food stores.

VARY IT! Swap out the Brazil nuts for cashews for a decadent taste. You can also add some dairy-free dark chocolate chips or cacao nibs to get your fix of chocolate.

TRAIL MIX: HEALTHY AND FULL OF FLAVOR

Trail mix. It's the easiest way to get a snack that's both sweet and salty. Beyond that, it's a good balance of protein, healthy fats, and carbs — even *superfoods* (foods that are densely loaded with a full spectrum of nutrients, such as vitamins, minerals, antioxidants, and protein). There's no reason, other than allergies to nuts and seeds, not to take a simple, homemade trail mix with you on the go. Keep it in your car, purse, bag, or desk. A container of trail mix is the easiest thing to make and eat.

Spicy Herb Roasted Mixed Nuts

PREP TIME: ABOUT 5 MIN	COOK TIME: 15 MIN	YIELD: 12 SERVINGS

INGREDIENTS

1 cup raw, unsalted almonds

1 cup raw, unsalted cashews

½ cup raw, unsalted hazelnuts

½ cup raw unsalted pecan halves

2 tablespoons pure maple syrup

2 tablespoons granulated coconut sugar

2 tablespoons finely chopped fresh rosemary

2 teaspoons sea salt, or to taste

¾ teaspoon garlic powder

¼ teaspoon freshly ground black pepper

¼ teaspoon cayenne, or to taste

DIRECTIONS

1 Preheat the oven to 325 degrees. Line a rimmed baking sheet with parchment paper and set aside.

2 In a large bowl, combine the almonds, cashews, hazelnuts, and pecans. Pour the maple syrup over the nuts and mix well to coat evenly.

3 In a small bowl, combine the coconut sugar, rosemary, salt, garlic powder, pepper, and cayenne and stir well to combine.

4 Pour the spice mixture over the nuts and mix well until evenly distributed.

5 Pour the nut mixture onto the prepared baking sheet in one even layer. Bake, stirring every 5 minutes to prevent burning, until they're a shade darker and smell nutty and fragrant, about 12 to 15 minutes.

6 Add another sprinkle of salt, if desired.

7 Let cool on the baking sheet. The nuts will continue to get crunchier as they cool.

8 When the nuts are completely cool, transfer them to an airtight glass jar for storage.

PER SERVING: *Calories 207 (From Fat 153); Fat 17g (Saturated 2g); Cholesterol 0mg; Sodium 314mg; Carbohydrate 10g (Dietary Fiber 3g); Protein 6g.*

VARY IT! Use your favorite combination of nuts for this recipe. Cut out the ones you don't care for and double up on the ones you love. Just make sure you have 3 cups of nuts overall.

Energizing Coconut Vanilla Chia Pudding

PREP TIME: ABOUT 15 MIN	COOK TIME: NONE	YIELD: 2 SERVINGS

INGREDIENTS

¼ cup chia seeds

2 tablespoons hempseeds

½ cup coconut milk

1 tablespoon vanilla-bean powder or pure vanilla extract

1 tablespoon goji berries or fresh raspberries

1 tablespoon pure maple syrup

DIRECTIONS

1 Place the chia seeds in a bowl with the hempseeds and add the coconut milk. Let the mixture stand for 5 to 10 minutes or longer so the chia seeds can gel and form a pudding.

2 Stir in the vanilla, goji berries or raspberries, and maple syrup.

3 Let the mixture stand for another 5 minutes to soften the goji berries. Then enjoy!

PER SERVING: *Calories 319 (From Fat 198); Fat 22g (Saturated 17g); Cholesterol 0mg; Sodium 24mg; Carbohydrate 19g (Dietary Fiber 9g); Protein 9g.*

NOTE: Chia seeds like to expand, so be sure to use a big enough bowl and enough liquid to let the chia seeds grow. You can add more coconut milk if you want a creamier consistency.

VARY IT! Instead of vanilla-bean powder, try adding cocoa or cacao powder with the raspberries for a chocolate raspberry flavor.

Mint Matcha Smoothie

PREP TIME: ABOUT 5 MIN	COOK TIME: NONE	YIELD: 2 SERVINGS

INGREDIENTS

1 frozen banana

½ avocado, peeled and pit removed

1 to 2 teaspoons matcha green tea powder

1 cup light coconut milk, oat milk, or hemp milk, plus more to thin as needed

½ teaspoon pure vanilla extract

¼ teaspoon peppermint extract

1 cup baby kale or spinach

1 to 2 tablespoons pure maple syrup (optional)

Handful of ice cubes

DIRECTIONS

In a high-speed blender, add all the ingredients and purée until smooth. Add more milk, as needed, to thin the smoothie to your desired consistency.

PER SERVING: *Calories 241 (From Fat 92); Fat 10g (Saturated 6g); Cholesterol 0mg; Sodium 55mg; Carbohydrate 26g (Dietary Fiber 8g); Protein 2g.*

MATCHA POWDER: THE MOOD BOOSTER

Matcha is a variety of green tea made from whole tea leaves. It has more antioxidants and more caffeine than traditional green tea. Even though it has quite a bit of caffeine, it actually has a milder effect and produces a longer buzz than coffee because of the high amounts of *L-theanine,* an amino acid that causes relaxation and helps fight stress. This could help improve your mood and concentration.

A good-quality matcha powder should be bright green and will taste grassy, creamy, and smooth. The best ones come from Japan. They can be a bit expensive but a little goes a long way.

Chocolate Banana Super Smoothie

PREP TIME: ABOUT 4 MIN	COOK TIME: NONE	YIELD: 2 SERVINGS

INGREDIENTS

2 cups water

3 tablespoons hempseeds

2 tablespoons goji berries, soaked in water for 10 minutes

1 tablespoon coconut oil or coconut butter

1 tablespoon cacao powder

1 tablespoon raw creamy almond butter

2 tablespoons cacao nibs

1 to 2 scoops plant-based protein powder or hemp powder

2 tablespoons chia seeds

1 tablespoon coconut nectar or pure maple syrup

1 cup ice

1 banana, frozen

DIRECTIONS

1 To make a quick hemp milk base, add the water and hempseeds to a high-speed blender and blend until smooth.

2 Add the remaining ingredients and blend until creamy and smooth.

PER SERVING: *Calories 559 (From Fat 297); Fat 33g (Saturated 23g); Cholesterol 0mg; Sodium 25mg; Carbohydrate 51g (Dietary Fiber 13g); Protein 23g.*

TIP: Coconut oil is a great addition to this smoothie, but it tends to clump up a bit when combined with ice. You can use coconut butter instead, which has a creamier texture (like a nut butter) with all the fiber intact. Either will work and both taste delicious.

NOTE: You can also use the Homemade Hempseed Milk from Chapter 9 in place of Step 1, or use another type of nut or seed for variation.

CACAO OR COCOA

There's a difference between cacao and cocoa. Cacao is the bean from which chocolate is made. It's chocolate's rawest form and often shows up in recipes as "cacao nibs." Cocoa is created when the cacao beans are processed. Although delicious, cocoa isn't as well rounded in nutrients as cacao, which is considered by many to be a superfood.

We suggest that you use cocoa in baking and other heated desserts and cacao in raw snacks that don't require any cooking, such as Chocolate Avocado Pudding (see Chapter 16) or a smoothie.

Apple Cinnamon Bites

INGREDIENTS

½ cup chopped pitted dates

½ cup ground flaxseeds or hempseeds

½ teaspoon ground cinnamon

½ cup dried apple pieces, finely chopped

2 tablespoons flax oil or coconut oil

2 tablespoons apple butter or raw honey

⅔ cup oat flakes

¼ cup crushed raw unsalted sunflower seeds, hempseeds, or pumpkin seeds

DIRECTIONS

1 In a food processor, place the dates and blend until they form a thick paste. Transfer to a large bowl. Stir in the flaxseeds or hempseeds, cinnamon, apple, oil, and apple butter or honey. Use a fork or your hands to combine. Then add the oats and stir again to combine.

2 Dampen your hands with water and form the mixture into small balls by the spoonful.

3 Put the crushed seeds on a plate or tray. Roll the date balls across the seeds, coating them well.

4 Place the balls on a plate and let them set in the refrigerator for 1 hour. Store them in a glass container for a quick snack.

PER SERVING: *Calories 143 (From Fat 63); Fat 7g (Saturated 2.5g); Cholesterol 0mg; Sodium 22mg; Carbohydrate 19g (Dietary Fiber 4g); Protein 3g.*

NOTE: These apple cinnamon bites keep for up to 2 months in the fridge or freezer. They taste extra great right out of the freezer!

Brown-Rice Crispy Bars

PREP TIME: ABOUT 30 MIN	COOK TIME: 10 MIN	YIELD: 9 SERVINGS

INGREDIENTS

½ cup chopped almonds

¼ cup raw, unsalted sunflower seeds

¼ cup raw, unsalted pumpkin seeds

¼ cup raw, unsalted sesame seeds

1 tablespoon virgin coconut oil

½ cup raw creamy almond butter

½ cup brown-rice syrup

½ cup raw honey or coconut nectar

2½ cups puffed-rice cereal

1¼ cups rolled oats

½ cup chopped unsulphured dried apricots

½ cup raisins

¼ cup dairy-free dark chocolate chips (optional)

DIRECTIONS

1 Preheat the oven to 200 degrees.

2 Spread the almonds, sunflower seeds, pumpkin seeds, and sesame seeds on a large baking pan and lightly toast in the oven for about 10 minutes.

3 In a large saucepan, warm the coconut oil, almond butter, and brown-rice syrup on low heat for 5 minutes. Turn off the heat, add the honey or coconut nectar, and stir over the residual heat until blended.

4 In a separate bowl, combine the rice cereal and oats and mix in the almond mixture until the grains are well coated.

5 Add the apricots, raisins, and chocolate chips (if desired); mix well.

6 Using lightly oiled hands, press the mixture evenly into an 8-inch square cake pan greased with coconut oil. Let stand for 15 minutes in the refrigerator until firm.

7 Cut into squares and serve.

PER SERVING: *Calories 423 (From Fat 180); Fat 20g (Saturated 3g); Cholesterol 0mg; Sodium 21mg; Carbohydrate 56g (Dietary Fiber 6g); Protein 10g.*

VARY IT! For an extra boost of protein, stir 1 tablespoon of Manitoba Harvest Hemp Yeah! Max Protein Unsweetened into the almond-butter mixture after removing it from the stove. You can find it at https://manitobaharvest.com/products/hemp-yeah-max-protein-unsweetened.

Sunflower Fig Balls

PREP TIME: ABOUT 5 MIN	COOK TIME: NONE	YIELD: 12 SERVINGS

INGREDIENTS

½ cup plus 2 tablespoons raw shelled sunflower seeds, divided

10 dried figs, stems removed

Zest and juice of 1 lemon

¼ teaspoon cardamom

DIRECTIONS

1   In a food processor, pulse 2 tablespoons of the sunflower seeds until the consistency is almost like flour. A few little chunks are fine. Don't overprocess because it'll become sticky. Pour into a small bowl and set aside.

2   In the same food processor bowl, place the remaining ½ cup of sunflower seeds, figs, lemon zest, lemon juice, and cardamom. Process until a sticky dough forms.

3   Roll about 1 tablespoon of dough into a ball and transfer to a large plate. Repeat with the remaining dough.

4   Roll each ball into the processed sunflower seed "flour."

5   Enjoy immediately or store in an airtight container in the fridge until ready to eat.

PER SERVING: *Calories 58 (From Fat 32); Fat 4g (Saturated 0g); Cholesterol 0mg; Sodium 1mg; Carbohydrate 6g (Dietary Fiber 1g); Protein 2g.*

TIP: This recipe could easily be doubled or tripled.

VARY IT! If you don't care for cardamom, try another warm spice like cinnamon or ginger.

Zesty Kale Crisps

PREP TIME: ABOUT 10 MIN	COOK TIME: 30 MIN	YIELD: 8 SERVINGS

INGREDIENTS

1 bunch kale, washed and torn

¼ cup tahini

2 to 3 tablespoons tamari

2 tablespoons apple cider vinegar

1 clove garlic

Juice of ½ lemon

¼ teaspoon sea salt

2 tablespoons nutritional yeast

DIRECTIONS

1 Preheat the oven to 200 degrees or your oven's lowest setting. Line a baking sheet with parchment paper. Place the kale in a large bowl and set aside.

2 In a blender, combine the tahini, tamari, vinegar, garlic, lemon juice, salt, and nutritional yeast. Blend until smooth to get a thick consistency. You may have to add a bit of water.

3 Pour the mixture over the kale and massage thoroughly with your hands to coat the kale. Make sure the mixture covers the kale well.

4 Place the kale on the baking sheet and bake for about 30 minutes. Keep an eye on it and turn it often to make sure they dry evenly.

PER SERVING: *Calories 71 (From Fat 45); Fat 5g (Saturated 0.5g); Cholesterol 0mg; Sodium 342mg; Carbohydrate 4g (Dietary Fiber 1g); Protein 4g.*

VARY IT! Add more nutritional yeast to give your crisps a cheesier flavor.

TIP: If you prefer, you can use a dehydrator instead of an oven. Just place the kale onto 2 dehydrator trays and dehydrate for 4 to 8 hours at 115 degrees. Rotate the kale occasionally to dry uniformly.

Happy Hemp Loaves

PREP TIME: ABOUT 20 MIN	COOK TIME: 20 MIN	YIELD: 6–8 SERVINGS

INGREDIENTS

6 tablespoons virgin coconut oil, warmed slightly to liquefy, plus extra for greasing

½ cup hemp flour

1 cup brown-rice flour

½ cup coconut flour

1 teaspoon baking soda

1 teaspoon baking powder

½ teaspoon sea salt

¼ cup pure maple syrup

½ cup unsweetened applesauce or pureed apples

1 banana, mashed

1 tablespoon ground flax mixed with 3 tablespoons water

1 teaspoon pure vanilla extract

¼ cup blueberries

DIRECTIONS

1 Preheat the oven to 350 degrees. Grease 6 to 8 mini loaf pans with coconut oil.

2 In a large bowl, combine the hemp flour, brown-rice flour, coconut flour, baking soda, baking powder, and salt. Set aside.

3 In another bowl, combine the 6 tablespoons of coconut oil, maple syrup, applesauce, and banana and beat until well mixed.

4 Add the flax mixture and vanilla to the wet mixture and mix well.

5 Add the wet ingredients to the dry ingredients; then add the blueberries. Mix until just blended.

6 Pour the batter into the loaf pans so they're half full. Press the batter down to flatten. Bake for 15 to 20 minutes.

7 Remove the loaves from the oven and allow them to cool on a baking rack.

8 Serve with a tablespoon of almond butter or apple butter and a glass of water or almond milk for a tasty, high-protein snack.

PER SERVING: *Calories 368 (From Fat 153); Fat 17g (Saturated 13g); Cholesterol 0mg; Sodium 379mg; Carbohydrate 50g (Dietary Fiber 11g); Protein 8g.*

TIP: These loafs tend to crumble a bit because they're gluten-free (the flours absorb more moisture). Be sure to press them into the loaf pans so that they don't crumble as much when they come out of the oven.

NOTE: The high fiber content is why you should serve these with something to drink. They need some liquid to move through your body.

VARY IT! Instead of blueberries, try mixing in raisins or dairy-free chocolate chips.

Hummus Tortilla Rollups

PREP TIME: ABOUT 15 MIN | COOK TIME: NONE | YIELD: 8 SERVINGS

INGREDIENTS

8 whole-grain or sprouted grain tortillas

1½ cups Creamy Oil-Free Hummus (see the recipe earlier in this chapter) or your favorite store-bought savory hummus

1 bell pepper, any color, cut into thin strips

2 carrots, peeled, halved crosswise, and cut into thin strips

3 radishes, halved and cut into thin slices

1 small cucumber, halved crosswise, and cut into thin strips

Several handfuls of arugula

DIRECTIONS

1 Lay a tortilla flat on a large plate or cutting board. Spread about 3 tablespoons of hummus over the whole tortilla, leaving a small space along the edges.

2 Place 3 or 4 bell pepper strips over half of the hummus, followed by 3 or 4 carrot strips, 4 radish slices, 3 or 4 cucumber strips, and a sprinkling of arugula leaves all on the same side.

3 Starting from the side with the vegetables, roll up the tortilla as tightly as possible.

4 Using a serrated knife, cut the tortilla into equal bite-size pieces.

5 Repeat with the remaining ingredients.

PER SERVING: *Calories 204 (From Fat 42); Fat 5g (Saturated 1g); Cholesterol 0mg; Sodium 319mg; Carbohydrate 35g (Dietary Fiber 6g); Protein 7g.*

TIP: These tortilla rollups make great party food. The recipe will feed about 16 as an appetizer.

NOTE: The ingredient amounts for the vegetables don't have to be exact. Use more or less of any of the veggies. Just don't fill the tortilla too much or it'll break apart or tear when rolling.

VARY IT! Instead of the Creamy Oil-Free Hummus, try these with the Roasted Carrot Bean Dip or White Bean Dip with Dill, both earlier in this chapter.

Loaded Avocado Toast

PREP TIME: ABOUT 5 MIN	COOK TIME: NONE	YIELD: 2 SERVINGS

INGREDIENTS

1 avocado, pit removed and peeled

2 slices sprouted-grain, whole-grain or gluten-free bread, toasted

4 teaspoons hempseeds

2 radishes, thinly sliced

Drizzle of balsamic vinegar

2 pinches sea salt

2 pinches freshly ground black pepper

DIRECTIONS

1 On a small cutting board or plate, mash the avocado flesh with the back of a fork.

2 Spread half the avocado on 1 slice of toast. Top with 2 teaspoons hempseeds, 1 sliced radish, a drizzle of balsamic vinegar, a pinch of salt, and a pinch of pepper.

3 Repeat with the remaining ingredients.

PER SERVING: *Calories 230 (From Fat 133); Fat 15g (Saturated 2g); Cholesterol 0mg; Sodium 268mg; Carbohydrate 19g (Dietary Fiber 7g); Protein 8g.*

VARY IT! Fresh sliced tomatoes would be delicious in place of the radishes, if you prefer. A few arugula leaves would be a nutritious and tasty addition as well.

Chapter **15**

Sauces and Dressings

The sauce makes the meal! Sauces and dressings have the ability to enhance the flavors and textures of a dish, add moisture, and bring visual appeal. These versatile recipes are the ones that will take your meals from good to great. They bring all the other components of a dish together and provide so much flavor.

Simple steamed or roasted vegetables are elevated with a savory sauce. Leafy greens become crave-worthy with a delicious dressing. Tofu and tempeh are restaurant-quality with tasty marinades. And grains and noodles are made into a meal with herbaceous pesto.

Seeing the Benefits of Whipping Up Your Own Sauces and Dressings

We all like things saucy. Sauces and dressings add texture and creaminess and can make whatever it is you sauced taste that much better. The creamy addition of a homemade sauce or dressing can be the missing link between your wrap, quinoa, or veggie burger and ultimate deliciousness. The right topping can make the boring brilliant. It can make the same old, same old sensational. You get the idea. But beware: It only works if you make them yourself.

Store-bought or prepackaged sauces and dressings are laced with extra calories, sugar, fats, and other random ingredients like corn oil, *maltodextrin* (a processed sugar derived from corn), and potato starches. Plus, they don't have the unique touch that you can only add at home.

Other benefits include the following:

>> **Cost:** You can make your own sauces and dressings from ingredients you already have at home.

>> **Portion control:** Especially for couples and individuals, sometimes a prepackaged sauce or dip is just too much to use. When you make your own, you determine the amount.

>> **Variety:** You don't get stuck working your way through that giant jar of marinara sauce until it's gone. When you make your own sauce, you can easily try different flavors — even during the same meal.

If you're taking all this time to make the rest of your meal healthy and delicious, why ruin it with a toxic store-bought sauce? Make sure all the ingredients in your gorgeous veggie-based dishes are complementary and enhance the flavors of the main event.

Here are the basic components of sauces and dressings:

>> **Base:** Whether it's bean, fruit juice, nut butter, oil, or tomato sauce, the base of your dressing or sauce should be thick and rich to act as the carrier for the other ingredients.

>> **Vinegar or acid:** Whether it's apple cider vinegar, balsamic vinegar, or lemon juice, most dressings require an acid (although not all sauces do).

>> **Oil:** A cold-pressed or pure oil can be an amazing addition to your sauce, dressing, or marinade. It adds the richness needed to round out the flavors. The best oil to use is olive oil. It lends good flavor and offers some health benefits.

>> **Thickener:** Try using Dijon mustard, miso, seeds, or tahini to thicken up your sauces and dressings. These also help bind together the ingredients, keeping everything smooth and creamy.

>> **Added flavors:** These can come in the form of spices, herbs, or even sweeteners such as pure maple syrup or raw honey. This is what pushes your dressing, sauce, or marinade over the edge, making it unique and distinguished.

Fixing Unbalanced Flavors in Sauces

Part of cooking is tasting and adjusting seasonings along the way. Before you drizzle, dollop, or slather a sauce or dressing all over your meal, be sure the flavors are balanced and complementary to the dish. Here are a few easy tweaks to common problems when combining ingredients:

>> **Too spicy:** If you've gone overboard on the heat, try toning it down by adding something acidic (a squeeze of citrus or a dash of vinegar), fatty (a tablespoon of nut butter or vegan yogurt), or sweet (pure maple syrup).

>> **Too sweet:** Sweetness is important for balancing flavors, but unless you're making a dessert sauce, too much will ruin your dish. Try adding something bitter, like tahini, to offset the sweet taste. Although, it may sound like a good idea, don't add salt, which can enhance the sweet flavors already there.

>> **Too salty:** If you overdid it on the salt, try adding more liquid or tang, like lemon juice or olive oil.

>> **Too bitter:** To offset a bitter flavor, add a little sweetness, like apple juice, pure maple syrup, or raw honey. Be careful of going overboard in the opposite direction, though. Start with a teaspoon or two and only add more after tasting.

>> **Too bland:** This is the easiest to fix! To punch up the flavors of a lackluster sauce, try balsamic vinegar; fresh herbs; garlic; hot sauce; spices; a squeeze of fresh lemon, lime, or orange juice; or salt and pepper.

Balsamic Maple Dressing

PREP TIME: ABOUT 5 MIN	COOK TIME: NONE	YIELD: 4 SERVINGS

INGREDIENTS

½ cup olive oil

¼ cup balsamic vinegar

1 tablespoon Dijon mustard

1 clove garlic, minced

1 tablespoon pure maple syrup

Pinch of sea salt

DIRECTIONS

1 In a bowl, blender, or glass jar, place all the ingredients and mix until combined to form a thick dressing.

2 Serve on a fresh bed of greens or on top of brown-rice pasta, farro, or quinoa.

PER SERVING: *Calories 267 (From Fat 243); Fat 27g (Saturated 3.5g); Cholesterol 0mg; Sodium 219mg; Carbohydrate 6g (Dietary Fiber 0g); Protein 0g.*

VARY IT! Swap apple cider vinegar for the balsamic vinegar, and raw honey for the maple syrup to make this a honey Dijon dressing.

Lemon Vinaigrette

PREP TIME: ABOUT 5 MIN	COOK TIME: NONE	YIELD: 6 SERVINGS

INGREDIENTS

¼ cup extra-virgin olive oil, plus more to taste

Zest of 1 lemon

¼ cup lemon juice (about 1 to 2 lemons)

1 tablespoon Dijon mustard

2 cloves garlic, minced

1 tablespoon Italian seasoning

¾ teaspoon sea salt, or to taste

¼ teaspoon freshly ground black pepper, or to taste

1 teaspoon pure maple syrup, to taste (optional)

DIRECTIONS

1 In a bowl, place all the ingredients and whisk until fully combined. If you prefer, you can place the ingredients in a jar with a fitted lid and shake vigorously until combined.

2 Add more olive oil, as needed, to reach your desired consistency.

PER SERVING: *Calories 88 (From Fat 82); Fat 9g (Saturated 1g); Cholesterol 0mg; Sodium 263mg; Carbohydrate 2g (Dietary Fiber 0g); Protein 0g.*

TIP: This vinaigrette is delicious on pasta salad!

NOTE: If you prefer a milder lemon flavor, start with just 2 tablespoons of lemon juice and work up from there.

NOTE: This vinaigrette should keep well in an airtight container in the fridge for up to 2 weeks.

Hempseed Ranch

INGREDIENTS

½ cup shelled hempseeds

¼ cup unsweetened, plain, dairy-free yogurt

Zest of 1 lemon

2 tablespoons freshly squeezed lemon juice

¼ teaspoon onion powder

¼ teaspoon garlic powder

⅛ teaspoon celery seed (optional)

½ teaspoon sea salt, or to taste

¼ teaspoon fresh ground black pepper, or to taste

2 to 3 tablespoons water

1 tablespoon chopped fresh parsley

1 tablespoon chopped fresh dill

DIRECTIONS

1 In a high-speed blender, add the hempseeds, yogurt, lemon zest, lemon juice, onion powder, garlic powder, celery seed (if using), salt, pepper, and water. Blend until smooth and creamy. Then transfer to a bowl or glass jar.

2 Using a small whisk, stir in the parsley and dill until incorporated throughout.

PER SERVING: *Calories 133 (From Fat 89); Fat 10g (Saturated 1g); Cholesterol 0mg; Sodium 238mg; Carbohydrate 5g (Dietary Fiber 1g); Protein 7g.*

TIP: Control the amount of water you use in order to reach your desired consistency. Use less water to make a thicker consistency that can be used as a dip, or use a little more water to make a pourable dressing.

Basil Spinach Pesto

PREP TIME: ABOUT 10 MIN	COOK TIME: NONE	YIELD: 8 SERVINGS

INGREDIENTS

¼ cup pine nuts, pumpkin seeds, or hempseeds

2 cups fresh basil, washed and stems removed

1 cup fresh spinach, washed and stems removed

¼ cup olive oil

1 to 2 cloves garlic

2 tablespoons freshly squeezed lemon juice

1 teaspoon white miso paste

1 tablespoon raw honey or coconut nectar

Sea salt to taste

Freshly ground black pepper to taste

DIRECTIONS

1 In a food processor or blender, place all the ingredients and pulse for a few minutes until well combined. Use a spatula to scrape down the sides.

2 Serve the pesto on top of brown rice, quinoa, or whole-grain pasta. You can even use it as the base for a pizza on either a sprouted-grain tortilla or a homemade pizza crust.

PER SERVING: *Calories 103 (From Fat 90); Fat 10g (Saturated 1g); Cholesterol 0mg; Sodium 87mg; Carbohydrate 4g (Dietary Fiber 1g); Protein 1g.*

TIP: If you use hempseeds, grind them separately first and then add the remaining pesto ingredients.

VARY IT! Instead of spinach, try using kale or arugula.

Creamy Avocado Dill Sauce

PREP TIME: ABOUT 5 MIN	COOK TIME: NONE	YIELD: 8 SERVINGS

INGREDIENTS

1 avocado, peeled and pit removed

2 cups fresh dill

3 cloves garlic

¼ cup cashews, soaked in hot water for 30 minutes

Juice of 1 lemon

Juice of 1 lime

½ teaspoon sea salt, or to taste

1 teaspoon spirulina (optional)

¼ to ½ cup water, as needed to thin

DIRECTIONS

1 In a high-speed blender, place the avocado, dill, cloves, cashews, lemon juice, lime juice, salt, and spirulina (if using), and blend until smooth.

2 Add ¼ cup water to thin. If needed, add another ¼ cup (a little at a time) to reach a thinner consistency.

PER SERVING: *Calories 56 (From Fat 40); Fat 4g (Saturated 1g); Cholesterol 0mg; Sodium 132mg; Carbohydrate 4g (Dietary Fiber 1g); Protein 1g.*

TIP: Serve this creamy sauce with raw veggies, roasted potatoes, or whole-grain crackers, or use it as a sandwich spread or sauce for grain bowls.

TIP: We love a strong dill flavor in this sauce. If you prefer milder dill flavor, start with just 1 cup and add more to taste.

NOTE: This sauce should keep well in an airtight container in the fridge for up to 2 days.

Orange Maple Marinade

PREP TIME: ABOUT 15 MIN	COOK TIME: NONE	YIELD: 3–6 SERVINGS

INGREDIENTS

¼ cup fresh orange juice

2 tablespoons tamari

2 tablespoons grapeseed oil or olive oil

1 tablespoon pure maple syrup

2 tablespoons diced onions (see Figure 15-1)

1 clove garlic, minced

DIRECTIONS

1 In a small glass bowl, mix all the ingredients and stir with a fork or spoon.

2 Let sit for at least 10 minutes to absorb the flavors.

3 Serve over tempeh or tofu, which will absorb the marinade's flavor.

PER SERVING: *Calories 118 (From Fat 81); Fat 9g (Saturated 0.5g); Cholesterol 0mg; Sodium 672mg; Carbohydrate 8g (Dietary Fiber 0g); Protein 2g.*

TIP: Warm the marinade in the oven before serving. The heat brings out the flavors, making it taste even better.

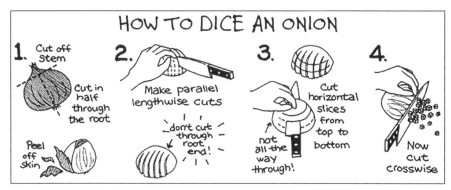

FIGURE 15-1: Knowing how to dice an onion comes in handy.

HOW TO DICE AN ONION

1. Cut off stem — Cut in half through the root — Peel off skin

2. Make parallel lengthwise cuts — don't cut through root end!

3. Cut horizontal slices from top to bottom — not all the way through!

4. Now cut crosswise

Illustration by Elizabeth Kurtzman

Tahini Miso Gravy

PREP TIME: ABOUT 5 MIN | COOK TIME: 5 MIN | YIELD: 4 SERVINGS

INGREDIENTS

¼ cup tahini

2 tablespoons brown-rice miso

1 tablespoon tamari

2 tablespoons brown-rice vinegar

2 to 4 tablespoons water

DIRECTIONS

1 In a small blender, place all the ingredients and blend until smooth and creamy. Or place the ingredients in a glass bowl and use a fork or whisk to combine.

2 Serve alongside steamed greens or roasted or mashed potatoes, or with any grain, such as brown rice, millet, or quinoa.

PER SERVING: *Calories 110 (From Fat 72); Fat 8g (Saturated 1g); Cholesterol 0mg; Sodium 632mg; Carbohydrate 5g (Dietary Fiber 1g); Protein 4g.*

NOTE: This sauce tastes especially good on Rosemary Cauliflower Mashed Potatoes (see Chapter 13).

VARY IT! For a tangy variation, swap out the brown-rice vinegar for apple cider vinegar or fresh orange juice.

Smoky Barbecue Sauce

PREP TIME: ABOUT 5 MIN	COOK TIME: 20 MIN	YIELD: 6 SERVINGS

INGREDIENTS

One 15-ounce can tomato sauce

¼ cup tomato paste

¼ cup regular molasses

¼ cup pure maple syrup or coconut sugar

¼ cup apple cider vinegar

2 tablespoons coconut aminos or tamari

1 tablespoon smoked paprika

2 teaspoons mustard powder or prepared yellow mustard

1 teaspoon chili powder

1 teaspoon onion powder

1 teaspoon garlic powder

½ teaspoon sea salt

¼ teaspoon freshly ground black pepper

Dash of liquid smoke (optional)

Pinch of cayenne pepper (optional)

DIRECTIONS

1 In a medium saucepan, place all the ingredients and whisk together. Cover with a lid offset to allow steam to escape, and bring the mixture to a boil.

2 Decrease the heat to medium-low and simmer, whisking frequently to prevent burning, until reduced and thick, about 15 to 20 minutes.

3 Taste and adjust the seasonings to your liking, adding a bit more maple syrup, vinegar, or liquid smoke.

PER SERVING: *Calories 106 (From Fat 2); Fat 0g (Saturated 0g); Cholesterol 0mg; Sodium 880mg; Carbohydrate 26g (Dietary Fiber 2g); Protein 2g.*

TIP: Serve with Vegan Burgers (see Chapter 12), Mushroom and Chickpea Loaf (see Chapter 12), or Garlic Oregano Yam Fries (see Chapter 13).

NOTE: Use a bigger saucepan than you think you need. This sauce tends to splatter when simmering, and a bigger pan will help prevent those splatters from escaping. Also, don't forget to set the lid on top slightly askew so that steam can escape but splatters stay inside.

Chapter **16**

Dreamy Desserts

If we didn't have desserts, the world would be a very sad place. Sometimes it seems we may be heading in that direction: People feel guilty after consuming a well-deserved delicious treat, or they don't consume desserts at all for fear of gaining weight or experiencing other negative health conditions. It's true that there is a lot of junk out there, so you have to be discerning. This chapter proves that you can enjoy every bite of your dessert — as long as you eat it in moderation and it's made with wholesome, plant-based ingredients.

Concerned about taste and satisfaction? You're not alone, but don't worry — plant-based desserts are just as yummy (we promise!), *and* they're loaded with fiber, minerals, and vitamins that actually fill you up, so you're not as tempted to eat that whole cake in one sitting (bye-bye, guilt).

Getting to Know Alternative Sweeteners

Sugar is sugar in any form, so you need to watch your intake of alternative sweeteners, even if they're plant-based. Be sure to eat your treats in moderation and with a conscious mind. That said, using sweetening agents that aren't as refined as white sugar is a key to healthy baking and tasty desserts, so get to know the ones you should start stocking in your pantry pronto:

WARNING

» **The liquids:** Agave, brown-rice syrup, coconut nectar, date syrup, local raw honey, molasses, and pure maple syrup. You can use these in place of regular sugar in most recipes, especially beverages. Experiment and see which flavors you like best.

Agave has substantial drawbacks, including a high fructose content. Some health experts even consider it worse for your health than high-fructose corn syrup, so use it sparingly or not at all.

» **The granules and crystals:** Coconut sugar, maple sugar, cane sugar, and Sucanat. These are all amazing in baked recipes, such as brownies, muffins, cakes, and cookies.

» **Low-glycemic:** Lakanto, stevia, and xylitol. These are great for people with blood-sugar disorders such as diabetes. They're easy to use, but they can produce an overpowering flavor, especially when baking, so use them sparingly.

TIP

WARNING

Be sure to look for green powdered stevia. Stevia is a plant leaf, so any white or liquid derivative is an overprocessed version. Keeping the leaf as whole as possible is better for you. When you use stevia, add it in very small increments because it's overpoweringly sweet. A little goes a long way.

Xylitol is not well absorbed in the intestines; it draws water into the colon and can have a laxative effect.

» **Fruits:** Apples, bananas, dates, dried fruit, and figs. These can be used to sweeten baked goods, porridge, and smoothies. They contain naturally occurring sugars and have the added benefit of fiber, vitamins, and minerals. Depending on the recipe, you may want to use these wholesome and natural sources of sugar.

TIP

To make dates into a liquid consistency, cover approximately ½ cup of dates with water and soak them overnight or in warm water for an hour and then puree in a high-speed blender. After you have a paste, you can then use it in place of sugar as a liquid ingredient.

WARNING

Artificial sweeteners, like the ones in those little colored packets at restaurants, are chemically derived and toxic to your health. Eliminate these completely from your diet.

You don't have to follow too many rules in terms of which sweeteners to use in which circumstance — you can use different types of sweeteners in various recipes. The real fun is in getting creative and experimenting, but Table 16-1 has some general matchups to get you started.

TABLE 16-1   ## Which Sweeteners to Use

Dessert	Sweetener(s)
Brownies	Coconut sugar, Sucanat
Cookies	Coconut sugar, maple sugar, pure maple syrup
Creams	Coconut nectar, dates, honey, pure maple syrup
Dark cakes	Coconut sugar, Sucanat
Dessert squares	Coconut sugar, Sucanat
Granola	Coconut sugar, maple sugar, pure maple syrup
Light cakes	Pure maple syrup
Muffins	Pure maple syrup
Puddings	Coconut nectar, dates, honey, pure maple syrup
Raw desserts	Coconut nectar, dates, honey, pure maple syrup

TIP

When substituting a liquid sugar for a granulated one, make sure to use ¼ cup less. For example, 1 cup of white sugar = ¾ cup of pure maple syrup.

No Eggs, No Dairy, No Problem!

It may seem strange to make a dessert without traditional ingredients such as eggs and dairy products, but plant-based desserts actually work quite well without butter, cream, eggs, or milk. You can use many natural substitutions.

For the sake of this book, we keep the desserts rather simple, focusing on plant-based ingredients that everyone can use and will love to eat!

Here's a quick rundown on how to make general substitutions for the foundation ingredients in the dessert world:

» **Butter:** To replace butter, use coconut oil, grapeseed oil, or sunflower oil in the same measurements.

» **Buttermilk:** To replace buttermilk, mix 1 cup of nondairy milk with 1 tablespoon of apple cider vinegar.

» **Cream:** To replace cream, use cashew milk or coconut milk in the same measurements.

» **Eggs:** To replace 1 egg, mix 1 tablespoon of ground flax or ground chia seeds with 3 tablespoons of water.

» **Milk:** To replace dairy milk, use almond milk, coconut milk, hempseed milk, or rice milk in the same measurements.

Chocolate Avocado Pudding

INGREDIENTS

2 ripe avocados, peeled and cut into small pieces

1 tablespoon vanilla extract

2 to 4 tablespoons pure maple syrup

5 Medjool dates (soaked overnight or in warm water for 20 to 30 minutes)

2 tablespoons pure, unsweetened cacao powder

1 to 2 tablespoons almond butter, coconut butter, or other seed-based butter

1 ripe banana, peeled

1 teaspoon cinnamon

Cacao nibs, coconut flakes, or raspberries, for garnish

DIRECTIONS

1 In a blender, place the avocados; vanilla; maple syrup; dates; cacao powder; almond butter, coconut butter, or other seed-based butter; banana; and cinnamon. Blend on high until well blended into a thick, creamy pudding.

2 Divide the pudding into two bowls.

3 Garnish with the cacao nibs, coconut flakes, or raspberries, and serve.

PER SERVING: *Calories 662 (From Fat 270); Fat 30g (Saturated 4g); Cholesterol 0mg; Sodium 56mg; Carbohydrate 98g (Dietary Fiber 18g); Protein 9g.*

Brown Rice Pudding

PREP TIME: ABOUT 15 MIN, PLUS 1 HR FOR COOLING	COOK TIME: 1 HR	YIELD: 10 SERVINGS

INGREDIENTS

Coconut oil, for greasing

1½ cups brown rice

3 cups water

2 tablespoons arrowroot powder

1½ cups vanilla rice milk, divided

¼ cup raisins

¼ cup pure maple syrup

1 teaspoon vanilla powder or vanilla extract

1 tablespoon ground cinnamon

½ teaspoon sea salt

1 teaspoon pistachios, for garnish

1 teaspoon almonds, for garnish

DIRECTIONS

1 Preheat the oven to 350 degrees. Grease a large baking dish with coconut oil.

2 In a heavy, medium saucepan, place the brown rice and water and bring to a boil.

3 Reduce the heat to low, cover, and simmer until very soft, about 40 to 50 minutes.

4 In a large bowl, dissolve the arrowroot powder in 1 cup of the milk. Add the cooked rice, raisins, maple syrup, vanilla, cinnamon, and salt; mix well to combine.

5 Transfer to the baking dish. Cover with foil and bake until browned and bubbly, about 1 hour.

6 Remove from the oven and stir in the remaining ½ cup of rice milk. Let cool for about 1 hour before serving. Garnish with pistachios and almonds.

PER SERVING: *Calories 161 (From Fat 9); Fat 1g (Saturated 0g); Cholesterol 0mg; Sodium 120mg; Carbohydrate 34g (Dietary Fiber 1.5g); Protein 2.5g.*

NOTE: If you use cinnamon sticks, remember to fish them out at the end so you don't crunch down on one.

Carob Fig Frozen Fudge

PREP TIME: ABOUT 10 MIN, PLUS 1 HR FOR SOAKING AND 3 HR FOR FREEZING TIME	COOK TIME: NONE	YIELD: 12 SERVINGS

INGREDIENTS

1 cup figs

1½ cups water

1 tablespoon pure vanilla

½ to 1 cup almond butter or sunflower butter

½ to 1 cup raw carob powder

½ cup hempseeds

DIRECTIONS

1 In a bowl, place the figs and water and soak until soft, about 1 hour. Drain, reserving the liquid.

2 In a blender, place the figs and vanilla and blend until smooth, slowly adding the water from the figs, as needed, to form a creamy consistency.

3 Transfer the fig mixture to a large bowl, add the almond butter or sunflower butter, and stir to combine.

4 In a separate bowl, mix the carob powder and hempseeds.

5 Gradually add the dry carob mixture into the wet fig mixture. Stir well.

6 Press evenly into an 8-x-8-inch baking pan and freeze until firm, about 3 hours.

7 To serve, cut into 1-inch squares.

PER SERVING: *Calories 115 (From Fat 45); Fat 5g (Saturated 0.5g); Cholesterol 0mg; Sodium 8mg; Carbohydrate 12g (Dietary Fiber 3g); Protein 4g.*

VARY IT! You can roll this mixture into bite-size balls instead of squares for little fudge bites on the go.

Smoothie Popsicles

PREP TIME: ABOUT 10 MIN, PLUS 4 HR FOR FREEZING	COOK TIME: NONE	YIELD: 10 SERVINGS

INGREDIENTS

1 medium ripe banana

2 cups frozen pineapple

2 cups loosely packed baby spinach or baby kale

1 cup full-fat coconut milk

1 to 2 tablespoons pure maple syrup or local raw honey (optional)

DIRECTIONS

1 Place all the ingredients in a high-speed blender and blend until smooth.

2 Pour into popsicle molds until each cavity is ¾ full (or until the fill line is reached if your molds have one). Cover and insert sticks through the holes.

3 Freeze until solid, about 4 hours.

4 To release the popsicles from the molds, run the bottoms of the molds under warm water for a few seconds; then gently pull up on the wooden sticks. If they still won't budge, run them under warm water for another few seconds and try again.

PER SERVING: *Calories 73 (From Fat 44); Fat 5g (Saturated 4g); Cholesterol 0mg; Sodium 8mg; Carbohydrate 8g (Dietary Fiber 1g); Protein 1g.*

NOTE: You need about 3 cups of smoothie in total to make 8 popsicles. If you're a little short, add a bit more coconut milk until you have 3 cups. Alternately, if you end up with more than 3 cups, simply drink the remainder after pouring it into the molds.

VARY IT! Try blueberries, mango, peaches, raspberries, or strawberries in place of the pineapple.

WHAT'S UP, HONEY?

Honey is a complicated topic, especially from a vegan's perspective. Because honey is sourced from an animal, it doesn't fit into a vegan lifestyle. Technically, however, it's derived from a plant, so it *is* a plant-based food.

We suggest that you make your own decision about what feels right for you. Choosing a local, organic, raw, or unpasteurized form of honey is, we believe, a healthy part of even a plant-based diet. However, other alternatives are available, so don't fret — you have plenty to choose from if you don't want to use honey. Because honey is a living food, it offers a slew of health benefits that other sweeteners don't, such as antiviral and antibacterial properties.

Chocolate Malted Shake

PREP TIME: ABOUT 2 MIN	COOK TIME: NONE	YIELD: 2 SERVINGS

INGREDIENTS

2 frozen bananas

3 tablespoons unsweetened cocoa powder

2 tablespoons maca powder

2 tablespoons raw cashews

¼ cup rolled oats

1¼ to 1½ cups cold almond milk, oat milk, or rice milk

1 to 2 tablespoons pure maple syrup (optional)

DIRECTIONS

In a high–speed blender, place all the ingredients and blend until smooth.

PER SERVING: *Calories 233 (From Fat 70); Fat 8g (Saturated 2g); Cholesterol 0mg; Sodium 30mg; Carbohydrate 43g (Dietary Fiber 8g); Protein 6g.*

TIP: Top with whipped coconut cream and cacao nibs or dairy-free chocolate chips for an indulgent treat.

NOTE: Maca is earthy and nutty with a caramel-like flavor reminiscent of malt powder. Turn to Chapter 4 for more information about superfood maca.

Cherry Chocolate Walnut Truffles

PREP TIME: ABOUT 15 MIN, PLUS 40 MIN FOR FREEZING	COOK TIME: NONE	YIELD: 12 SERVINGS

INGREDIENTS

1 cup raw walnuts

2 tablespoons unsweetened cocoa powder

½ teaspoon sea salt

8 ounces dried cherries, soaked in hot water for 15 minutes

1 cup dairy-free chocolate chips

1 tablespoon unsweetened almond milk, plus more as needed

DIRECTIONS

1 Line a baking sheet or large plate with parchment paper and set aside.

2 In a food processor, place the walnuts and pulse until the consistency of a fine crumb.

3 Add the cocoa powder and salt and pulse a few times to combine.

4 Drain the dried cherries and add them to the food processor. Process until the dough starts to come together in 1 big sticky ball.

5 Form the dough into balls by taking 1 to 2 tablespoons at a time and rolling in the palm of your hand.

6 Place the balls on the baking sheet or plate and transfer to the freezer for 20 to 30 minutes.

7 In a small pot, warm the chocolate chips and milk over low heat. Stir constantly until smooth. This will only take a few minutes — don't walk away or it'll burn. If you want it a bit thinner, add more milk 1 tablespoon at a time until the desired consistency is reached. Turn off the heat.

8 Remove the truffles from the freezer and dip them in the chocolate, 1 or 2 at a time, turning them so they're coated evenly. Using a fork, lift them out of the chocolate and place them back on the baking sheet or plate. Transfer back to the freezer to set the chocolate, about 10 to 15 minutes.

9 Enjoy them straight from the freezer after they're set.

PER SERVING: Calories 216 (From Fat 110); Fat 12g (Saturated 1g); Cholesterol 0mg; Sodium 78mg; Carbohydrate 28g (Dietary Fiber 4g); Protein 3g.

TIP: After the truffles are completely frozen, transfer them to a freezer-safe container or resealable bag to store.

NOTE: Any leftover dipping chocolate can be used to double-coat the truffles or use it for drizzling on ice cream, cookies, brownies, and so on.

Jam Dot Cookies

PREP TIME: ABOUT 20 MIN	COOK TIME: 20 MIN	YIELD: 20 COOKIES

INGREDIENTS

1 cup ground almonds

2 cups light spelt flour

¼ teaspoon ground cinnamon

½ cup melted coconut oil

½ cup pure maple syrup

Pinch of sea salt

1 jar of no-sugar-added raspberry or apricot jam

DIRECTIONS

1   Preheat the oven to 350 degrees. Line 2 baking sheets with parchment paper.

2   In a medium bowl, combine the almonds, flour, and cinnamon. Mix well to combine.

3   In a separate bowl, blend the oil, maple syrup, and sea salt. Add to the flour mixture and stir to combine.

4   Roll into walnut-size balls. Place on the baking sheets and press down with your thumb.

5   Fill the indentations with jam and bake for 15 to 20 minutes.

PER SERVING: *Calories 154 (From Fat 72); Fat 8g (Saturated 4.5g); Cholesterol 0mg; Sodium 1mg; Carbohydrate 19g (Dietary Fiber 2g); Protein 2g.*

Chewy Oatmeal Raisin Cookies

PREP TIME: ABOUT 20 MIN | COOK TIME: 14 MIN | YIELD: 24 SERVINGS

INGREDIENTS

¾ cup spelt flour

½ teaspoon baking soda

½ scant teaspoon salt

½ teaspoon cinnamon

½ cup Sucanat or maple sugar

¼ cup coconut sugar

2 tablespoons pure maple syrup

¼ cup unsweetened applesauce

¼ cup melted coconut oil

½ teaspoon vanilla

1½ cups rolled oats

½ cup raisins

DIRECTIONS

1 Preheat the oven to 350 degrees. Line two cookie sheets with parchment paper.

2 In a medium bowl, mix together the flour, baking soda, salt, and cinnamon. Set aside.

3 In a medium bowl, mix the Sucanat or maple sugar, coconut sugar, maple syrup, applesauce, oil, and vanilla. Add the flour mixture and stir until blended.

4 Stir in the oats followed by the raisins. Let sit for 10 minutes.

5 Drop by rounded teaspoonful onto the cookie sheets about 1 inch apart. Bake for 12 to 14 minutes. Let cool for 2 to 5 minutes on the cookie sheets; then carefully use a spatula to transfer the cookies onto a wire rack.

PER SERVING: *Calories 92 (From Fat 27); Fat 3g (Saturated 2g); Cholesterol 0mg; Sodium 76mg; Carbohydrate 15g (Dietary Fiber 1); Protein 1g.*

TIP: You can use just 1 type of granulated sweetener if desired — Sucanat, maple sugar, or coconut sugar. We provide the option of a few for variety, but the recipe works fine with ¾ cup of just one of them.

Chocolate Chocolate Chip Cookies

PREP TIME: ABOUT 10 MIN	COOK TIME: 8 MIN	YIELD: 15 SERVINGS

INGREDIENTS

1¼ cups almond flour

¼ cup unsweetened cocoa powder

½ teaspoon baking soda

¼ teaspoon sea salt

½ cup pure maple syrup

¼ cup raw almond butter

1 teaspoon pure vanilla extract

1 teaspoon almond extract

¼ cup dairy-free chocolate chips

DIRECTIONS

1   Preheat the oven to 350 degrees. Line a baking sheet with parchment paper and set aside.

2   In a medium bowl, whisk the flour, cocoa powder, baking soda, and salt to combine and break up any lumps.

3   In a large bowl, whisk the maple syrup, almond butter, vanilla extract, and almond extract.

4   Add the dry ingredients to the wet and stir with a wooden spoon or spatula until well incorporated.

5   Mix in the chocolate chips.

6   Drop the batter onto the baking sheet. The batter will be sticky. It helps to use 1 spoon to scoop the dough and another spoon to help scrape the batter off the first spoon onto the baking sheet.

7   Bake for 8 minutes. Let cool on the baking sheet for 1 or 2 minutes before transferring to a cooling rack to cool completely. The cookies will firm up as they cool.

PER SERVING: *Calories 133 (From Fat 78); Fat 9g (Saturated 1g); Cholesterol 0mg; Sodium 51mg; Carbohydrate 13g (Dietary Fiber 2g); Protein 3g.*

NOTE: We like Trader Joe's Raw Creamy Almond Butter because the consistency is loose and runny. If your almond butter is thicker, you may need to heat it up a bit and stir well to create a runny texture, which will help the cookies spread.

NOTE: The cookie dough should be sticky, not like traditional cookie dough. It helps to gently moisten the spoon used to scoop the dough so it slides off more easily.

Dreamy Lemon Bars

PREP TIME: ABOUT 10 MIN PLUS 2 HR FOR COOLING	COOK TIME: 40 MIN	YIELD: 24 SERVINGS

INGREDIENTS

1 cup almond flour

1 cup oat flour

3 tablespoons coconut sugar

⅓ cup coconut oil, softened to room temperature

One 16-ounce package silken tofu

2 tablespoons arrowroot powder

1 tablespoon fresh lemon zest

½ cup fresh lemon juice

½ cup powdered sugar, plus more for dusting

¼ teaspoon sea salt

¼ teaspoon turmeric

DIRECTIONS

1 Preheat the oven to 350 degrees. Gently spray an 8-x-8-inch baking dish with cooking spray and set aside.

2 In a food processor fitted with the S-blade, add the almond flour, oat flour, coconut sugar, and coconut oil, and pulse just until it starts to come together and a dough forms. Press the dough evenly into the bottom of the baking dish. Bake until browned and set, about 20 minutes.

3 Rinse out the food processor. Add the tofu, arrowroot powder, lemon zest, lemon juice, powdered sugar, salt, and turmeric. Process until completely smooth.

4 When the crust is done baking, pour the filling evenly over the top. Bake until the filling is set, about 20 minutes. It will still be soft but shouldn't be liquidy.

5 Cool in the pan on a wire cooling rack for about 1 hour. Transfer to the fridge to continue cooling completely, about 1 to 2 hours or overnight.

6 Dust with extra powdered sugar, cut into squares, and enjoy.

PER SERVING: *Calories 117 (From Fat 63); Fat 7g (Saturated 3g); Cholesterol 0mg; Sodium 22mg; Carbohydrate 9g (Dietary Fiber 1g); Protein 4g.*

TIP: Make sure the coconut oil is just softened to room temperature and not melted.

NOTE: Don't try to remove the bars from the pan until they've cooled completely in the fridge or they won't set up properly. Store any leftovers in the fridge.

Apricot Fig Bars

INGREDIENTS

½ cup coconut oil, plus extra for greasing

1 cup chopped unsulphured dried apricots

1 cup chopped dried figs

Juice of 1 orange or 1 lemon

½ cup water

½ cup Sucanat, maple sugar, or coconut sugar

1¾ cups light spelt flour

¼ teaspoon sea salt

½ teaspoon baking soda

1 cup rolled oats

DIRECTIONS

1 Preheat the oven to 350 degrees. Grease an 8- or 9-inch square baking pan with coconut oil.

2 In a saucepan, combine the apricots, figs, juice, and water. Cover and cook over low heat, stirring occasionally, for 10 minutes. Remove from the heat and set aside.

3 In a large bowl, add the coconut oil, Sucanat, and maple sugar or coconut sugar and cream together. Stir in the flour, salt, and baking soda. Add the oats and mix using your hands. The dough will be crumbly but will hold together when squeezed.

4 Press ⅔ of the dough into the baking pan.

5 Stir the apricot mixture and spread it over the dough. Crumble the remaining dough on top.

6 Bake for 30 minutes; then allow to cool completely. Cut into bars and serve.

PER SERVING: *Calories 252 (From Fat 90); Fat 10g (Saturated 8g); Cholesterol 0mg; Sodium 89mg; Carbohydrate 37g (Dietary Fiber 4g); Protein 4g.*

TIP: The best way to cut these into clean squares, especially for serving, is to allow the pan to cool completely, refrigerate it for a few hours or overnight, and then cut the dessert into squares.

Apple Pie Bars

PREP TIME: ABOUT 5 MIN	COOK TIME: 20 MIN	YIELD: 12 SERVINGS

INGREDIENTS

3 cups pitted dates, soaked in warm water for 20 minutes, then drained

1 cup raw walnuts

1 teaspoon ground cinnamon

½ teaspoon ground ginger

¼ teaspoon sea salt

2 cups rolled oats, divided

1½ cups peeled, diced apples

DIRECTIONS

1 Preheat the oven to 350 degrees. Line an 8-x-8-inch baking dish with parchment paper. Let the ends of the parchment paper hang over the sides of the dish so you can use them as handles later to easily pull the bars out of the pan. Set aside.

2 In a food processor, add the dates, walnuts, cinnamon, ginger, salt, and 1 cup of the oats just until a dough is formed. The mixture should be sticky; don't overprocess.

3 Add in the remaining 1 cup of oats and the apples and pulse a few times to mix. Don't overmix. If the oats and apples don't incorporate easily and quickly, turn the dough out into a mixing bowl and mix everything with a wooden spoon or spatula just until incorporated.

4 Slightly dampen your clean hands (so the batter doesn't stick to them) and press the batter into the prepared baking dish evenly.

5 Bake until the edges start to get browned and firm, about 20 minutes.

6 Let cool in the pan on a cooling rack before removing the whole square from the pan. Cut into bars.

PER SERVING: *Calories 125 (From Fat 55); Fat 6g (Saturated 1g); Cholesterol 0mg; Sodium 67mg; Carbohydrate 17g (Dietary Fiber 3g); Protein 3g.*

TIP: These bars can be served warm, at room temperature, or cold straight from the fridge.

Fudgy Chickpea Blondies

PREP TIME: ABOUT 10 MIN | COOK TIME: 30 MIN | YIELD: 9 SERVINGS

INGREDIENTS

One 15-ounce can chickpeas, drained and rinsed, or 1½ cups cooked chickpeas

½ cup cashew butter

¼ cup old-fashioned rolled oats

⅔ cup coconut sugar

¼ cup pure maple syrup

1½ tablespoons ground cinnamon

1 teaspoon pure vanilla extract

½ teaspoon baking powder

¼ teaspoon baking soda

¼ teaspoon sea salt

DIRECTIONS

1 Preheat the oven to 350 degrees. Lightly spritz an 8-x-8-inch baking dish with cooking spray or line with parchment paper.

2 In a food processor, place all the ingredients and puree until smooth.

3 Pour the batter into the baking dish and smooth it out evenly.

4 Bake until the sides start to pull away from the sides of the pan and the top is firm, about 30 minutes.

5 Cool the blondies in the pan on a wire cooling rack. They'll continue to firm up as they cool.

6 Cut into squares and serve.

PER SERVING: *Calories 185 (From Fat 71); Fat 8g (Saturated 1g); Cholesterol 0mg; Sodium 142mg; Carbohydrate 19g (Dietary Fiber 3g); Protein 5g.*

Vegan Coconut Cake

PREP TIME: ABOUT 10 MIN	COOK TIME: 35 MIN	YIELD: 16 SERVINGS

INGREDIENTS

1½ cups white whole-wheat flour

2 tablespoons arrowroot powder

1 teaspoon baking soda

¼ teaspoon sea salt

¾ cup cane sugar

1 cup full-fat canned coconut milk

2 teaspoons apple cider vinegar

1 teaspoon coconut extract

½ teaspoon pure vanilla extract

Coconut Frosting (see the following recipe)

1 cup shredded coconut flakes (optional)

DIRECTIONS

1 Preheat the oven to 350 degrees. Line an 8-x-8-inch baking dish with parchment paper and set aside.

2 In a small bowl, whisk together the flour, arrowroot powder, baking soda, and salt. Set aside.

3 In a large bowl, whisk together the sugar, coconut milk, vinegar, coconut extract, and vanilla extract.

4 Pour the dry ingredients into the wet and stir until just combined and no white flour remains.

5 Pour the batter into the baking pan and bake until a toothpick inserted in the center comes out clean, about 30 to 35 minutes.

6 Let cool in the pan on a wire cooling rack for about 10 minutes before removing the cake from the pan and continuing to cool completely on the cooling rack.

7 When the cake is completely cool, spread the Coconut Frosting all over the top using an offset spatula. Sprinkle evenly with coconut flakes.

Coconut Frosting

½ cup vegan butter

2 cups powdered sugar

1 teaspoon coconut extract

1 to 2 tablespoons full-fat canned coconut milk, divided

1 In an electric mixer, beat the vegan butter until smooth. With the mixer on low, slowly add the sugar a little at a time, turning up the speed only after the sugar is mostly incorporated.

2 Add the coconut extract and 1 tablespoon of the milk. Add more milk only as needed to reach the desired consistency.

PER SERVING: *Calories 270 (From Fat 135); Fat 15g (Saturated 12g); Cholesterol 15mg; Sodium 76mg; Carbohydrate 35g (Dietary Fiber 1g); Protein 2g.*

NOTE: Store leftovers in an airtight container on the counter for 1 day; then transfer any remaining leftovers to the fridge.

Carrot Pineapple Layer Cake

PREP TIME: ABOUT 15 MIN | **COOK TIME: 40 MIN** | **YIELD: 10 SERVINGS**

INGREDIENTS

½ cup grapeseed oil, plus extra for greasing

1½ cups spelt flour, plus extra for dusting

1 cup pure maple syrup

2 teaspoons apple cider vinegar

¼ cup rice milk

1 teaspoon vanilla

1 cup grated carrot

1 cup chopped pineapple, canned crushed (and drained) or fresh

½ cup dried unsweetened coconut flakes

¼ teaspoon sea salt

½ teaspoon cinnamon

1 teaspoon baking powder

½ cup chopped walnuts

Cashew Cream (see the following recipe)

Walnuts, chopped pineapple, or coconut flakes, for garnish

DIRECTIONS

1 Preheat the oven to 350 degrees. Grease two 9-inch round pans with grapeseed oil and dust with spelt flour.

2 In a medium bowl, add the oil, maple syrup, vinegar, milk, and vanilla and mix together for about 2 minutes. Add the carrot, pineapple, and coconut and stir until combined. Set aside.

3 In a large bowl, combine the flour, salt, cinnamon, baking powder, and walnuts. Make a well in the center of these dry ingredients and pour the wet ingredients into the well. Stir gently until all the ingredients are thoroughly combined.

4 Scoop the mixture into the 2 pans. Bake for 40 minutes. Poke a toothpick, fork, or skewer into the center of the cake to make sure it's done; the toothpick should come out clean.

5 When the cakes are cool, run a knife around the inside edge of the pans to loosen the cakes from the sides. Turn them onto plates.

6 Spread Cashew Cream on top of the bottom cake, add the top cake, and continue to spread the remaining cream over the top and sides.

7 Garnish with walnuts, pineapple, or coconut.

Cashew Cream

1 to 2 cups cashews, soaked overnight in 1 to 2 cups water and drained

1 tablespoon almond butter or coconut butter

2 tablespoons brown-rice syrup

1 teaspoon cinnamon

1 teaspoon pure maple syrup (optional)

In a food processor, place all the ingredients and blend until well combined and creamy.

PER SERVING: *Calories 476 (From Fat 261); Fat 29g (Saturated 5.5g); Cholesterol 0mg; Sodium 127mg; Carbohydrate 49g (Dietary Fiber 4.5g); Protein 7g.*

TIP: The Cashew Cream makes an absolutely yummy addition to fruit salad!

NOTE: Make sure you let the cakes cool thoroughly on a rack before trying to remove them from the pans (otherwise, they may stick because of the pineapple).

NOTE: This cake has a wet, thick consistency from the pineapple, carrot, and coconut. Don't expect this to be your typical dry carrot cake — you'll be pleasantly surprised.

PRECISE MEASUREMENTS: WHY THEY'RE IMPORTANT

Precise measurements in baking are important for optimal results. Scooping flour straight from the container versus spooning it from the container into a measuring cup can yield quite different results. The correct way to measure flour is to fluff up the flour with a spoon, then gently spoon it into a measuring cup and level it off with the back of a knife or other straight edge without pressing or packing it down at all.

It's also important to use dry measuring cups for dry ingredients and liquid measuring cups for wet ingredients.

Amazing Banana Bread

PREP TIME: ABOUT 10 MIN	COOK TIME: 40 MIN	YIELD: 8–12 SERVINGS

INGREDIENTS

⅓ cup unsweetened applesauce

1 tablespoon ground flaxseeds

2 large ripe bananas, peeled and mashed

½ cup rice milk

¼ cup coconut oil, melted, or grapeseed oil

¼ cup maple syrup

2 cups spelt flour

1 teaspoon baking soda

1 teaspoon baking powder

¼ teaspoon cinnamon

½ teaspoon sea salt

1 cup blueberries or dairy-free dark chocolate chips

DIRECTIONS

1 Preheat the oven to 350 degrees. Grease a loaf pan with coconut oil or line two 12–cup muffin tins with parchment paper cups.

2 In a bowl, mix the applesauce and flaxseeds. Allow to set for 2 minutes.

3 Add the bananas, rice milk, oil, and maple syrup to the applesauce and mix. Set aside.

4 In a large bowl, combine the flour, baking soda, baking powder, cinnamon, and salt. Slowly fold the wet ingredients into the dry ingredients. Mix until there are no lumps. Stir in the blueberries or chocolate chips.

5 Drop by spoonsful into the prepared muffin tins or pour the batter into the loaf pan.

6 Bake for 20 minutes for muffins or 30 to 40 minutes for a loaf.

PER SERVING: *Calories 166 (From Fat 54); Fat 6g (Saturated 4g); Cholesterol 0mg; Sodium 243mg; Carbohydrate 28g (Dietary Fiber 3g); Protein 3g.*

Banana Walnut Snack Cake

PREP TIME: ABOUT 10 MIN, PLUS 15 MIN FOR COOLING	COOK TIME: 35 MIN	YIELD: 16 SERVINGS

INGREDIENTS

1½ cups whole-wheat flour or spelt flour

¼ cup flaxseed meal

2 teaspoons baking powder

1 teaspoon baking soda

¼ teaspoon sea salt

2 medium spotty ripe bananas, mashed really well (about 1 cup)

½ cup coconut sugar

1 tablespoon apple cider vinegar

1 teaspoon pure vanilla extract

1 cup unsweetened almond milk or rice milk

½ cup chopped raw walnuts

DIRECTIONS

1 Preheat the oven to 350 degrees. Line an 8-x-8-inch baking dish with parchment paper. Allow the parchment paper to hang over 2 opposite sides of the dish to use as handles later when lifting out the cake.

2 In a small bowl, whisk the flour, flaxseed meal, baking powder, baking soda, and salt.

3 In a medium bowl, whisk together the bananas, coconut sugar, vinegar, vanilla, and milk.

4 Whisk the dry ingredients into the wet just until combined. Don't overmix. Make sure there is no white flour visible. (A few lumps are fine and expected because of the bananas.)

5 Stir in the chopped walnuts.

6 Pour the batter into the baking dish. Bake until a toothpick inserted in the center comes out clean, about 30 to 35 minutes.

7 Let cool in the pan for 10 to 15 minutes before lifting out and continuing to cool on a cooling rack.

8 Cut into squares and enjoy.

PER SERVING: *Calories 111 (From Fat 32); Fat 4g (Saturated 0g); Cholesterol 0mg; Sodium 31mg; Carbohydrate 19g (Dietary Fiber 3g); Protein 3g.*

VARY IT! Use the same amount of chocolate chips instead of walnuts for a fun twist. You can also add a pinch of ground cinnamon to the batter for an extra kick.

Gingerbread Cupcakes

PREP TIME: ABOUT 10 MIN	COOK TIME: 22 MIN	YIELD: 12 SERVINGS

INGREDIENTS

1½ cups spelt flour or white whole-wheat flour

1 teaspoon baking soda

½ teaspoon salt

1½ teaspoons ground ginger

1 teaspoon ground cinnamon

½ teaspoon allspice

¼ teaspoon ground nutmeg

¼ teaspoon ground cloves

½ cup brown sugar

½ cup dark or robust molasses, not blackstrap

¼ cup grapeseed oil

1 teaspoon pure vanilla extract

½ cup water

Dusting of powdered sugar (optional)

DIRECTIONS

1 Preheat the oven to 350 degrees. Line a 12-cavity cupcake pan with paper liners or gently spray with cooking spray.

2 In a medium bowl, whisk together the flour, baking soda, salt, ginger, cinnamon, allspice, nutmeg, cloves, and brown sugar.

3 In a large bowl, whisk together the molasses, oil, vanilla, and water.

4 Stir the dry ingredients into the wet until just combined and no white flour remains.

5 Pour the batter into the cupcake pan until each cavity is ½ full.

6 Bake until a toothpick inserted into the center comes out clean, about 18 to 22 minutes.

7 Let cool on a wire rack in the pan for 2 to 3 minutes; then transfer each cupcake to the cooling rack to continue cooling completely.

8 When cool, dust with powdered sugar, if desired.

PER SERVING: *Calories 155 (From Fat 44); Fat 5g (Saturated 0g); Cholesterol 0mg; Sodium 201mg; Carbohydrate 27g (Dietary Fiber 2g); Protein 2g.*

Vegan Grasshopper Pie

PREP TIME: ABOUT 15 MIN, PLUS 2 HR FOR SOAKING AND 1 HR FOR FREEZING	COOK TIME: NONE	YIELD: 16 SERVINGS

INGREDIENTS

1 cup raw almonds

1 cup raw pecans

3 tablespoons cacao powder or unsweetened cocoa powder

¼ cup flaxseed meal

6 to 7 pitted Medjool dates, soaked for 15 to 30 minutes in warm water

1 to 2 tablespoons water, if needed

1½ cups raw cashews, soaked in hot water for 2 hours and drained

¾ cup coconut cream (not coconut milk)

¼ cup brown-rice syrup

¼ cup powdered cane sugar

1 teaspoon pure vanilla extract

1 teaspoon mint extract

1 teaspoon matcha green tea powder

DIRECTIONS

1 Line an 8-x-8-inch baking dish with parchment paper, letting the ends on 2 opposite sides hang over to use as handles later. Set aside.

2 In a food processor, place the almonds and pecans and pulse until the mixture has a coarse flourlike consistency.

3 Add the cacao powder or cocoa powder and flaxseed meal and pulse a few times to combine.

4 Add the dates and process until the mixture comes together into a sticky ball. Add the water, if needed, to reach this consistency.

5 Press the dough evenly into the prepared pan and transfer it to the freezer while you make the mint cream filling.

6 Meanwhile, in a high-speed blender, place the soaked cashews, coconut cream, syrup, powdered sugar, vanilla extract, mint extract, and matcha green tea powder, and blend until smooth. You may need to use the tamper to push the ingredients down and blend properly.

7 Pour the mint cream filling over the frozen brownie crust and transfer back to the freezer for about 1 hour to set.

8 When the filling is set, run a sharp knife along the edges to loosen it from the pan and lift the whole 8-x-8-inch square out by the parchment paper handles, cut into squares, and enjoy.

PER SERVING: *Calories 229 (From Fat 125); Fat 14g (Saturated 3g); Cholesterol 0mg; Sodium 27mg; Carbohydrate 26g (Dietary Fiber 3g); Protein 4g.*

NOTE: We prefer the regular mint extract over peppermint extract for this recipe.

TIP: Garnish with mini chocolate chips and a dusting of powdered sugar for even more indulgence.

Warm Peach Crisp with Maple Coconut Whip

INGREDIENTS

7 to 8 ripe peaches, peeled, pitted, and sliced

¼ cup plus 3 tablespoons coconut sugar, divided

1 tablespoon fresh lemon juice

2 tablespoons cornstarch

1 cup raw old-fashioned oats, divided

⅓ cup brown rice flour

¼ cup raw shelled pecans

1 teaspoon ground cinnamon

¼ cup solid coconut oil

1 can full-fat coconut milk, refrigerated overnight

1 tablespoon pure maple syrup

DIRECTIONS

1   Preheat the oven to 375 degrees. Lightly spray an 8-x-8-inch baking dish with cooking spray.

2   In the baking dish, place the peaches, 3 tablespoons of the coconut sugar, lemon juice, and cornstarch and spread out evenly.

3   In a food processor, place ½ cup of the oats, flour, pecans, cinnamon, and the remaining ¼ cup of coconut sugar. Pulse until a fine crumb is formed. Add the coconut oil and pulse until combined and the mixture is moistened throughout. Pour into a mixing bowl and stir in the remaining ½ cup of the oats, mixing well so the entire mixture is moistened.

4   Sprinkle the topping evenly over the peaches.

5   Bake until the peaches are soft and bubbly and starting to caramelize on the edges and the topping is crisp, about 35 to 40 minutes.

6   Transfer the pan to a cooling rack.

7   In the meantime, scoop out the solid part only of the coconut milk into a medium bowl. There will be liquid at the bottom of the can, but be careful not to transfer any of that to the bowl.

8   With a handheld electric whisk, beat the coconut cream until fluffy. Add the maple syrup and whisk again to incorporate.

9   Serve the peach crisp with a dollop of maple coconut whip.

PER SERVING: *Calories 398 (From Fat 201); Fat 22g (Saturated 16g); Cholesterol 0mg; Sodium 8mg; Carbohydrate 38g (Dietary Fiber 5g); Protein 7g.*

TIP: Try using your clean hands to ensure that the topping mixture gets sufficiently moistened throughout after adding the last of the oats.

4

Plant Based for All Stages of Life

Get tips for sticking to your plant-based diet when dining out and attending or hosting holiday celebrations.

Discover how to get children of any age to try (and maybe even like!) plant-based foods.

Keep up with your nutritional needs as you age.

Chapter **17**

Navigating Restaurants and Special-Occasion Dining

Getting together with your friends or family to share a meal, whether at someone's home or at a restaurant, and finding nothing you can eat is awful. What should be a happy and enjoyable experience quickly turns into a frustrating one.

Although eating out when you're on a special diet can be challenging, finding plant-based options may be easier than you think — certainly a lot easier than it was 30 years ago. More and more restaurants are able to accommodate plant-based diets. Some places go beyond simply accommodating and produce some really stellar, complex dishes that are entirely plant based. And then there are restaurants that are *entirely* plant based! In many ways, this is the golden age for plant-based eaters — stigma is down, availability is up.

We can offer some tricks of the trade to help you leave the party with a belly full of yummy food, not one that's growling. This chapter outlines how to successfully navigate meals you eat outside of your own kitchen. It also covers what you can do when hosting a dinner party for non-plant-based eaters.

REMEMBER

When eating out, just make the best choices you can in the moment. You may need to accept that your meal will be more processed and contain more saturated fat and sodium than something you would cook at home. Just don't make a habit out of it, and you'll be fine.

The Ins and Outs of Dining Out: Being a Proactive Plant-Based Eater

When eating a plant-based diet, preparing the majority of your meals yourself is typically the easiest way to make sure you get enough to eat. Plus, it's nice to become self-sufficient, enjoy the cooking process, and save some money, too!

Sometimes, however, dining out is on the agenda. Sometimes these meals are on your terms, and sometimes they're not. Either way, you can find ways to make sure your plant-based needs are met. In the following sections, we offer suggestions on enjoying a restaurant meal while sticking to your plant-based lifestyle.

Finding plant-friendly establishments

Good places for plant-based eaters to eat do exist — and you can find them. If you happen to live in a big city, finding amazing little cafés and restaurants that feature specialty vegetarian delights is probably easy. If you live in a small town, you may have to be a little extra savvy, but you can still do your research and find places to eat that suit your lifestyle.

REMEMBER

A restaurant doesn't have to be a hippie, veggie-loving café to be plant-based friendly — you can find options almost anywhere. You actually may end up frequenting mainstream restaurants because they typically have more options that can accommodate many types of diets.

TIP

Here are some good ways to discover plant-friendly restaurants that can meet your dietary needs:

>> **Go online.** One of the best ways to find restaurants that can accommodate your needs is to search the Internet before venturing out. Several websites provide resources for restaurants, markets, cafés, and other stores that are accommodating. One example is HappyCow (www.happycow.net), an online resource that displays all the vegetarian and health-inspired eateries and stores in a city. It's searchable by region and diet (vegan, vegetarian, or veg-friendly), gives you price ranges, and includes user reviews. No website

can provide an exhaustive list — just because a restaurant isn't listed on the site doesn't mean the restaurant doesn't have a plant-based option or two.

>> **Ask around at restaurants.** When you find a place, don't be shy about asking about other places to try. Not only will the restaurant owner and staff members know about similar restaurants in the area, but regular patrons will know other good places to eat.

>> **Pick up local newspapers and free health magazines.** Pay attention to the newspaper racks on the street and in public places. Look for a local magazine or newspaper that lists all the restaurants in the area; these listings are often categorized by food type, making it easier to find places that cater to plant-based eaters. You may even find some discounts!

>> **Visit farmers markets, trade shows, and other local fairs and festivals.** Attending local events is a great way to sample good food and get to know the owners of restaurants that serve the type of food you're looking for. Chat up your neighbors and get to know your area in a whole different light.

>> **Tap into social media and folks you know.** Don't forget about the old adage, "It's not what you know — it's who you know." You may know people in your circle who are experts on veggie dining — you just may not know it yet. Do you have a coworker who seems to eat healthfully and is into fitness? Ask them if they have any suggestions. What about parents or teachers at your kids' school? If you're on social media, make sure to ask for suggestions there.

Navigating menus

When you're in the restaurant, it's time to navigate the menu and see what's in it for you.

The first step is to ignore the sections the menu is divided into. It doesn't so much matter where the item is listed, only that it's listed at all. As long as the item is listed on the menu, you can typically order it in any format you like. Knowing how to work with what you've got is your key to dining as a plant-based pro.

REMEMBER

You're the customer, and there's nothing wrong with ordering what you want in the way you want it. Although some restaurants won't accommodate special requests (there's usually a note on the menu indicating this), most restaurants will be happy to accommodate you and see to it that you feel just as important as anyone else.

TIP

If you have any doubts about a particular restaurant, call ahead to ask whether it has plant-based options. Some of the best plant-based meals we've had were at meat-heavy restaurants where we called ahead and asked if the chef would be willing to accommodate our dietary preferences. A good chef is usually excited to experiment and make you something amazing. The key is calling *days* ahead (not minutes), and maybe even placing a reminder call on the day of, so the chef can prep in advance. It may seem like more work on your end, but trust us, it's worth it! The chef and staff will be appreciative of the advance notice and much more willing to work with you.

Making entrees work for you

Anything on the menu is fair game for your entree. The dishes may be listed in the entree section or as a salad, soup, or appetizer. Learn to read the menu without sections, and you won't have to despair if all the entrees contain meat.

Some entrees are easier to modify than others. You can swap out meat or fish in most stir-fries, salads, and pastas. Depending on the options the restaurant has, you can usually substitute extra veggies, beans, tofu, avocado, or even nuts. For steak and fish dishes, you can possibly swap for a portobello mushroom or grilled tofu. Of course, this all depends on the type of restaurant you're in and what else it has available.

WARNING

Some restaurants may offer veggie burgers as an entree. Note that most veggie burgers served in restaurants are frozen and not freshly made, and some of those varieties may contain dairy and/or egg. Ask as many questions as you like so you can use your educated discretion. Sometimes a veggie burger is the closest thing you can find on the menu to a plant-based meal, so if you order it, don't feel guilty! Just enjoy it and know that your next meal at home will be filled with healthy whole plant foods.

Sticking with sides

At restaurants that aren't 100 percent plant-based, your best bet is sometimes going with sides. If you can't find a main dish on the menu that suits your needs, sides may become your best friend. You can eat only so many pastas and stir-fries before you get bored with the same meals. At least you can get creative with sides!

Any of the following items may show up in the sides section of a menu, so be on alert that any combination of at least three of them can make up your dinner. (And this is certainly not an exhaustive list!) Just ask for some olive oil and lemon juice or, if you're lucky, a delicious plant-based sauce that's already on the menu.

>> **Veggies:** Steamed greens; side salads; steamed, grilled, or roasted veggies; shredded beets or carrots; sauerkraut; cucumber slices; or veggie sticks

>> **Fruits:** Any fresh fruit

>> **Cooked grains:** Brown rice, quinoa, or wild rice

- **Starches:** Baked potatoes or sweet potatoes; sweet-potato french fries; whole-grain or gluten-free pasta with olive oil; or whole-grain bread, crackers, or wraps

- **Proteins:** Baked tofu or grilled tempeh, plain beans, baked beans or bean salads, edamame, tofu scrambles, nuts, or seeds

- **Soup:** Pureed or chunky veggie soup

- **Hummus**

Note: Some restaurants have a menu section dedicated to side dishes and building a combo plate. Be sure to look for it on the menu!

WARNING

Always be sure to ask what these side items are cooked in. Some restaurants regularly use butter, cream, or milk. You can ask for yours plain or with another option (such as garlic, lemon, and olive oil).

Asking for what you want

Sometimes you have to ask questions to figure out whether a food listed on the menu meshes with your needs. If you're assertive but polite, your server should be willing to help you put together a satisfying meal. One idea to break the ice when it's your turn to order is to announce in a jovial manner, "I apologize in advance — I'm the difficult one!" You can also go the earnest route: "I have special dietary restrictions, but I don't want to make it hard on you — can you help me order?" Just be sure to be clear and concise — no one likes the nitpicky person at the table. And always remember to thank them for taking the time to help accommodate you!

Depending on the restaurant, you may have many or just a few options to get creative with, but either way, you're probably going to have to ask some questions.

Ask these questions about the ingredients:

- Is there chicken or beef stock in this soup?

- Is there fish sauce or stock in this?

- Is there anchovy paste in this salad dressing or sauce?

- Is there butter, cream, dairy, or milk in there?

- Is there egg in that bread or pasta?

- Is there anything not on the menu that I can order?

TIP

You probably shouldn't ask all these questions at once; use them sparingly. Remember to be assertive, not annoying.

Ask these questions about preparation and serving:

>> Is a different grill, pan, or pot used for tempeh, tofu, and veggies?

>> Is this deep-fried in the same fryer as meat?

>> Can you serve that on the side?

>> Can you hold the dressing or put the dressing on the side?

>> Can you steam this for me?

>> Can you substitute avocado for cheese?

>> Can I have gluten-free or whole-grain bread instead?

>> Can you bring olive oil and balsamic vinegar on the side?

>> Can I have just sides?

>> Can you make my pasta without meat sauce?

>> Can you make my pizza without cheese?

>> Can I get steamed greens or grilled veggies instead?

>> Can I get a salad instead of potatoes, rice, pasta, or meat?

>> Do you have tofu or beans to put into my stir-fry or pasta?

You may decide that some of these issues, like using the same grill pan or fryer for meat and veggies, don't matter so much to you when you're eating out. Stress isn't good for anyone, so just do the best you can in each situation and don't worry about being perfect.

Eating Delivery and Takeout, Veggie Style

Depending on your lifestyle, you may often order food for delivery or takeout. However, as a plant-based eater, you may have difficulty with ordering health-fully and in a way that provides you with a well-rounded meal. Because most takeout food is categorized by culture, we give you a little guide to the best plant-based items to order, based on cuisine. (*Note:* Any of these suggestions is valid for dining at a restaurant, as well.)

Chinese

Chinese food is one of the most common forms of takeout. People just love their noodles and rice! However, be mindful of the oils and sauces, because many Chinese restaurants use poor sources of both. Feel free to ask for low sauce and oil. Most restaurants should accommodate you.

Here's what we suggest the next time you order Chinese food:

» Green vegetables and mushrooms

» Sautéed eggplant

» Steamed brown rice

» Steamed greens

» Steamed tofu

» Stir-fried green beans

» Vegetable chow mein

» Vegetable consume

Japanese

Japanese food tends to be pretty safe for plant-based diners; however, watch out for preservatives, monosodium glutamate (MSG), and added sugars. Typically, you can eat a plant-based, gluten-free meal that's loaded with veggies.

Try the following items:

» Brown rice

» Brown rice vegetarian rolls

» Miso soup (made with vegetable stock, not fish stock)

» Seaweed salad

» Steamed edamame

» Steamed greens

» Steamed tofu

» Tofu stir-fry

Some seaweed salads are made with octopus, so be sure to ask beforehand.

Italian

Italian food can be limited in terms of plant-based options, but you can usually find something. More and more, Italian restaurants have gluten-free and/or whole-grain options for pizzas and pastas, so be sure to ask or look for the fine print, asterisks, and parentheses on the menu.

Look for these options:

» Garden salad or other green salad with vinaigrette

» Whole-grain or gluten-free pasta with tomato sauce, olive oil and garlic, or vegan pesto sauce

» Whole-grain or gluten-free pizza with veggies

Be sure to ask whether the pasta noodles are made with eggs.

Mediterranean

Mediterranean is one of the easiest cuisines from which to order. You have so many options, especially when doing delivery or takeout, because you can supplement the meal with your own fresh salad and whole-grain or gluten-free breads or crackers for dips.

Here are some good items to try:

» Baba ghanoush (tahini-based, not mayonnaise-based)

» Baked beans

» Falafel

» Grilled vegetable skewers

» Hummus

» Lentil soup

» Rice with lentils

» Roasted cauliflower or potatoes

» Stuffed grape leaves (sometimes called dolmas)

Mexican

Mexican restaurants are definitely popular — people love their guacamole! Watch out for cheese, meet, and sour cream. You may also want to ask whether the refried beans are made with lard. Other than that, you should be safe with beans, rice, and tortillas.

Luckily you can choose some of these plant-based options:

>> Black bean soup

>> Guacamole or salsa with corn chips

>> Tortilla salad with beans and rice

>> Vegetable burrito, fajitas, taco, or quesadillas (without cheese or sour cream)

>> Veggie nachos (without cheese or sour cream)

Thai

Just as with Japanese cuisine, you can usually find lots of plant-based options on a Thai menu. Many Thai restaurants offer white noodles and rice as a default, which is totally plant-based (ask for brown rice as a healthier option, if you prefer). Also, look out for sauces that are oily, are fish- or oyster-based, or have added sugars and preservatives.

Otherwise, here are some good choices:

>> Brown rice

>> Green salad

>> Mango salad

>> Marinated eggplant

>> Raw rice-paper rolls with fresh veggies

>> Steamed greens or other vegetable stir-fries

>> Vegetable curry

>> Vegetable pad Thai with tofu or extra veggies (without egg or meat)

TIP

Spring rolls are healthier than fried egg rolls, but both *may* be vegan. Egg-roll wrappers sometimes contain egg, so be sure to ask.

Celebrating Holidays and Special Occasions

When it comes to holidays and parties, you may think you have to give in and go with the flow. You may think it's too much effort or not worth it to stay on your plant-based diet, because no one wants to eat what you're eating, or maybe you just want an excuse to indulge and cheat a little. But stay true to yourself — not only is this the perfect time to impress friends and family with your new skills, interest, and lifestyle, but you can also experiment with new recipes that may be different from everyone else's day-to-day cuisine.

This isn't a time to fall off track! Stick to the choice you made to be a plant-based eater and be a plant-based partier. You'll be thanking yourself later when everyone else is in a food coma and you're not!

The following sections explain how to eat plant-based at parties, whether you're attending an event hosted by someone else or throwing your own get-together.

Being a gracious guest

The best way to be a great guest is to bring something. Not only do you cover your own needs by making sure you have something to eat, but most people love it when you bring something to share. You can do this even when you're not asked to bring something.

REMEMBER

This suggestion is best for informal gatherings and potluck-style parties and may not be a good idea for formal dinner parties unless you communicate your intentions with the host beforehand. The last thing you want to do is offend someone who has spent a great deal of time putting together an amazing meal. At the very least, make sure the host knows your dietary restrictions — maybe they have a perfect meal already planned for you!

Plan ahead and maybe eat a little something before you go to a party. Or bring a small snack that no one will notice if you step out for a few moments to eat. The bottom line is that you need to feed yourself good plant-based food.

So, what dishes work best for parties and dinners? Here are some of our favorites:

>> **Green salad:** Don't just make a boring green salad — load it up with avocado, colorful vegetables, dried fruits, nuts, and seeds, and make an interesting dressing that takes your salad to a whole new level. Or, make Kale and Cabbage Slaw Salad (see Chapter 10) — it's always a party pleaser!

>> **Guacamole or bean dip:** This hearty dish is simple to make and bring to any dinner or party. You can bring a variety of crackers or flatbreads, along with cut-up veggies, for dipping. Add fun, unique ingredients to your dips or garnish them with herbs and spices to make them look fancy. (Turn to Chapter 14 for great guacamole and hummus recipes.)

>> **Quinoa salad:** Quinoa is an easy vessel for adding familiar vegetables like broccoli, cucumbers, green beans, peas, or tomatoes. Top it with a tasty vinaigrette, and you've got a flavorful, satisfying dish that works as a side or an entree. (The Quinoa Tabbouleh Salad recipe in Chapter 10 will get you started.)

>> **Vegetarian nori rolls:** Use brown rice and pack these full of veggies. This is a great, easy-to-make appetizer for any party. Most people like sushi, so they'll be more willing to try (and like) a new plant-based food.

Being a host with the most

Okay, so you're having people over for dinner — people who eat all sorts of things, including meat. Don't panic. This is your time to shine! You can make a balanced plant-based meal that everyone will love, from appetizers to desserts. But how?

First, know your crowd — make things they're going to like (or alternatives to their preferred dishes). Whether it's a hearty "meaty" meal of tempeh burgers, something with Asian flair like a stir-fry, or something light and refreshing, try to accommodate your guests.

You can be upfront with folks and let them know your menu will be fully plant-based so they can prepare and decide ahead of time if they want to come. Or, of course, you can just make it a nonissue, no different than any other dinner.

If you're putting the whole meal together yourself, you may want to choose a simple menu that you can execute alone. If you're new to plant-based cooking, select either easy recipes or ones you've made before. That way, you take out the stress of trying something new. If you want a bit of help, enlist a willing friend or family member. Even if they've never cooked plant-based foods, as long as they can follow directions, they can be of service.

Here's a sample dinner-party menu that's simple to make, with enough variety and balance that you're sure to please many palates. (Just keep allergies in mind!)

>> Citrus Wild Rice and Broccoli (see Chapter 13)

>> Black Bean Cumin Burgers (see Chapter 12)

>> Sweet Pea Guacamole (see Chapter 14)

>> Fresh fruit with cashew cream or Apricot Fig Bars (see Chapter 16)

TIP

Make your dessert ahead of time if it requires baking or freezing. It saves you time the night of your dinner, makes the dessert easier to cut, and even gives you time to decorate it.

If you're not up for doing the whole thing yourself (or you just want to try something different), try these unique takes on the typical dinner party:

>> **Host a potluck.** This is the best way to take the pressure off of yourself and have everyone contribute to the meal. However, you must direct your guests well; otherwise, you leave some dishes open to chance and may have non-plant-based ingredients lurking in your home without knowing it. One idea is to design a menu and give everyone a recipe to make. That way, you know exactly what's coming. Or, if you don't want to seem like a control freak, just give gentle guidelines about what to bring. Or be even more flexible: Make a few plant-based dishes that you can eat and have other people bring the rest of the food.

>> **Offer a cooking class.** This is a fun and creative way to get your guests involved in the creation of the meal in real time. Of course, this only works if your guests are willing to take this on, or if you're willing to take a chance and surprise them. You can buy all the ingredients ahead of time, get everything organized, and set up stations, and then when people come, have them group up at a station to make part of the meal. This can be a fun way to engage and socialize with one another before you eat, and the meal is that much more meaningful because everyone becomes part of the experience. The food will taste that much better to your guests because they're involved in making it.

Showing People Just How Fun Veggie Dining Can Be

If you choose to, you can make it your mission to inspire people to learn about plant-based diets and eat the way you do. Here are some ways to do it:

>> **Take interested people to a delicious plant-based restaurant** that serves a hearty (and maybe even upscale) meal that will impress them.

>> **Impress people by sharing something homemade with them** that's really exciting and yummy, such as Chocolate Avocado Pudding (see Chapter 16).

>> **Share inspiring stories of some of the health benefits** you've noticed from being on a plant-based diet.

>> **Talk about some of the new foods or recipes you've discovered.** Offer to share recipes when people express an interest.

>> **Invite meat-eating folks to come over for a night of taste testing.** Make your best meat-like and dairy-like dishes and dare people to notice the difference!

>> **Buy anyone who shows resistance a copy of your favorite plant-based book (this one!).** Or, if you want to go the more economical route, email links to particularly poignant articles, videos, and the like.

And, of course, here are some things *not* to do:

>> **Don't make fun of or judge anyone else's food in any way.** You may feel all high and mighty in the moment, but you should never judge what anyone else is eating. You don't want to be that person. Just think about how you'd feel if someone did that to you.

>> **Don't talk about how much better your food is.** You don't want to be a plant-based food elitist. You likely know when you have a more delicious and healthful plate of food in front of you than someone else does. But just silently acknowledge it and don't brag about it. No one will be interested in the way you eat if you do that!

>> **Don't preach; instead, lead by example.** To be honest, the less you say, the more people will be drawn to you and want to know or ask more.

>> **Don't get discouraged.** It may take a couple of occasions (or even years) for friends and family to fully get it. In fact, they may never get it, and you just have to accept that. But some of them will come around and not only want to try what you've made but also ask you all kinds of health questions. Sometimes plant-based eaters become the health gurus of the family, and people start to confess their ailments and ask for advice.

Chapter **18**

Raising Children on a Plant-Based Diet

W e can't think of a better way to raise children than infusing their little bodies with the best nature has to offer. When you start feeding a plant–based diet to your young children, you train their palates, their brains, and their bodies to become accustomed to the taste, texture, and benefits of plants (in other words, you teach them lifelong healthy habits). The infusion of nutrition that plants give to a growing body is beyond any other category of food. Here are some of the benefits of feeding your child plants at a young age:

» It makes it more likely that your children will build strong immunity right from the beginning, which will help them build a healthy constitution for the rest of their lives.

» It greatly increases the chance that they'll get all the recommended daily allowances of macronutrients and micronutrients.

» It significantly reduces their intake of saturated fats, cholesterol, preservatives, and additives.

» It takes away the risk of meat-borne illness.

» It prepares their palate to enjoy fruits and vegetables for the rest of their life.

KNOWING WHAT TO WATCH OUT FOR

One of the biggest concerns that parents seem to have is that their children won't get the right or enough vitamins and nutrients to grow strong and healthy. To do this successfully, you have to be on top of things and make sure that your child gets a healthy variety and balance. Luckily, the plant world is loaded with vitamins and minerals (for a refresher, flip back to Chapter 3), but here are some tips to keep in mind:

- Make sure that your pediatrician or naturopath knows and supports your decision so they can be on the lookout for any deficiencies that may pop up. Common deficiencies in plant-based kids are iron, zinc, and vitamin B12. One way to address this is to give them more foods that are rich in these sources. Nuts, seeds, and seaweeds are a great place to start. We highly recommend a good-quality B12 supplement because it's difficult to get enough from food intake alone.

- **Don't overfeed your kids the bad stuff.** Many parents worry that children aren't getting enough protein, for example, so they stuff them full of saturated fats and sugars. Be sure to look into all the healthy sources of plant-based protein from beans, lentils, nuts, seeds, plant-based protein powders, and fermented soy, all of which provide a healthy dose of protein.

Despite these concerns, making the choice to base your kids' diets around plants is one of the best decisions you can make.

Raising children on a plant-based diet is more doable than ever! This chapter takes you from birth through the teenage years and outlines different strategies for and benefits of feeding your kids plant-based diets.

Nurturing a Plant-Based Baby

None of us can grow up without being a baby first, and that's where a plant-based diet begins. Because a baby's food typically comes directly from their mother in the form of breast milk, it's up to her to maintain a well-balanced, healthy diet. However, you may also need to consider using formula, and eventually you'll introduce solid foods. The following sections help you move from breast milk to plant-based solids.

Understanding why breastfeeding is essential for your baby

There is no better food for an infant than breast milk. The makeup of a mother's milk offers the perfect ratio of nutrients for a growing child, especially if the mother is eating a high-quality plant-based diet. No formula can replace what the body makes on its own. Breast milk is the most essential source of nutrition, so if you're able to breastfeed with ease, do so for as long as possible. The ideal standard is six months to a year; some mothers go as long as two years. Plant-based solid foods can be introduced during that time, but a healthy mom's breast milk should ideally be the only milk your baby gets unless you face breastfeeding challenges.

REMEMBER

Some women simply can't breastfeed for various reasons, whether health concerns, cultural expectations, job constraints, or the like. Consider your own individual situation when deciding whether to breastfeed (see more later in this chapter), and don't beat yourself up about it if breastfeeding just isn't working for you.

Although some folks contend that breast milk is still milk and isn't technically vegan, this position is just not accurate. Human breast milk is meant for human babies, and there is no exploitation happening to get it. Breastfeeding your infant or using donor milk is a morally and ethically sound decision.

Here's why breastfeeding is essential:

>> **Better brain:** A child's brain grows most quickly during infancy, doubling its volume and reaching about 60 percent of its adult size by the baby's first birthday, so this is a critical time of development. Children who are breastfed are known to have higher IQ scores. A key ingredient called *docosahexaenoic acid* (DHA), along with other fats, contributes directly to brain growth by providing the right substances for manufacturing myelin so the brain's pathways can carry information. Breast milk is also rich in cholesterol; formula contains none. Cholesterol is used for building the brain and manufacturing hormones and vitamin D.

>> **Good sugar:** The predominant sugar in breast milk is lactose, which breaks down into glucose and galactose. Galactose is a valuable nutrient for brain tissue development.

>> **Smarter connections:** During rapid brain growth, neurons proliferate and connect with other neurons to make circuits throughout the brain. The more circuits, and the better the quality of these circuits, the smarter the baby. Interaction with caregivers increases these connections. Breastfed babies feed more often and are held more closely, with more skin-to-skin contact, so each

feeding encourages the growing brain to make the right connections, adding more circuits with the right nutrients.

» **Better breathing and hearing:** Breastfed babies develop a larger nasal space and a larger U-shaped dental arch that doesn't infringe on the nasal passages above. Breastfed babies are also likely to have fewer ear infections and fewer allergies.

» **Intestinal health:** Breast milk is easier to digest and easier to pass in stools. Reflux occurs less often in breastfed babies because breast milk is emptied twice as quickly from the stomach and because breastfed babies tend to eat smaller meals.

» **Reduced risk of diabetes:** Breastfeeding, plus the delayed introduction of cow's milk, reduces the risk of type 1 diabetes.

» **Higher immunity:** One drop of breast milk contains around a million white blood cells. These cells (called *macrophages*) gobble up germs. Babies have a limited ability to produce antibodies to germs. Especially from six months to a year, when the placental antibodies are gone and the baby can't yet make their own antibodies, breast milk is important.

» **Better general health:** While babies breastfeed, they're protected from a variety of illnesses, and when they do become ill, they're less likely to become dehydrated.

Loading breast milk with nutrients

It's one thing to just eat a good, wholesome, plant-based diet for healthy breast milk, and it's another thing to kick it up a notch. Here are some helpful hints for producing healthy plant-based breast milk:

» Consume more of these foods to promote nutrient-rich milk:

- Apricots
- Asparagus
- Carrots
- Grains
- Green beans
- Leafy greens
- Parsley
- Sweet potatoes

>> Drink plenty of pure, filtered water.

>> Get plenty of rest (or as much as you can with a newborn!). Lack of sleep produces milk shortages.

Understanding the ins and outs of formula

Although breast milk is best, mothers may not be able to breastfeed for all kinds of reasons:

>> Personal discomfort with breastfeeding

>> Difficulty with the baby latching onto the breast

>> Difficulty producing milk

>> A blocked duct in the breast

>> A busy work schedule and no time to feed

>> Presence of mercury or alcohol in the blood

>> A medical condition requiring certain treatments or medications

>> Breast surgery or reduction, which can prevent milk flow

As far as we know, there are no 100 percent plant-based vegan infant formulas on the market today due to the sourcing of vitamin D. You can find several soy-based options for dairy-free formulas, though. If you're thinking about going the soy route, be sure to talk with your child's pediatrician first and choose an organic formula.

WARNING

Don't use a homemade plant-based formula or plain milks of any kind for an infant.

REMEMBER

If you're unable to breastfeed, rest assured that all infant formulas on the market are developed with the nutrition to ensure proper development and growth. Now is not the time to push the vegan diet.

Starting on solids

Deciding when (and how) to put your infant on solids can be overwhelming and sometimes stressful. Typically, infants start on solids somewhere in the range of six to nine months of age.

Don't jump the gun before the baby is ready and hasn't fully developed the right enzymes to digest solid food. Feeding your child anything but breast milk in the first six months can increase the risk of allergies, gastroenteritis, infections, iron deficiency, and sudden infant death syndrome (SIDS).

Wait as long as possible and be extremely methodical about your approach to introducing solid foods. Some foods should be introduced earlier than others.

Reasons to wait on solids include the following:

>> The baby's intestines are immature.

>> The baby's tongue thrust reflex hasn't developed, and the swallowing mechanism is immature.

>> The baby needs to be able to sit up.

The old-school schedules of feeding your child rice cereal, then vegetables and meats, then cheese, and so on aren't very useful anymore (or applicable to plant-based eaters). Instead, you can introduce them to simple, soft fruits and cooked vegetables as soon as they show an interest in solid foods — often by watching what you're eating or making chewing motions. This usually happens by the time they have their first couple of teeth, around seven months. Here's a suggested timeline:

>> **At seven months,** start your baby on soft, nutrient-dense foods like apple-sauce, avocados, bananas, peaches, and steamed broccoli.

>> **Around eight or nine months,** introduce a few more foods, such as mashed sweet potatoes or rice cereal, mashed peas or green beans, or tofu. (If you feed tofu, watch for any signs of allergies or intolerance to soy.)

Introduce one new food at a time for three to four days before trying another one. That way, if any allergies develop, you can determine the offending food.

Babies, when breastfed, don't need a lot of variety when they start eating solids. The food acts as a supplement, more for the experience and exposure to new things than for the nutrition (because most of their calories and nutrients come from the breast milk).

>> **Around one year,** add things like nondairy yogurt and beans. Puffed rice, puffed millet, and gluten-free toasted oat cereals are also great foods for older babies. Brown rice cakes are great, too.

Avoid feeding your child these foods until they're at least 12 to 18 months old:

>> **Citrus fruits:** A drop of lime or lemon is okay.

>> **Honey:** Can cause botulism.

>> **Kiwi:** Allergenic.

>> **Nuts:** Allergenic, but a lot depends on your family's history.

>> **Strawberries:** Allergenic.

>> **Tomatoes:** Too acidic, which can cause a rash on their faces and little baby bums!

>> **Wheat (gluten):** Introduce gluten-free grains first, and watch for signs of celiac disease.

Introducing solid foods can seem like a chore sometimes. Try these hints as you embark on this phase:

>> Remember that it takes a baby 8 to 12 times of trying a new food before they adapt to a new flavor, so be patient and don't get too discouraged.

>> Feed solid food when milk supply is low.

>> Feed one new food at a time.

>> Skip introducing something new if your baby is cranky or sick.

>> Leave plenty of time for feeding; it's a long process.

Whipping up your own baby food

When feeding your children solid foods, you want to give them the best quality organic food. Even extremely low doses of pesticides are linked to cancer, birth defects, and more — particularly during fetal development, infancy, and childhood.

One way of introducing the foods listed earlier in this chapter (aside from offering them to your baby as they are) is to make your own baby food. It's actually fast and easy, and it saves money! You can choose exactly what goes into your baby and customize the food combinations to create new tastes and textures to suit your child as they grow. Just cut up a few extra veggies for baby and prepare them the same way (but without any spices) at the same time you're making your own dish.

Make the food in bulk and then freeze in small portions of 1 to 2 tablespoons (an ice cube tray works great for this!). Then you can pull out just what you need at mealtime.

Here's how to do it:

1. **Peel, core, and chop fruits or vegetables into smaller cubes so they steam more quickly.**

2. **Fill a saucepan with enough water to steam and not evaporate; heat over high heat until boiling.**

3. **When the water is boiling, put the fruit or vegetable into a steamer basket and place it on top of the water; steam on medium heat.**

TIP

Dried fruits, such as apricots or prunes, must be boiled with enough water to cover them in the saucepan until they become soft.

4. **Steam until the fruit or vegetable is tender.**

A knife should slide through them easily, and you should be able to mash them without resistance. Denser vegetables will take longer.

5. **Empty the contents into a bowl and mash by hand, in a blender, or in a food processor before adding any water.**

6. **Add water by very small amounts until you get the consistency you want.**

TIP

Add a little breast milk to the puree for palatability and ease of digestion because of the rich source of probiotics.

7. **Puree until it's the texture of smooth, thick soup.**

As your baby gets older, reduce the water and leave a few lumps in the food.

TIP

If needed for the sake of giving a variety of nutrients, frozen organic fruits and vegetables (with nothing added) can be convenient and are a great way to have out-of-season foods all year.

REMEMBER

Never stop feeding children the fruits and veggies they get as baby food. Don't stop when they start eating finger foods, or you'll never get them to eat broccoli when they're 5 years old!

Navigating the Toddler Years

Start your children on healthy, wholesome foods as young as possible. The younger they are, the more likely they are to know no different. If you wait until, say, pre-school begins, you may find it challenging to introduce the plant-based foods you want your child to eat. The following sections outline some foods that you may not think to introduce. We also list some of the healthiest foods for toddlers and give you ideas on how to serve them.

Introducing a variety of foods

Toddlers (ages 1 to 3) have gums that can "chew," and the enzyme production in their mouths has also become more active, so you can cut food into a size they can handle. Typically, a toddler requires approximately 4 to 10 tablespoons a day of solid food, in addition to breast milk.

Here are some foods to introduce at this age:

>> **Fruits (one to two servings per day):** Mangos, melons, nectarines, papaya, peaches, pineapples, and plums.

>> **Veggies (one to two steamed servings per day):** Asparagus, bell peppers, collards, eggplant, green peas, kale, lima beans, onions, spinach, split peas, Swiss chard, and turnips.

>> **Grains (six servings per day):** Buckwheat, millet, quinoa, rice, and teff. *Note:* You can try barley and oats after 15 months, and you can try wheat at 18 months, but watch for an allergy!

>> **Legumes (¼ to ½ cup per day):** Chickpeas and kidney beans.

Gradually, you can add more foods, such as amaranth, beans, figs, lentils, raisins (soaked and pureed), seeds (pumpkin and sunflower), and tofu one to two times per week, and you can start introducing spices.

Choosing nutrient-dense foods

You can find so many wonderfully healthy options when it comes to feeding plant-based foods to your kid. You truly can't go wrong, but if you need a little help knowing where to start, here are some of the most nourishing plant-based foods for feeding your child in the early years:

>> **Amaranth:** Most kids eat more than their fair share of white bread and pasta. If your child falls in the carb-loving camp, try serving them amaranth (a complex carbohydrate) instead. Compared to wheat, it has more calories, iron, and protein, and it has the most calcium, folic acid, and vitamin E of any grain.

Amaranth seeds have a sweet, nutty flavor and can be popped like popcorn, added to soups or stews, and used to make hot cereal. It's also sold as flour and can be used to make healthy homemade bread.

>> **Avocado:** Full of B vitamins, fiber, folic acid, potassium, and vitamin E, avocado is the ultimate nutrient-rich food. It's also sodium and cholesterol free. Per cup, avocado has 235 calories and 22 grams of fat — most of which is monounsaturated (the good kind).

Avocado is super easy to serve. For infants, mash it up or scoop bites straight from the shell. For older children, make guacamole or drizzle slices with olive oil, balsamic vinegar, and a pinch of salt for a nutrient-rich salad.

>> **Blueberries:** Often referred to as a superfood, blueberries have more antioxidants — health-enhancing vitamins and enzymes — than any other fruit or vegetable. They're also high in fiber; just 1 cup delivers 14 percent of the daily recommended amount.

Serve a bowl of blueberries as a snack; add them to muffins, pancakes, or fruit salads; or blend them with plain yogurt and ice for a nutrient-rich smoothie.

>> **Lentils:** They may be small, but lentils pack a big nutritional punch. With 230 calories per cup, lentils have high levels of both soluble and insoluble fiber and are rich in iron and protein.

Mash up and blend lentils with pureed apples, carrots, or sweet potatoes.

>> **Nut butters:** With 166 calories and 14 grams of fat in a 1-ounce serving, almonds provide plenty of calcium, fiber, iron, protein, vitamin E, and zinc. However, if your child has a nut allergy, opt for sunflower-seed butter instead.

The best way to serve nut butters is on toast, on a sandwich, or as a dip for fruits and veggies.

>> **Pumpkin seeds:** Compared to other seeds, the ones we dig out of our pumpkins each year — and often throw away — are among the most nutritious. A good source of magnesium (which strengthens nerves, muscles, and bones), pumpkin seeds contain immune-boosting zinc and a good amount of protein.

With 186 calories per ¼ cup, pumpkin seeds can add a sweet and nutty flavor to your child's favorite hot or cold cereal, homemade granola, muffins, pancakes, or yogurt. They're delicious on their own, too.

WARNING

Whole seeds of any kind are a possible choking hazard and should not be given to children under the age of 4. To serve them to younger children, grind them up in a food processor or small coffee grinder and add them to muffins, pancakes, oatmeal, or yogurt. You can also make seed butter to spread on toast or crackers.

>> **Sweet potato:** Touted as one of the healthiest vegetables you can eat, sweet potatoes are complex carbohydrates that pack a nutritional punch. Rich in beta-carotene, which the body converts to vitamin A, this root vegetable is easily digested and is a good source of iron, potassium, and vitamin C.

Serve sweet potato puree (keep the skins on for additional nutrients), add cinnamon to spice it up, or mix with applesauce, mashed bananas, or pureed carrots. For children 1 year or older, roasted sweet potatoes make a great side dish, finger food, or on-the-go snack. Cut sweet potatoes into cubes and drizzle with olive oil, which adds healthy fats and calories, before roasting in a 350-degree oven for 45 minutes or until soft.

Raising Healthy Kids and Teens

Kids and teens are potentially the most difficult age group to deal with when it comes to transitioning to healthier foods — that is, of course, if you didn't get them started young. Even if you did, you may find that they're exposed to all kinds of things you can't control at school or through friends.

The truth is, you don't have much control at this age (unless you want to be *that* parent). And if you do, your child may resist you, and you'll end up doing more damage than good. Just do your best to raise them on good principles and healthy eating and hope (with fingers crossed) that they make wise choices when it comes to food outside the home.

In the following sections, we offer some suggestions on how to help older kids give plant-based foods a chance. We also give you some ideas for guiding your kids through situations like eating lunch during the school day and attending birthday parties.

Overcoming resistance

There is no doubt that the more you push a lifestyle on your kids, the more they may push back, and — at all costs — you want to avoid this resistance. You can take many approaches with your family to get everyone on board in a fun and innovative way that's cool enough for them to want to be part of it.

Every family is unique, and there is no cookie-cutter approach to do this, so you may have to try a few different things to see what sticks.

Getting your kids involved

Get everyone involved in the process of preparing plant-based foods. Your kids are more likely not only to try new things but also to be empowered or inspired to experiment and create their own recipes. Here are some suggestions for getting the whole family involved:

>> **Treat eating healthy as an exciting adventure.** Make an experiment out of it, and have your kids track the different tastes and preferences of everyone in the family.

>> **Have the kids help pick the recipes, and get them involved with shopping and food prep.** They're more likely to want to eat meals when they take part in or maybe even control the creation of them. You can even involve toddlers by offering them several healthy options and letting them select which foods they'd like to eat.

>> **Compromise with them — especially when they're younger than 10 years old.** Make up a chart of foods you know they like (for example, pizza and dessert). They can earn stars for trying new foods during the week, and when they've earned enough stars, you can make them a healthy version of their favorite food. This practice gets them to try things they wouldn't otherwise try and gives you peace of mind knowing they at least have some of the healthier food in their bellies.

>> **For older kids, show them the evidence about the benefits of eating a plant-based diet, and let them make their own decisions.** That way, you're not the enemy or unilaterally deciding for them.

>> **Encourage an interest in fruits and vegetables by growing a garden together and harvesting your own foods.**

Compromising to make everyone happy

To make things work with your kids, you often have to compromise. For example, when you make a new recipe, always ask your kids to give it a fair chance with a positive attitude by trying at least one bite. If they don't care for it, let it be and don't force it on them. Of course, this approach can potentially create more resistance down the line when they figure out all they have to do is eat one bite to get off the hook. So, instead of totally giving in, letting them have what they want, or making a whole other meal, make at least one thing at each meal that you know they like, and let them have as much as they want. That way, everybody wins.

Another approach is to make the same recipe at least three or four times before you call it a wash. Sometimes the kids will come around, and sometimes they won't. Think of it this way: If you don't like to be asked to eat something you don't like, then don't do that to your kids.

If your child decides not to eat plant-based, don't freak out — just do your best to work with them. You may have to meet them halfway by letting them have their pick of some non-plant-based foods while still providing them with enough plant-based things that they'll eat. *Remember:* It doesn't have to be all-or-nothing.

REMEMBER

As the parent, you control what foods are in your house. But maybe you can let your kids choose whatever they want when you eat out or if they go to a friend's house. They may end up eating chips, candy, meat, or cheese. Try to be comfortable with this — after all, you know that what they eat at home (the majority of their diet) is healthy, whole, and plant-based.

Providing balanced meals and snacks

In your hectic life, it can be difficult to always make and eat balanced meals and snacks. With school, extracurricular activities, and homework, your kids can easily miss out on proper nutrition. Here are some ideas to help *you* help your kids eat well:

>> **Whether you or your kids do it, pack lunches the day before.** You already experience enough chaos in the morning — you can minimize the chaos (or at least not add to it) by doing it in the evening.

>> **Fill water bottles.** Have them in the fridge, ready to tote.

>> **Cook things in batches that make good leftovers to take for lunch and heat up for future dinners.**

>> **Pack plenty of fresh fruit in your kids' lunches, and make it easy for them to eat.** Yes, it feels like a nuisance sometimes to peel those mandarins or cut oranges into bite-size pieces and pop them into a container. Why not just pack the whole fruit? Well, kids have very little time to eat at school, that's why. So, make it easy for them to eat that fruit. Peel and slice or cut it into small pieces and pack it in a container along with a fork. Kids are far more likely to eat it that way.

>> **Pack occasional treats.** Healthy truffles or cookies seem indulgent, but they can be loaded with fiber and nutrients. (Turn to Chapter 16 for recipes.)

>> **Don't forget about weekends and after school!** Have on hand plenty of healthy snacks that are ready to eat when hunger strikes.

>> **Keep sweet treats around.** Examples include Apple Cinnamon Mini Muffins (see Chapter 9) or Apple Cinnamon Bites (see Chapter 14). They can be kept frozen and pulled out on demand for a delicious treat.

Handling occasions outside of your control

Although you get to be in control as a parent when kids are young, when your kids turn 12 or 13, look out! That's about the time when they'll decide that they are in control. Add to that the situations they encounter outside the house at school and with friends, and now you're even further removed. You have to find ways to work with these social situations that not only put you at ease but, more important, allow your children to make their own healthy decisions.

The school cafeteria and special events

Making a lunch for your child to take to school is the best way to avoid the cafeteria. If you make plentiful dinners at home, leftovers are the best bet. Other than that, you can create new lunches with your kids so they're excited about what they're taking and there are no surprises in their lunch boxes.

If your kids are on board with the plant-based lifestyle, they may not let other kids or the food served at school influence them. This may be hard to believe, but I have many friends with kids who have proven this to be true. My advice is not to fall victim to what you think their influences are; don't serve them anything less than what you make at home.

If you're encountering some challenges or resistance from your child, be innovative with lunches so your kid has something cool or comparable to what's served or what their friends may have.

Ultimately, you're trying to create healthy behaviors that will stay with your kids at any age. The goal is that they're satisfied with (and maybe even proud of) the foods they eat so they don't feel deprived or embarrassed. If you're really lucky, they'll end up feeling like they have the best lunches ever!

Here are some healthy foods you can try in your kids' lunches:

>> A hearty sandwich

>> Leftover pasta with tomato sauce

>> Hummus Tortilla Rollups (see Chapter 14)

>> Black Bean Cumin Burgers (see Chapter 12) and Garlic Oregano Yam Fries (Chapter 13)

>> Arame Soba Noodle Salad (see Chapter 10)

If your kid eats school lunches and you're unhappy with what's being served, don't be afraid to take it up with the school board. Maybe you can even be part of a committee to advocate for healthier school lunches. You can make changes to the system!

Birthday parties and sleepovers

Social situations call for a little bit of flexibility. Kids encounter many situations that challenge them (and you). Especially after you've spent years trying to mold their eating habits and palates, birthday parties, sleepovers, and other occasions present tempting treats. Your children may stick to their well-formed habits even when out, or (more likely) they'll have what their friends are having or what's being served. Many times, you just have to let these situations roll off your back and do the best you can, but here are some tips that can prevent some of this from happening:

>> Try to make sure that they eat something nourishing before going somewhere like a birthday party or sleepover.

>> Encourage your children to participate in the activities at a party but not the food (especially if they're going on a full belly).

>> Encourage them to select the plant-based options that are available (or, at the very least, the vegetarian options). If you're there with them, you can guide them.

>> Send your children with their own food. Make sure to pick fun snacks that are similar to what's being offered so they don't feel left out. Maybe the other kids will even ask them what they're eating!

Check first with the party host to make sure that none of the party guests is allergic to the foods you're planning to send.

>> Talk to the parents ahead of time to find out what they're serving or whether you can offer to make a few things for everyone to enjoy.

Once in a while, you may want to let your kids eat what's offered — things like cake, candy, ice cream, nuggets, pizza, and soda — so they can experience for themselves how they feel. They're more than likely to come home with a stomachache, which is their chance to see how their own choices impact them. It gives you a segue to talk about how unhealthy foods make you feel.

HOSTING HEALTHY HALLOWEEN CELEBRATIONS

The best way to do Halloween is to do it in reverse! Instead of allowing your kids to go out and trick-or-treat on toxic (and most definitely *not* plant-based) candy, hand out healthier versions of snacks and treats at home while letting your kids make and eat healthy desserts like chocolate cake, cookies, and "ice cream" sundaes, all from natural, dairy-free sources. They can eat as much as they want, and you may notice that when you let them control with amounts, they actually stop sooner than you'd expect. Plus, that healthy dessert also has some nutrients (and not just empty calories).

Or, what about throwing a big plant-based Halloween party so your kids can invite friends over? It's a great way to help your kids to not feel left out and introduce their friends to how normal this diet can be. Plus, you know they're sticking to the menu!

Chapter **19**

Getting Older, Getting Wiser about Your Plant-Based Diet

G rowing older can be fraught with unwelcome changes: Your body isn't as strong as it once was, you may develop a lifelong or life-altering condition or disease, or you may not have as much energy as you once did. For those reasons, you want to make sure that everything you consume is good for you. As you age, your body doesn't handle junk food or heavy foods the same way it did when you were younger, so it's critical to know the nutrients you need and to avoid foods that don't contribute to your well-being.

The physiological changes that occur with aging alter nutrient needs. As a result, packing more nutrition into fewer calories becomes a challenge for older adults, which means you must focus on quality food choices. The senior population can really benefit from a plant-based diet. This chapter outlines the positive effects a plant-based diet can have on older folks.

Knowing How Plants Contribute to a Longer Life

Eating more plants can lead to a longer life. The power they have to prevent disease and boost immunity and overall health is just amazing. In the following sections, we provide you with some of the research that proves the remarkable benefits of following a plant-based diet as you age.

Pondering how plants protect your cells

Sometimes a little hard research is all it takes to prove (or at least highlight) a point. People who follow a plant-based diet are generally less prone to obesity and disease. A small pilot study concluded in 2013 found that switching to a health-conscious diet and lifestyle can actually reverse cell aging.

The Preventive Medicine Research Institute and the University of California, San Francisco, conducted a study of 35 men in their 50s and 60s. Ten of the men switched for five years to a mostly vegan diet rich in plant-based protein, fruits, vegetables, unrefined grains, and legumes. They also exercised for a minimum of 30 minutes a day, six days a week, and did some type of stress management (such as meditation, yoga, or stretching) for an hour every day. At the end of the five-year study, the ten men who made healthy lifestyle changes showed a 10 percent *lengthening* of their cells' *telomeres* (the parts of chromosomes that impact cell aging; see the nearby sidebar), implying that the cells would have a longer life span. The 25 men who hadn't made any lifestyle changes showed a 3 percent *shortening* in cell telomeres. The study indicates that by making lifestyle changes such as exercising, shifting to a plant-based diet, and reducing stress, you can increase the relative length of telomeres.

TECHNICAL STUFF

UNDERSTANDING TELOMERES

Telomeres are the sequences at the end of a chromosome that protect that chromosome from deterioration. During chromosome replication, the enzymes that duplicate DNA can't continue the duplication all the way to the end of the chromosome, so in each duplication, the end of the chromosome is shortened. The telomeres are disposable buffers that protect the genes on the chromosome from being cut off. With each cell division, the telomere ends become shorter. The small study we mention in this chapter, conducted by the Preventive Medicine Research Institute and the University of California, San Francisco, shows that a plant-based diet can help lengthen telomeres, giving cells a longer life span, although larger studies are needed to confirm this finding.

Eating a plant-based diet lowers your risk for some chronic diseases and health conditions, including heart disease, diabetes, and some forms of cancer, according to the Boston University School of Public Health. People who eat a plant-based diet also tend to exercise more and smoke less than *omnivores* (people who include animal-based products in their diet).

Slowing down diseases

These days, it sometimes seems like a given that we're all going to contract some major disease or health condition. Many seniors suffer from myriad health problems, but if you're a plant-based eater, you may be able to avoid or reverse some of the conditions of aging.

Convincing evidence shows that plant-based diets can slow, prevent, and treat numerous chronic diseases, including heart disease, high blood pressure, stroke, cancer, obesity, diabetes, gallbladder disease, arthritis, kidney disease, gastrointestinal disorders, and asthma. There are several reasons for this. Plant-based eaters

>> **Tend not to be overweight compared to non-plant-based eaters.**

>> **Consume less saturated fat.** Saturated fat may increase the amount of LDL cholesterol, the bad kind that can increase the risk of heart disease and stroke.

>> **Consume much higher amounts of fiber (especially soluble fiber).** Fiber improves blood-glucose response in the blood; poor blood-glucose response is linked to diabetes and obesity.

>> **Consume more magnesium.** Insufficient magnesium may lead to insulin resistance, which can lead to diabetes.

>> **Consume more unrefined foods, such as whole grains, legumes, vegetables, nuts, and seeds.** These foods help improve digestion and gut health because of their fiber and help keep the cells strong and healthy.

>> **Consume a lot of foods that are rich in antioxidants.** Antioxidants are powerful protectors against *free radicals* (unstable atoms that can damage cells and cause premature aging and other disease) and are linked to a reduced risk of cataracts, macular degeneration, heart disease, various forms of cancer, and even wrinkles.

If you want specifics, here are some common health conditions that many individuals, including seniors, face, along with details about how a plant-based diet can slow or reverse these conditions:

>> **Heart disease and high cholesterol:** Heart disease is the number-one cause of death in the United States and worldwide. Of all dietary groups, plant-based eaters have the lowest intakes of saturated fat, trans fatty acids, and cholesterol, all of which are bad for the heart. The most powerful cholesterol-lowering agents are soluble fiber, plant protein, polyunsaturated fats, and phytochemicals, all of which are found exclusively or primarily in plant foods. It comes as no surprise that plant-based eaters have the lowest total and LDL cholesterol levels of all dietary groups.

>> **Cancer:** Experts estimate that improving diet and exercise alone could prevent 30 percent to 40 percent of all cancers. Consuming fruits and vegetables, in addition to eliminating animal products, is associated with a lower risk of almost all types of cancer.

>> **Obesity:** Heart disease and high blood pressure are both associated with excessive body weight. A plant-based diet can keep weight in check because of its high fiber content (which improves *satiety,* or the sense of being full), lower fat content (which reduces caloric density), and higher glucagon secretion (glucagon increases blood-glucose concentration, promotes appetite control, and increases fat oxidation).

>> **Diabetes:** Diabetes is the seventh-leading cause of death in the United States. Approximately 80 percent of those suffering from type 2 diabetes are overweight. Excess body weight is the single most important risk factor for type 2 diabetes. Worldwide, the lowest frequency of type 2 diabetes is found among populations eating plant-based diets.

>> **Strokes:** Plant-based eaters have a reduced risk for stroke because of their high-fiber, low-saturated-fat, cholesterol-free, phytochemical-rich diets.

>> **High blood pressure:** The risk of both coronary artery disease and stroke is increased by high blood pressure. Although plant-based populations have slightly lower blood pressures than omnivores, rates of hypertension are even lower because of a diet higher in fiber, magnesium, potassium, and phytochemicals; lower in total and saturated fat consumption; and possibly lower in sodium intake.

Ensuring That You're Getting the Right Nutrients

As you age, it becomes even more important to make sure that you're getting the most nutritional mileage out of every bite and sip. And that starts with making sure you're eating the right foods and avoiding ones that lack nutrients and contain empty calories.

Getting enough of special nutrients

As you age, you need to pay greater attention to and make a bigger effort to get enough of certain nutrients. Of course, which vitamins and minerals are critical depends on the health status of each individual, but some of the most important are the following:

» **Calcium:** As you age, your body doesn't absorb calcium as easily as it once did. Increased calcium excretion accompanies decreased absorption. Age-associated loss of bone density increases the risk for fractures and osteoporosis. The loss of skeletal calcium in postmenopausal women can reach more than 40 percent. Because bone fractures are a significant contributor to morbidity and mortality in older people, achieving daily calcium needs is critical, yet only 5 percent of older women and 10 percent of older men consume the daily recommended amount (1,200 milligrams per day). Make sure you get yours!

» **Fiber:** Because constipation may affect up to 20 percent of people over age 65, foods rich in dietary fiber become increasingly important for older adults. Additional causes of constipation among this age group may include side effects of medications and lack of appropriate hydration. Low fiber intake may also contribute to other gastrointestinal diseases common among older adults, including diverticulosis.

» **Fluids:** Drinking enough fluids not only eases constipation but it also helps avert dehydration, a serious threat to the elderly. Causes of impaired fluid and electrolyte balance include physiological impairments in renal function and thirst perception, reduced body fluid, and blunted medication effects. Severe dehydration in the elderly can lead to cognitive impairment and functional decline.

>> **Sodium:** Because many people develop high blood pressure at some point — typically, the higher their salt intake, the higher their blood pressure — older adults should aim to consume no more than 1,500 milligrams of sodium per day (about ¾ teaspoon of sea salt). As a group, older adults tend to be more salt sensitive than others.

>> **Vitamin B12:** Most individuals over age 50 have a reduced ability to absorb naturally occurring B12 and, therefore, must consume it in its crystalline form (through fortified foods or supplements). Vitamin B12 deficiency can cause cognitive dysfunction and neurological problems in older people.

>> **Vitamin D:** Evidence suggests that vitamin D, best known for its role in bone health, may have a function in preventing a number of diseases. According to dietary guidelines, the need for the "sunshine vitamin" increases from 600 IU to 800 IU per day after age 70 as blood levels of vitamin D decline. For the elderly, higher amounts (800 IU per day) from both fortified foods and supplements are recommended.

>> **Other nutrients:** The role of antioxidants in the aging process is worth mentioning. Zinc, along with vitamins C and E and the phytochemicals beta-carotene, lutein, and zeaxanthin from food sources or supplements, may help prevent or slow the onset of age-related macular degeneration, the leading cause of blindness in people over age 55.

Figuring out nutrition shakes

Nutrition drinks (like Boost and Ensure) have become the go-to "healthy" drink for the elderly population (and even for younger people who are in a compromised state of digestion or who aren't getting a full spectrum of nutrients). However, these well-marketed milkshakes contain low-quality ingredients, including milk powder, sugar, and preservatives.

The marketers of these nutritional drinks claim that these products meet all your nutrition requirements in one beverage, but this is far from the truth. With ingredients like canola oil, corn, maltodextrin, and milk protein, these products aren't even plant-based! They can actually be harmful to your health, causing gas, bloating, constipation, and — in some cases — rashes and other discomforts.

TIP

The good news is that there's an easy solution: You can make your own well-rounded beverages from protein powders based on brown rice or hemp. These are easy to digest and absorb and can be blended with nondairy milks for an easy drink to sip. Check out Chapters 9 and 14 for some healthy smoothie ideas.

Training caregivers on the plant-based approach

If you have limited mobility, you may rely on someone else to do your grocery shopping or deliver or prepare your meals. Maybe a relative or a caregiver helps. But you still want to stick to your plant-based diet. So how do you make sure that you get the foods you want? Here are some tips for making sure other folks understand the importance of buying and preparing plant-based foods for you:

>> If needed, conduct thorough interviews so you can select a trained caretaker or live-in aide who can shop for, prepare, and cook wholesome, healthy, plant-based meals. Don't settle for someone who doesn't support or understand this diet.

>> Research different food-delivery services that can customize or provide healthy meals or fresh groceries to your door. Many seniors use Meals on Wheels (www.mealsonwheelsamerica.org), but if you've got extra funds, you can use a plant-based food-delivery service, like Purple Carrot (www.purplecarrot.com), Splendid Spoon (https://splendidspoon.com), or Veestro (www.veestro.com). Make sure to inquire about plant-based menus before committing to any service. Don't be afraid to stand up for yourself (or get a loved one to make the call for you).

>> Keep your eyes and ears open for other plant-based seniors who are in a similar situation and find out what they do, or maybe team up with them for group meals or recipe exchanges.

>> If someone else does your shopping, give them a crash course on how to navigate nutrition labels (see Chapter 8 for a refresher).

Preparing plant-based foods for easier consumption

Traditional chewing may become more difficult over the years. Mouths, teeth, and metabolism all change. The way you crunched or munched on a salad or sandwich in the past may no longer be appealing or possible. But the good news is that you can always modify foods by mincing and pureeing in order to minimize the amount of chewing necessary, while allowing you to get the nutrients you need.

You can get excellent nutrition on a soft-food or cut-up diet. If eating crunchy fruits and vegetables is difficult, try softer options! Use ripe fruits, such as bananas, berries, kiwi, mangos, melons, nectarines, papaya, peaches, and pears. You may also find cooked or steamed vegetables easier to eat, so try soft-cooked eggplant, potatoes, squash, sweet potatoes, yams, zucchini, and other veggies, and don't forget about a nicely marinated or seasoned serving of tofu.

Here's a quick list of plant-based soft foods:

>> Applesauce

>> Fruit or green smoothies

>> Fruit purees

>> Homemade vegetable juices

>> Soft grains, such as porridge (see the recipes in Chapter 9)

>> Soft proteins, such as tofu or pureed or blended beans

>> Soft, ripe fruits

>> Steamed or cooked vegetables

>> Vegetable soup purees

TIP

Invest in a good juicer, blender, and/or food processor so you can easily make nutritious juice blends and pureed foods at home.

Working with Prescriptions and Diet

Your diet accounts for most of the health benefits you reap from a healthy life-style, so staying on (or even starting) a plant-based diet throughout your senior years can make a huge positive impact — naturally.

Many members of the aging population take at least one prescription drug. Doctors prescribe medications for seniors at an alarmingly high rate. And although *some* of these medications are no doubt warranted, many are not. Unfortunately, this overreliance on medication has taken a toll on seniors' health. Consider how many times a prescribed pill causes another ailment or condition as a side effect, prompting the doctor to prescribe another pill, and it turns into a vicious cycle.

Over the years, this perpetual medicating can drastically age someone and cause more harm than good. Although we're in no position to tell anyone to stop taking their medications, we do suggest that the more you work with your diet to increase the nutrients you get from whole foods, the more likely it is that you'll boost your health naturally. The good news is that, in time, you and your doctor may find that you can gradually wean off of the pills you thought you would have to take for the rest of your life!

Don't stop taking any prescribed medication without first consulting with your healthcare provider.

Taking fewer pills, getting more health

If you want to live a long and healthy life, avoiding drugs as much as possible — even those that are prescribed to you — is a good idea. Of course, you should always consult with your healthcare provider if you want to go this route.

You probably don't expect your medications to harm you — after all, they're usually prescribed for a reason — but keep in mind that taking drugs, especially painkillers or multiple drugs, can pose great risks to your health.

Now, we're not telling you to throw out all your pills. That would be reckless. Instead, we recommend that you take time to understand the risks and benefits of a drug *before* you opt for treatment. You have to make the right choice for yourself and work with your healthcare practitioner to come to the best solution. You may need to take certain medications in spite of your plant-based diet, and that's okay.

Your health doesn't have to be dependent on drugs. Instead, you can ease (or avoid) health complications when you commit to a healthy, active lifestyle — including a plant-based diet. And if there are one or two medications you *have* to take, that's okay. *Remember:* It's your body, not your doctor's or your pharmacist's, so it's up to you to decide which drugs to take, if any.

You can find so many wonderful ways to offset the use and effects of drugs. The world of natural medicine, if approached in a balanced way, includes therapies like supplements, homeopathic remedies, acupuncture, chiropractic care, and dietary protocols that are 100 percent plant-based. These methods have been known to lessen, or in some cases even reverse, the effects of conditions like diabetes and cancer, and people can often stop taking their medications over a period of time (with the guidance of their healthcare practitioner, of course).

Staying well naturally, without the use of drugs or even frequent conventional medical care, is not only possible, but it may be the most successful strategy you can employ to increase your longevity. If you adhere to a healthy lifestyle, you may not ever need medications in the first place.

Search online for nutritionally oriented physicians who avoid prescribing pharmaceuticals, or ask around to find a physician like this in your area.

Table 19-1 shows a few common medical conditions and potential plant-based treatments.

TABLE 19-1 **Natural Treatment Alternatives for Common Ailments**

Health Condition	Natural Alternative
Acid reflux	Lose weight and avoid heavy meals after 6 p.m. Eat alkaline foods like fruits, green veggies, nuts, seeds, and whole grains.
Arthritis	Try daily stretching exercises, pool workouts, and physical therapy. Eat sulfur-containing foods like asparagus, garlic, and onions. Flaxseeds, pineapple, and rice bran are also known to be helpful.
Common cold	Have confidence in the knowledge that colds are caused by viruses, and antibiotics kill only bacteria. Consume fresh vitamin C from broccoli and other green vegetables, citrus fruits, and strawberries.
High blood pressure	Engage in *biofeedback* (a process in which different instruments give you information on and help you improve your health) or try yoga. Eat foods like apples, bananas, broccoli, cabbage, and squash, along with grains like buckwheat and millet.
High cholesterol	Lose weight, exercise regularly, and eat nutritious and high-fiber plant foods like apples, bananas, carrots, dried beans, garlic, and grapefruit.
High blood sugar	Engage in regular vigorous exercise and work with a nutritionist to get the weight off. Eat a diet rich in fiber from beans, leafy vegetables, and whole grains.

A key reason doctors prescribe so many medications is that (understandably) the vast majority of patients want a quick fix. After all, who likes being sick or in pain? However, you can do a lot to help yourself through diet.

TIP

Good health requires lifestyle changes and a few dollars spent out of pocket. The truth is, many seniors should meet with a nutritionist or fitness trainer (you don't have to wait until you're older to do that!). Sometimes people reject this option because their health insurance won't pay for it, but see if you can save up a little so you don't have to allow your insurance company to control your health and, ultimately, your longevity. Sock away some money so you can access the care you want and need.

Recognizing dangerous interactions between medicines and foods

Healthy eating is critical for people who are battling long-term diseases. In fact, it can help reverse a condition or reduce the need for medication. But even healthy foods, including fruits and vegetables, can cause unintended and possibly dangerous interactions with certain medications.

Perhaps the best-known example is grapefruit, which, along with pomegranate, can alter the way certain cholesterol medications work. An enzyme in grapefruit juice blocks the wall of the intestine and prevents many drugs, including cholesterol medications, from being absorbed into the body.

Other examples include leafy green veggies, such as kale and spinach. Their high vitamin K levels pose risks for patients being treated with blood thinners to prevent strokes. The following foods have also been known, anecdotally, to interfere with blood thinners; however, the scientific research is inconclusive:

>> Avocados

>> Cranberry juice

>> Flaxseeds

>> Garlic

>> Ginger

>> Mangos

>> Papayas

>> Seaweed

>> Soy

REMEMBER

To minimize your risk, make sure that you keep your healthcare provider up to date about the medications and natural products you're taking. This includes vitamins, minerals, and herbal products.

If you're eating a plant-based diet, tell your doctor or pharmacist so they can help you avoid interactions like the ones we mention.

5

The Part of Tens

Find out which foods are surprisingly not always plant based.

Explore how you can boost your immune system with super-nutritious plant-based foods.

Discover reasons you won't ever want to eat meat again.

Chapter **20**

Ten Foods That Are Surprisingly Not Plant Based

Don't be fooled — some non-plant-based foods present themselves as plant-based. Look closely at labels on these innocent-looking foods, and you may find ingredients you don't want in your body. Some of the foods you think are safe actually aren't. This chapter gives you a rundown of some common foods that may be fooling you.

Bread

This supermarket aisle is usually a disappointment for plant-based eaters. Many well-known national brands use non-plant-based ingredients. Many whole-wheat breads contain milk products, for example, and some traditional Italian breads contain lard. But better supermarkets also stock bread from a local bakery — you have to check the ingredients, but locally baked bread is frequently vegan. (Oddly, these local breads are often kept in a different aisle than the national brands.)

The solution? Look for breads that are made from 100 percent whole grains and have either active cultures (for sourdough bread) or other added ingredients like nuts, seeds, or even legumes. You should be able to recognize every ingredient in your bread. If you're savvy in the kitchen, make your own bread instead. (Check out *Bread Making For Dummies* by Wendy Jo Peterson, MS, RDN [Wiley], for lots of great recipes and bread-making tips.)

WARNING

Don't confuse locally baked breads with ones from the supermarket's in-house bakery, which typically bakes some of the most compromising bread ever produced. Check the ingredients and you'll see what we're talking about.

Veggie Burgers or Sausages

It's funny to think that a veggie burger may have non-plant-based ingredients in it. That's why you have to be extremely vigilant about reading labels. Many brands contain trace amounts of milk or eggs.

The solution? Be sure to look for brands that are made exclusively from organic soy (and not isolated soy protein, which is extremely processed), tempeh, whole grains, or nuts and seeds, with just veggies and herbs added.

Worcestershire Sauce

Worcestershire sauce contains anchovies, which are certainly not suitable for plant-based eaters.

The solution? Annie's and The Wizard's both have vegan versions of Worcestershire sauce. Or just grab a bottle of *tamari* (fermented soy sauce). Tamari is completely vegan and can be used in place of Worcestershire sauce, both in recipes and as a condiment.

Alcoholic Beverages

The one item that we're sure you don't want to know contains non-plant-based ingredients is alcohol. Unfortunately, most filtering practices use some kind of animal product, particularly in the production of beers, wines, and ciders.

The solution? Vegan wines do exist! Of course, when you buy one, you're probably getting a beverage that's also organic or local (and will therefore likely taste better). Do some exploring and try something new. You can usually find alternatives at your local liquor store, bar, or winery. Just ask!

Noodles and Pasta

Many noodles in restaurants and stores are made with eggs, which is fair, because traditional pasta includes eggs as part of the recipe.

The solution? Most dried pasta varieties that are whole-grain and gluten-free are suitable for plant-based eaters, because they're made with just the whole grain and water. If you're dining out, ask your server about the pasta to make sure it's egg-free (turn to Chapter 17 for more ideas about how to navigate restaurant dining).

Dairy-Free Cheese

Although you may assume that soy-, nut-, and rice-based "cheeses" are non-dairy, they often contain some form of casein or whey protein.

The solution? To be safe, look for products labeled "vegan," which indicates that they are, in fact, dairy-free. Be sure to read all the ingredients, searching for words like *rennet, evaporated milk powder,* or *casein,* and make sure to avoid them. You can also try making your own dairy-free cheeses from cashews. Nutritional yeast is also a great solution, along with avocado. See Chapter 7 for a list of alternatives to cheese.

Granola

Granola is traditionally prepared with a mixture of raw grains, dried fruits, nuts, and seeds that are tossed with a sweetener and either butter or oil. Although there's no rule of thumb about which granolas use which fats, oil-based granola is often labeled as such. However, if you're at a buffet, resort, or restaurant, there's no way of knowing where the granola was sourced or what it's made of if it's not made in-house.

The solution? Luckily, granola is incredibly easy to prepare and makes your home smell wonderful as it bakes. Try out our Morning Millet Granola recipe in Chapter 9 and see for yourself!

Boxed Cereal and Cereal Bars

More boxed cereals than you'd ever suspect contain some form of dairy, even "health food" and "natural" cereals. Usually they contain casein, nonfat milk powder, whey protein, or whey protein isolates.

Aside from the obvious yogurt varieties, many cereal bars contain some form of dairy — typically butter fat, casein, milk powder, or whey.

The solution? Many varieties of cereal are now made from whole grains with no added traces of dairy. Look for brands that are relatively plain so you can upgrade them yourself at home with almond milk, rice milk, and other toppings, such as coconut and fruit. Making oatmeal from scratch is another safe solution to make sure that your breakfast is clean and plant based.

Orange Juice

Orange juice that is enriched with omega-3 fatty acids can have traces of fish oils. Not something you expected to hear, right? Most omega-3-enriched drinks or foods (such as bread, margarine, and olive oil) also may contain fish-based rather than plant-based sources of omega-3 fatty acids.

The solution? Don't buy boxed juices. Instead, make your own fresh-pressed juices or, if you must buy premade juice, look for juices that are 100 percent from fruit sources and not enriched with other nutrients.

Veggie Soups and Curries

Be wary of some seemingly vegetarian stocks in restaurants and even on store shelves. They may contain traces of animal fats or other animal products. Thai vegetable curries often contain fish stock or shrimp paste, and Indian-based curries may contain *ghee* (clarified butter).

The solution? Always double-check with your server in a restaurant to make sure the soup or curry is vegan and always read labels when shopping for products in the grocery store. The other option is to make your own stocks from leftover veggie scraps, sea vegetables, and herbs. This is the cleanest way to enjoy a broth, and you know exactly what's going into it!

Chapter **21**

Ten Plant-Based Foods That Boost Your Immunity

The plant world contains a natural army of foods that are ready to fight — infections, that is! Getting a steady supply of the following foods helps you build up immunity so that, when that cold comes for you, you may be able to block it entirely — or, at the very least, not be affected as much. In addition to eating these ten foods regularly, you can use them to make home remedies at the first sign of a cold or flu!

Garlic

One of the most pungent of the plant kingdom inhabitants, garlic contains the immune-stimulating compound *allicin*, which promotes the activity of white blood cells to destroy cold and flu viruses. It also stimulates other immune cells, which fight viral, fungal, and bacterial infections. Garlic kills with near 100 percent effectiveness the human rhinovirus, which causes colds, common flu, and respiratory viruses.

Because allicin is released when you cut, chop, chew, or crush raw cloves, allow freshly chopped garlic to stand for 10 minutes and then cook it, sprinkle it over foods, drop it into soup, or swallow bits of garlic with some water like a pill.

Onions

Onions, like garlic, contain allicin. They also contain *quercetin,* a nutrient that breaks up mucus in your head and chest while boosting your immune system. Additionally, the pungency of onions increases your blood circulation and makes you sweat, which is helpful during cold weather to help prevent infections. Consuming raw onion within a few hours of the first symptoms of a cold or flu produces a strong immune effect.

TIP

Adding chopped onions to your favorite soup or cooked recipe is a great way to enjoy them.

Ginger

Spicy, pungent, and delicious, ginger reduces fevers, soothes sore throats, and encourages coughing to remove mucus from the chest. Anti-inflammatory chemicals like *shogaol* and *gingerol* give ginger that spicy kick that stimulates blood circulation and opens your sinuses. Improved circulation means more oxygen is getting to your tissues to help remove toxins and viruses. Research has indicated that ginger can help prevent and treat the flu. Ginger is also extremely helpful for stomachaches, nausea, and headaches.

TIP

If you're feeling a little sickly, a homemade ginger tea is one of the best things you can drink. Slice some fresh ginger root, place it into a pot with water, and bring to a boil. Then drop in a bit of lemon juice or cayenne, which makes the tea that much more effective at nourishing and purifying your system.

Cayenne

The cayenne family of hot peppers (cayenne, habanero, Scotch bonnet, and bird peppers, to name a few) contains *capsicum,* a rich source of vitamin C and bioflavonoids, which aid your immune system in fighting colds and flus. It does this by increasing the production of white blood cells, which cleanse your cells and tissues of toxins. Cayenne pepper is also full of beta-carotene and antioxidants that support your immune system and help build healthy mucus membrane tissue that defends against viruses and bacteria. Spicy cayenne peppers raise your body's temperature to make you sweat, increasing the activity of your immune system.

You can use the cayenne you find in the spice aisle, but the ground cayenne isn't as potent as a fresh pepper. The fresher the pepper, the more effective it is. However, fresher also means spicier, so choose accordingly.

TIP

When you're sick, add organic cayenne powder to some warm water with lemon juice for an intense immune boost.

Squash

Squash is a good source of vitamin C and carotene. The six carotenoids (out of the 600 found in nature) found most commonly in human tissue — and supplied by squash and other gourds — decrease the risk of various cancers, protect the eyes and skin from the effects of ultraviolet light, and defend against heart disease. One of them, alpha-carotene, helps slow down the aging process. Butternut squash is the strongest source of these nutrients, but you can also try acorn, calabaza, delicata, Hubbard, and spaghetti squash.

TIP

Whether roasted in the oven or pureed into a soup, butternut squash is sweet and delicious and will warm your body from the inside out! Any of the items in this chapter can be combined to make a delicious squash soup on days you're feeling less than 100 percent.

Almonds

Almonds offer up a good dose of vitamin E. This immunity-boosting antioxidant is known for increasing the production of *B cells,* those white blood cells that kill unwanted bacteria. Enjoy chopped or sliced almonds in salads or oatmeal, or just grab a few whole almonds as a snack.

Citrus Fruits

Adding a bit of citrus to your diet goes a long way toward fending off your next cold or flu. Packed with vitamin C, oranges and grapefruits help increase your body's resistance to nasty invaders.

TIP

The best way to enjoy citrus fruits is to eat them whole. Otherwise, you can make fresh juice yourself (stay away from the premade stuff in cartons or in the freezer section of your supermarket). You can also squeeze some fresh lemon juice into some water, either warm or at room temperature, for a healing beverage. Lemon juice is pretty sour, so add it gradually to avoid making it undrinkable.

Green Tea

Green tea is a potent source of antioxidants called *polyphenols* — especially catechins. Some studies have found that catechins can destroy the influenza and common cold viruses.

TIP

Sipping a hot cup of green tea when you're feeling under the weather can really help you come alive again. Try adding a squeeze of fresh lemon to kick it up a bit.

Miso Soup

Miso soup is the plant-based version of chicken noodle soup. It has wonderful healing properties that are amazing at boosting immunity. As a living food, miso is loaded with enzymes and healthy bacteria that help fight infection and keep your cells thriving.

TIP

All you need is 1 teaspoon of miso paste stirred into a mug or bowl of warm water, and you're set. Sip it down, especially at the first sign of a cold or when you're just feeling "off" with a stomachache or headache. This is sure to hit the spot and make you feel good all over.

Mushrooms

For centuries, people around the world have turned to mushrooms for a healthy immune system. Contemporary researchers now know why. Studies show that the anti-inflammatory effect of mushrooms increases the production and activity of white blood cells, making them more aggressive at defeating foreign bodies and making you less susceptible to serious illness. This is a good thing when you have an infection.

TIP

Chaga, maitake, reishi, and shiitake mushrooms appear to pack the biggest immunity punch. Experts recommend eating ¼ ounce to 1 ounce a few times a day for maximum immune benefits. If you're sick, having mushrooms in tea form or as an extract is the best way to go for immediate results.

Chapter **22**

Ten Bad Things about Eating Meat

E ating meat creates health concerns not only for consumers but also for the environment and (of course) the farmed animals, and it's unfortunate that people overlook so many of these problems. Animals are taken advantage of, our environment suffers, and ultimately, we suffer, as well. Throughout this book, we explain why eating plants is the way to go, but in this chapter we explicitly outline the negatives of eating meat.

Meat Production Wastes Natural Resources

The world is a diverse place that offers many natural resources. Sadly, people tend to take advantage of these resources without any real concern for how their use impacts the abundance of the resources. The meat industry is one of the ugliest examples of this. It places extreme stress on natural resources, causing reduction and depletion of the following:

>> **Water:** It takes more than 1,800 gallons of water to produce 1 pound of meat, whereas it takes less than 200 gallons of water to produce 1 pound of wheat. Additionally, toxins, pesticides, and other residues from the extreme amount of animal waste produced by meat farms end up in nearby water supplies and cause pollution.

>> **Land:** According to the United Nations, raising animals for food now uses over 30 percent of the Earth's land mass (including land used for grazing and land used to grow feed crops). More than 260 million acres of U.S. forests have been cleared to grow grain to feed farmed animals, and every minute more land is cleared to produce more feedlots. Additionally, the destruction of habitats for farming and livestock grazing is one of the main reasons that plant species in North America become threatened and go extinct, and it also leads to soil erosion and barren land. Finally, cattle raising is a primary factor in the destruction of the world's remaining tropical rainforests.

>> **Food:** Raising animals for food is extremely inefficient. Animals eat large quantities of grain, soybeans, oats, and corn, but they produce comparatively small amounts of meat, dairy products, or eggs in return. More than half of the grain and cereals grown in the United States are fed to farmed animals. It takes up to 13 pounds of grain to produce just 1 pound of meat, and even fish on fish farms must be fed up to 5 pounds of wild-caught fish to produce 1 pound of farmed fish flesh. Imagine the impact on world hunger if we ate the plants directly — we'd have 13 times more food available to feed people.

>> **Energy:** Raising animals for food scoops up precious energy. It takes more than 11 times as much fossil fuel to make 1 calorie from animal protein as it does to make 1 calorie from plant protein. To get a feel for this, all you need to do is add up the energy-intensive stages of raising animals for food:

1. Grow massive amounts of corn, grain, and soybeans (with all the required tilling, irrigation, crop dusting, and so on).

2. Transport the grain and soybeans to feed manufacturers on gas-guzzling 18-wheelers.

3. Operate the feed mills (requiring massive energy expenditures).

4. Transport the feed to the factory farms (again, in gas-guzzling vehicles).

5. Operate the factory farms.

6. Truck the animals many miles to slaughter.

7. Operate the slaughterhouses.

8. Transport the meat to processing plants.

9. Operate the meat-processing plants.

10. Transport the meat to grocery stores.

11. Keep the meat refrigerated or frozen in the stores until it's sold.

Meat Isn't as Rich in Nutrients as Plants

An animal-based diet isn't as diverse in terms of nutrients as a plant-based diet is. You pretty much get two main macronutrients — protein and fat — with essentially no vitamins or minerals and no fiber. What most people don't know is that the body needs vitamins and minerals to digest and assimilate protein efficiently. You also need fiber to help the body push things through so you can assimilate nutrients.

The body can take two to three days to be fully digest meat, causing you to feel tired and undernourished. Whereas plants, which are full of fiber, can be digested easily within a day. Going plant-based ensures that your body at least gets the nutritional baseline it requires to thrive on a day-to-day basis. For example, eating kale instead of meat provides your body with fiber, vitamins, minerals, and even protein, while also giving you energy without weighing you down with excess fat or calories.

Animals Are Fed Poor-Quality Feed

Most conventionally raised animals are fed bottom-of-the-barrel feed that isn't in any way natural to them. This not only leaves animals unsatisfied on many levels but also affects their biological makeup. Many animals are starved of the nutrients they require to be healthy because they're fed an unnatural diet. This affects not only *their* well-being but ultimately the well-being of meat consumers.

Here are some of the top things animals are fed but should not be eating:

>> Parts from other animals (even within their own species)

>> High-grain diets, including genetically modified corn and soy (even though most animals are meant to eat grass)

>> Unnatural feed (garbage and human leftovers)

In the United States, up to 70 percent of antibiotics are fed to farm animals that aren't even sick. This injudicious use of antibiotics presents a serious and growing threat to human health because the practice creates new strains of dangerous antibiotic-resistant bacteria.

If these animals were living in the wild, they would be eating a diet that contributed to a more natural life and to the composition of their genetics. But unfortunately, their diets are manipulated by humans to whom they're merely a commodity. This food, in turn, goes into your body when you consume their meat. *They* get trashy feed; *you* get trashy feed.

If you're in the midst of transitioning or choosing to keep meat as part of your diet, make plants the priority on your plate and choose wild, organic, or naturally raised meat, poultry, eggs, and fish (local, if possible). One option is to look for products that are "certified humane" by Humane Farm Animal Care. Visit https://certifiedhumane.org for more information.

Meat Is Acidic

Meat is one of the major foods in the standard American diet that triggers an acidic reaction when metabolized. It's difficult for the body to break down and digest and requires extra work from the kidneys. As a result, it produces too much acid in the body. Too much acid not only weakens the body's immune defenses, which increases the risk of infection, but also contributes to chronic diseases.

The other consideration to look at is the *quality* of meat that a majority of people eat: Often it's fried, overcooked, and not eaten alongside green vegetables. This not only creates acidity in the body but also does nothing to help neutralize it. Choosing to eat more plants throughout the day can help balance this ratio.

Meat Is Loaded with Toxins

Animals are sponges that soak up toxicity. Because a majority of their biological makeup is fat, their bodies can accumulate an excessive amount of toxins. So, when the animals eat a toxic diet, these toxins get carried with them for life, and they end up in the foods you eat. According to the U.S. Food and Drug Administration (FDA), studies suggest that exposure to these toxins can lead to a variety of health issues, like cardiovascular disease, increased risk of cancer and diabetes, and reproductive problems.

For example, livestock can ingest toxins such as pesticides from the conventional produce they eat (that is, of course, if they're not raised organically). Because the cost of organic produce is so much higher, a majority of farmers choose to save money when it comes to animal feed.

Finally, the sea life that swims in polluted oceans and waterways has incredibly absorbent skin and fat, which is why fish and other seafood are often tainted with mercury and other heavy metals.

Meat Is High in Saturated Fat

It's one of the things we hear a lot these days: "Be mindful of the amount of saturated fat you eat!" Unfortunately, many people get confused about the sources of this unhealthy fat and don't realize that a majority of it is from animals. Saturated fat is healthy for the living animal, but the human body can't break it down in a healthy way.

Eating the amount of saturated fat from animals that most people do can lead to major health problems. Additionally, many people are eating fried meats, fatty cuts, and skin — all of which contribute to plaque buildup, heart disease, and other diseases such as obesity and diabetes.

Eating Meat Can Increase Your Risk for Cancer and Osteoporosis

In addition to causing heart disease, excess meat consumption leads to other health-degrading conditions, such as osteoporosis and even cancer. The excess protein — despite what people may think — isn't good for the body. Eating a very high-protein diet stresses the kidneys, which can lead to dehydration and an increased risk of kidney stones.

All in all, choosing an all-natural plant-based diet can have an incredible impact on your health and help prevent and arrest chronic degenerative diseases (see Chapter 2).

Eating Meat Impacts Climate Change

The impact that meat consumption continues to have on climate change is quite intense. Although most people wouldn't associate the two, here's a bit of the picture: To keep up with the demand for meat, cows are fed an incredible amount of food, which produces waste. This waste gives off methane gases, which contribute to ozone depletion by trapping heat in the atmosphere. Take the number of feedlots that exist across the world and multiply that by the amount of waste made each day by farm animals and you've got a lot of gases making the world a scarier place by the minute. In addition, enormous amounts of carbon dioxide stored in trees are released during the destruction of vast acres of forest to provide pastureland and to grow crops for farmed animals.

Additionally, manufacturing 1 calorie from animal protein requires 11 times as much fossil fuel input as producing 1 calorie from plant protein. Why is this bad? Burning fossil fuels (such as oil and gasoline) releases carbon dioxide, the primary gas responsible for climate change.

REMEMBER

By choosing to eat more plants over meat, you're choosing not to contribute to this vicious cycle. Not only that, but the more plants are farmed, the more beneficial gases (such as oxygen) are produced for the atmosphere.

Eating Meat Is Cruel

As a result of the increase in demand for meat, *factory farms* (large, industrialized farms on which large numbers of livestock are raised indoors in conditions intended to maximize production at minimal cost) are on the rise.

What this means is that animals are treated with no respect. How would you feel being crowded into a small space with no room to run around, lift your hand, or even sit down? This is truly the case for most animals these days, and it's all for the purpose of fast, cheap, moneymaking production. Very little care is taken for the animals' welfare. They're given antibiotics to combat the infections they get from living in such close quarters and growth hormones to increase their size and weight in an unnaturally short period of time (and both of these things eventually wind up in your food).

An old saying goes, "If slaughterhouses had glass walls, everyone would be vegetarian." You can find many ways to inform yourself about some of these actions; check out resources such as documentaries, books, and websites. These are some of our favorites:

>> **Documentaries:** *Cowspiracy* (2014), *Death on a Factory Farm* (2009), *Earthlings* (2005), *Food, Inc.* (2009), *Food Matters* (2008), *Forks over Knives* (2011), *Seaspiracy* (2021), *Vegucated* (2011), and *What the Health* (2017)

>> **Websites:** Farm Sanctuary (www.farmsanctuary.org), The Humane Society of the United States (www.humanesociety.org), Meat.org (www.meat.org), The Meatrix (www.themeatrix.com), NutritionFacts.org (https://nutritionfacts.org), and People for the Ethical Treatment of Animals (www.peta.org)

>> **Books:** *The China Study* by T. Colin Campbell, PhD, with Thomas M. Campbell II (BenBella Books), *Eating Animals* by Jonathan Safran Foer (Back Bay Books), *That's Why We Don't Eat Animals* by Ruby Roth (North Atlantic Books), and *Whole: Rethinking the Science of Nutrition* by T. Colin Campbell, PhD, with Howard Jacobson, PhD (BenBella Books)

The Meat Industry Is Getting Worse

The more control mankind has had over food, the worse it has gotten. This is apparent with packaged foods but especially with animal-based foods. Obviously, an increased demand for meat has strained the supply chain. To put enough meat on the shelves at inexpensive prices, farmers have put into place often-unsustainable practices. This can mean manipulating the environments in which animals are raised, which can lead to contamination of the animal feed, the soil, the land, and ultimately the meat on your plate. It's no wonder that every couple of years we hear about some bacteria, such as salmonella or *E. coli*, that has found its way into food.

Here are just a few more things happening in the animal industry that affect not only animals' lives but humans' lives as well:

>> Contamination of animal feed ultimately infects the food supply with super-bugs, *E. coli,* and mad cow disease.

>> Farmers are using more growth hormones to raise animals.

>> Organic farming practices are underused because they aren't as economically efficient.

Appendix A
Metric Conversion Guide

Note: The recipes in this book weren't developed or tested using metric measurements. There may be some variation in quality when converting to metric units.

Common Abbreviations

Abbreviation(s)	What It Stands For
cm	Centimeter
C., c.	Cup
G, g	Gram
kg	Kilogram
L, l	Liter
lb.	Pound
mL, ml	Milliliter
oz.	Ounce
pt.	Pint
t., tsp.	Teaspoon
T., Tb., Tbsp.	Tablespoon

Volume

U.S. Units	Canadian Metric	Australian Metric
¼ teaspoon	1 milliliter	1 milliliter
½ teaspoon	2 milliliters	2 milliliters
1 teaspoon	5 milliliters	5 milliliters
1 tablespoon	15 milliliters	20 milliliters
¼ cup	50 milliliters	60 milliliters
⅓ cup	75 milliliters	80 milliliters
½ cup	125 milliliters	125 milliliters
⅔ cup	150 milliliters	170 milliliters
¾ cup	175 milliliters	190 milliliters
1 cup	250 milliliters	250 milliliters
1 quart	1 liter	1 liter
1½ quarts	1.5 liters	1.5 liters
2 quarts	2 liters	2 liters
2½ quarts	2.5 liters	2.5 liters
3 quarts	3 liters	3 liters
4 quarts (1 gallon)	4 liters	4 liters

Weight

U.S. Units	Canadian Metric	Australian Metric
1 ounce	30 grams	30 grams
2 ounces	55 grams	60 grams
3 ounces	85 grams	90 grams
4 ounces (¼ pound)	115 grams	125 grams
8 ounces (½ pound)	225 grams	225 grams
16 ounces (1 pound)	455 grams	500 grams (½ kilogram)

Length

Inches	Centimeters
0.5	1.5
1	2.5
2	5.0
3	7.5
4	10.0
5	12.5
6	15.0
7	17.5
8	20.5
9	23.0
10	25.5
11	28.0
12	30.5

Temperature (Degrees)

Fahrenheit	Celsius
32	0
212	100
250	120
275	140
300	150
325	160
350	180
375	190
400	200
425	220
450	230
475	240
500	260

Index

B

babies, plant-based, 310–316

bacon, substitutions for, 120

Baked Veggie Potato Fritters recipe, 226

bakeware, 103

baking goods, stocking, 99

Balsamic Maple Dressing recipe, 172, 258

Balsamic Roasted Beet Salad recipe, 172

Banana Walnut Snack Cake recipe, 289

bananas, 123, 125–126, 128, 132–133, 246–247, 252, 268, 271, 274–275, 288–289

Barbecue Jackfruit Tacos recipe, 213

Barbecue Ranch Chickpea Salad recipe, 173–174

barley, as a carbohydrate source, 37

basil, 42, 157, 165, 196, 200–201, 229, 237–238, 261

Basil Spinach Pesto recipe, 186, 210–211, 261

bay leaves, recipes using, 145, 196, 198

beans, 33, 75, 99, 305. *See also specific types*

beets

  heart disease/high blood pressure and, 25

  peeling, 172

  recipes using, 162, 172, 179, 218, 227

  on salads, 142

bell peppers

  heart disease/high blood pressure and, 26

  recipes using, 137, 151, 153, 155, 173–174, 182, 199, 200, 204–205, 207–211, 227, 253

  on salads, 142

berries, recipes using, 123, 124, 133, 167. *See also specific types*

beta-carotene, requirements for, 330

bioflavonoids, 63–64

Black Bean Breakfast Tacos recipe, 138

Black Bean Cumin Burgers recipe, 193

Black Bean Quinoa Chili recipe, 208–209

black beans

  heart disease/high blood pressure and, 25

  recipes using, 138, 173–174, 187–188, 193, 204–205, 208–209, 238

  on salads, 142

black olives, recipes using, 185

blackberries, 26, 167

bladderwrack, 59, 61

blender, 105

blood pressure. *See* high blood pressure

blood-sugar controlling foods, 22

blueberries

  heart disease/high blood pressure and, 26

  recipes using, 123, 125, 126, 252, 274, 288

  for toddlers, 318

Blueberry Buckwheat Pancakes recipe, 126

bok choy, recipes using, 146, 199

brain health, breastfeeding and, 311

Brazil nuts, recipes using, 122, 243

bread crumbs, recipes using, 195, 219

breads, 339–340

Breakfast Quinoa Bowl recipe, 136

breastfeeding, 311–313

breathing, breastfeeding and, 312

broccoli, 25, 152, 198, 199, 221, 225

brown rice

  as a carbohydrate source, 37

  heart disease/high blood pressure and, 25

  recipes using, 154, 155, 178, 229, 272

  on salads, 142

brown rice noodles, recipes using, 145

Brown Rice Pudding recipe, 272

brown rice vermicelli, recipes using, 146

brown sugar, recipes using, 290

Brown-Rice Crispy Bars recipe, 249

brown-rice flour, recipes using, 193, 219, 252, 292

brown-rice miso, recipes using, 264

brown-rice syrup. 268, 287, 291

Brussels sprouts, recipes using, 166, 210–211

buckwheat, as a carbohydrate source, 38

buckwheat flour, recipes using, 126

buckwheat soba noodles, recipes using, 159

Buffalo Cauliflower Dip recipe, 240

burger buns, recipes using, 194, 207

burgers, veggie, 340

Butler Soy Curls, 158

butter, 33, 270. *See also specific types*

Butter Lettuce Salad recipe, 170

buttermilk, substitutions for, 270

butternut squash, 26, 145, 148, 153, 163, 198, 203, 227
Butternut Squash Apple Soup recipe, 148

C

cabbage, 142, 162, 213

caçao/caçao nibs/caçao powder
   about, 12, 247
   recipes using, 132, 243, 245, 247, 271, 291
   as a superfood, 56

calcium, 14, 27, 28, 49, 329

calories, 83–85

Campbell, T. Colin (author), 33, 355

Campbell, Thomas M., II (author), 355

cancer, 21, 328, 353

cane sugar, 268, 284–285

cannellini beans, recipes using, 152

cantaloupe, heart disease/high blood pressure and, 26

carbohydrates, 34–42

cardamom, recipes using, 250

caregivers, training, 331

Carob Fig Frozen Fudge recipe, 273

Carrot Pineapple Layer Cake recipe, 286–287

carrots
   heart disease/high blood pressure and, 26
   recipes using, 146, 150–151, 154, 157–159, 162, 166, 178–179, 182, 195–196, 198–199, 207–209, 212, 218, 223, 226, 242, 253, 286–287
   on salads, 142

cashew butter, recipes using, 133, 283

Cashew Cream recipe, 286–287

cashew milk, ecipes using, 148

cashews, recipes using, 204–205, 206, 240, 243, 244, 262, 275, 287, 291

cauliflower, recipes using, 156, 198, 199, 218, 240

cayenne, for boosting immunity, 345

celery, recipes using, 145, 146, 150, 152, 154, 158, 180, 181, 183–184, 196, 198, 199

celiac disease, gastrointestinal illnesses and, 24

cell aging, 326–327

cereal/cereal bars, 342

cheese, 74, 101–102. *See also specific types*

Cheesy Chili Mac recipe, 204–205

cherries, recipes using, 130, 276

Cherry Baked Oatmeal Muffins recipe, 130

Cherry Chocolate Walnut Truffles recipe, 276

Chewy Oatmeal Raisin Cookies recipe, 278

chia seeds, recipes using, 132, 133, 245, 247

chicken, eliminating, 74

chickpea flour, recipes using, 226

Chickpea Walnut Bolognese recipe, 202

chickpeas
   as an iron source, 50
   recipes using, 138, 151, 158, 160, 165, 167–168, 173–174, 181, 185, 190, 195–196, 202, 212, 238, 241, 283
   on salads, 142

children, 309–323

The China Study (Campbell and Campbell II), 33, 355

Chinese delivery/takeout, 301

chipotle peppers in adobo, Creamy Oil-Free Hummus, 241

chlorella, 56

chocolate, 26, 130, 243, 249, 252, 276, 279, 288, 289

Chocolate Avocado Pudding recipe, 271

Chocolate Banana Super Smoothie recipe, 247

Chocolate Chocolate Chip Cookies recipe, 279

Chocolate Malted Shake recipe, 275

Chocolate Nice Cream Breakfast Parfait recipe, 125

Chunky Miso Soup recipe, 146

cilantro, recipes using, 138, 153, 173–174, 204–205, 208–209, 213, 230, 241

cinnamon, recipes using, 132, 133, 134, 239, 248, 250, 271, 272, 283

citrus fruits, for boosting immunity, 346. *See also specific types*

Citrus Wild Rice and Broccoli recipe, 221

Clean Fifteen, 109

climate change, impact of eating meat on, 354

cloves, recipes using, 134

cocoa powder, 125, 208–209, 245, 247, 275, 276, 279, 291

jalapeño peppers, recipes using, 138, 194, 204–205, 213, 224, 236, 237

Jam Dot Cookies recipe, 277

Japanese delivery/takeout, 301–302

Japanese eggplant, recipes using, 199

K

kale
  as an iron source, 50
  recipes using, 124, 152, 162, 166, 172, 210–211, 246, 251, 261, 274
  on salads, 142

Kale and Cabbage Slaw Salad recipe, 162

kamut, as a carbohydrate source, 37

kamut flour, recipes using, 129

kelp, 59, 62

ketchup, recipes using, 207

Kidney Bean Salad recipe, 161

kidney beans
  heart disease/high blood pressure and, 25
  recipes using, 145, 161, 198, 204–205, 238
  on salads, 142

kids, plant-based, 319–323

kitchen, 95–105

kitchen experience, 77–78

kitchen tongs, 103

knives, 103

kombu, 59, 61, 62, 146, 238

kombucha, 233

kosher salt, 51

kuzu, 59, 62

L

lacto-ovo vegetarian, 8

lacto-vegetarian, 8

lakanto, 268

L-arginine, 27

leeks, recipes using, 196

leftovers, 188

legumes
  about, 11

as an antioxidant source, 65

as a calcium source, 49

cancer and, 21

as a carbohydrate source, 40

diabetes and, 22

food guide for, 18–19

for toddlers, 317

Lemon Vinaigrette recipe, 169, 259

lemons/lemon juice, recipes using, 132, 134–136, 147, 152, 154, 156, 158, 160, 162, 168, 170–171, 179–181, 185, 189, 194, 201, 206, 221–222, 229, 235–236, 238, 240–241, 250–251, 259–262, 280, 281, 292

length conversions, 359

Lentil Rice Soup recipe, 154

lentils
  adding-in, 75
  as an iron source, 50
  recipes using, 154, 155, 165, 207, 212, 238
  on salads, 142
  for toddlers, 318

lettuce, recipes using, 152. *See also specific types*

limes/lime juice, recipes using, 138, 153, 167, 187–188, 200, 204–205, 208–209, 213, 225, 230, 236, 241, 262

Liquid Nutrition Smoothie recipe, 123

liquid smoke, recipes using, 155

liquifying dates, 268

list runner shopper category, 88

Loaded Avocado Toast recipe, 254

lucuma, as a superfood, 57

lutein, requirements for, 330

M

maca powder
  about, 275
  recipes using, 275
  as a superfood, 57

macadamia nuts, recipes using, 122

macaroni noodles, recipes using, 164, 204–205

macronutrients, 31–46, 90

magnesium, 27

mango, recipes using, 123, 274

as a calcium source, 49

cancer and, 21

heart disease and, 25

high blood pressure and, 25

as a protein source, 33

recipes using, 134–135

stocking, 99

as superfoods, 55

O

oat bran, recipes using, 131

oat flour, recipes using, 127, 129, 280

oat milk, recipes using, 206, 246, 275

oats

  as a carbohydrate source, 37

  heart disease/high blood pressure and, 25

  recipes using, 128, 129, 130, 131, 132, 195, 248, 249, 275, 278, 281, 282, 283, 292

obesity, plant-based diet and, 328

oils. *See* fats and oils

olives, recipes using, 185

omega-3/-6 fatty acids, 27, 44–45

one-pot dishes, 188–190

One-Pot Hummus Pasta recipe, 189

onions. *See also* green onions

  for boosting immunity, 344

  dicing, 263

  recipes using, 136, 139, 145–148, 150–156, 158, 160–161, 163, 168, 173–174, 180, 182, 185–186, 190, 193–196, 198–200, 202–213, 219, 225, 227–228, 237, 240, 242, 263

on-the-fly shopper category, 88

Orange Maple Marinade recipe, 263

Orange Maple Marinated Tempeh recipe, 139

Orange Spinach Salad recipe, 167

oranges/orange juice

  about, 342

  heart disease/high blood pressure and, 26

  recipes using, 124, 139, 165, 167, 190, 199, 221, 223, 237, 263, 264, 281

  on salads, 142

oregano, 142, 179, 196, 223

organic foods, 82, 113–115

organizer shopper category, 87–88

Orzo with Cherry Tomatoes and Basil recipe, 229

osteoporosis, 27–28, 353

Oven-Roasted Carrots recipe, 223

ovo-vegetarian, 8

P

panko bread crumbs, recipes using, 206

pans and pots, 104

pantry staples, 99–100, 110

papaya, heart disease/high blood pressure and, 26

Parmesan cheese, recipes using, 203

parsley, 142, 147, 151, 154, 157–158, 160–161, 164, 168, 170–172, 181, 185, 196, 198, 206, 212, 236, 260

parsnips, recipes using, 145, 218

pasta and noodles, 100, 341

pea shoots, recipes using, 179

peaches, recipes using, 123, 165, 237, 274, 292

peanut butter, recipes using, 125

pears, recipes using, 123, 132, 134, 172

peas, recipes using, 152, 153, 157, 164, 228, 236

pecans, 166, 221, 244, 291, 292

peeling, 172, 200, 236

People for the Ethical Treatment of Animals (website), 355

pescatarian, 8

Pesto Sauce recipe, 201

phytonutrients, 21, 62–63

Pickled Onion Pesto Grilled Cheese recipe, 186

pickles, recipes using, 207

pine nuts, recipes using, 159, 163, 190, 201, 261

pineapple, recipes using, 237, 274, 286–287

pinto beans, recipes using, 138

pistachios, recipes using, 272

pita bread, recipes using, 180, 185

pitting avocados, 236

plant-based diet
about, 7–8
aging and, 325–335
benefits of, 17–30
calories, 83–85
children and, 309–324
common pitfalls of, 77–79
diseases and, 327–328
FAQ, 13–15
food guide, 17–19
grocery shopping, 87–88
hydration, 85
inclusions, 9–12
meal planning, 86–87
not included, 12–13
organic *vs.* nonorganic, 82
organization for, 86–92
preparing foods for, 331–332
proportions, 82–83
support from others for, 75–77
transitioning to a, 15–16, 69–75
whole-foods plant-based diet *vs.*, 9, 82
polyunsaturated fats, 43
portobello mushrooms, recipes using, 163, 220
potassium, 27
potatoes, recipes using, 158, 171, 226, 227. *See also* sweet potatoes
potluck, 306
pots and pans, 104
poultry, eliminating, 74
powdered sugar, recipes using, 280, 285, 290, 291
power foods, 53–65
premenstrual syndrome (PMS), 34
prescriptions, 332–335
processed foods, diabetes and, 23
produce, 97–98, 108–109. *See also* fruits; vegetables
proportions, 82–83
protein powder, 33, 123, 125, 133, 247
protein(s), 14, 16, 25, 32–34, 91, 142, 176, 299
pseudo grains, 55, 100
puffed-rice cereal, recipes using, 249

pumpkin, recipes using, 127, 153
pumpkin seeds
heart disease/high blood pressure and, 25
recipes using, 131, 132, 133, 149, 166, 203, 217, 242, 243, 248, 249, 261
on salads, 142
for toddlers, 318
Purple Carrot, 331

Q
quinoa
as an iron source, 50
as a carbohydrate source, 39
heart disease/high blood pressure and, 25
recipes using, 131, 136, 157, 160, 166, 190, 208–209, 229
on salads, 142
Quinoa and Chickpeas with Spinach recipe, 190
Quinoa Tabbouleh Salad recipe, 160

R
radishes, recipes using, 136, 161, 170, 182, 230, 253, 254
rainbow chard, recipes using, 163
raisins, 128, 129, 130, 131, 134, 142, 166, 190, 249, 252, 272, 278
raspberries, 26, 245, 271, 274
raspberry jam, recipes using, 277
Raw Corn and Radish Salad recipe, 230
raw foods, 57–58
raw honey, 268, 269, 274
raw vegan, 8
recipes, modifying to be plant-based, 92–93. *See also specific recipes*
Recommended Dietary Allowance (RDA), 32–33
Red Lentil White Bean Stew recipe, 212
red meat, eliminating, 73
Red Pepper Carrot Soup recipe, 151
refrigerated items, stocking, 98
restaurants, 295–303
rheumatoid arthritis, 29
rice

white wine, recipes using, 203

whole foods/grains, 9, 18, 21, 75, 82, 100

Whole: Rethinking the Science of Nutrition (Campbell and Jacobson), 355

whole-wheat flour, recipes using, 284–285, 289, 290

wild rice, 39, 150, 221

wine, recipes using, 203

wire whisk, 104

Worcestershire sauce, 340

X

xylitol, 268

Y

yams, recipes using, 217

yogurt, 120, 167, 181, 240, 260

Z

zeaxanthin, requirements for, 330

Zesty Kale Crisps recipe, 251

Zesty Pesto Pasta with White Beans recipe, 201

zinc, 50, 330

zucchini, recipes using, 145, 147, 157, 173–174, 182, 195, 198, 204–205, 226, 228

About the Authors

Jenn Sebestyen: Jenn Sebestyen is the founder of the popular blog *Veggie Inspired* (www.veggieinspired.com), which features easy and flavorful plant-based recipes. She is the author of *The Meatless Monday Family Cookbook* (Fair Winds Press) and coauthor of *The Meat-Free Kitchen* (Fair Winds Press). Jenn has appeared on CBS's *The Doctors,* and her work has been featured in a variety of media outlets such as *Women's Health, Better Homes & Gardens, Fitness* magazine, *SELF, Country Living, Vegan Food & Living, The Washington Post, Buzzfeed, HuffPost,* MSN, *Parade,* www.peta.org, and more. She is a mom of three and lives with her husband and family in the Chicago area.

Marni Wasserman: As a culinary nutritionist, health strategist, and owner of Toronto's first plant-based food studio, Marni is dedicated to providing people with balanced, nutritious choices through organic, fresh, whole, and natural foods. Marni is a graduate of the Institute of Holistic Nutrition in Toronto and the Natural Gourmet Culinary School in New York, and she is the founder of Marni Wasserman's Food Studio & Lifestyle Shop in Midtown Toronto, where she teaches her signature cooking classes and offers collaborative workshops and urban retreats. Marni is also the coauthor of *Fermenting For Dummies* (Wiley) and several well-received e-books. You can learn more about Marni by visiting her on Facebook (www.facebook.com/marniwassermanpage), following her on Twitter (@ marniwasserman), checking out her Pinterest page (www.pinterest.com/fullynourished), or visiting her website (https://marniwasserman.com).

Dedication

Jenn Sebestyen: For Meghan. I hope you always see it.

Marni Wasserman: This book is dedicated to anyone who wants to adopt a healthier way of eating and living.

Authors' Acknowledgments

Jenn Sebestyen: This book would not have been possible without the support and collaboration of many people. Thank you to my husband and children for your love, support, and encouragement and for always being my best taste-testers and being willing to help out in the kitchen when needed; I love you forever and always. I'm so grateful to my friends and extended family for your continued support and for always being willing to try my recipes, visit my blog, and buy my books, even when you wouldn't necessarily choose this way of eating for yourself. Thank you to Kelsey Baird, Tracy Boggier, Elizabeth Kuball, Kristie Pyles, and the entire team at Wiley for entrusting me with this project and for your guidance, insights, and feedback along the way — it was a pleasure working with all of you. Thank you to Rachel Nix for further testing the recipes and providing nutritional insights and technical edits. Finally, to my Veggie Inspired blog readers, it is because of your continued support and interest in my plant-based recipes that I am lucky enough to have the opportunity to turn my love of food and passion for healthy cooking into a career and write books such as this one. I will be forever grateful!

Marni Wasserman: I would like to express thanks to the team at Wiley for asking me to be the author of the first edition of this book, *Plant-Based Diet For Dummies*. The core team with whom I worked to make that book come to life includes Sarah Sypniewski, Vicki Adang, and Tracy Boggier. They helped keep me going every step along the way. In addition, I would like to acknowledge Ashley Petry, Emily Nolan, and Tracey Eakin for making sure that everything I wrote makes sense and looks and tastes good!

Publisher's Acknowledgments

Senior Acquisitions Editor: Tracy Boggier

Project Editor: Elizabeth Kuball

Copy Editor: Elizabeth Kuball

Technical Editor: Rachel Nix, RD

Recipe Tester: Rachel Nix, RD

Nutrition Analyst: Rachel Nix, RD

Production Editor: Tamilmani Varadharaj

Photographers: Wendy Jo Peterson and Grace Geri Goodale

Cover Photos: Courtesy of Wendy Jo Peterson and Grace Geri Goodale

Take dummies with you everywhere you go!

Whether you are excited about e-books, want more from the web, must have your mobile apps, or are swept up in social media, dummies makes everything easier.

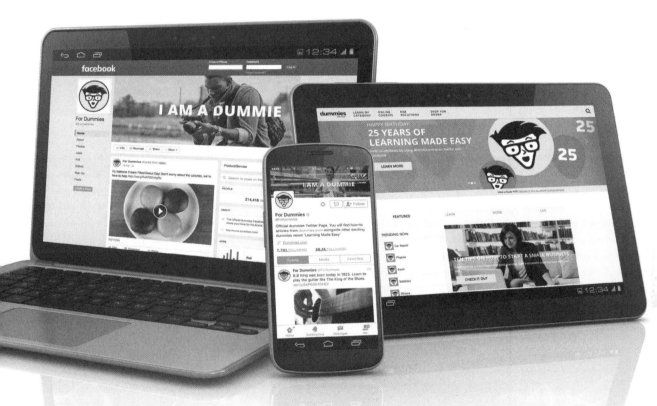

Find us online!

  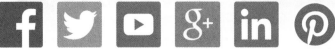

Leverage the power

Dummies is the global leader in the reference category and one of the most trusted and highly regarded brands in the world. No longer just focused on books, customers now have access to the dummies content they need in the format they want. Together we'll craft a solution that engages your customers, stands out from the competition, and helps you meet your goals.

Advertising & Sponsorships

Connect with an engaged audience on a powerful multimedia site, and position your message alongside expert how-to content. Dummies.com is a one-stop shop for free, online information and know-how curated by a team of experts.

- Targeted ads
- Video
- Email Marketing
- Microsites
- Sweepstakes sponsorship

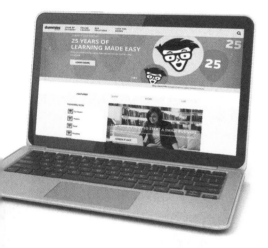

20 **MILLION** PAGE VIEWS **EVERY SINGLE MONTH**

15 MILLION **UNIQUE** VISITORS PER MONTH

43% OF ALL VISITORS ACCESS THE SITE VIA THEIR MOBILE DEVICES

700,000 NEWSLETTER SUBSCRIPTIONS TO THE INBOXES OF

300,000 UNIQUE INDIVIDUALS EVERY WEEK

# of dummies

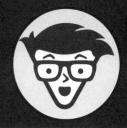

Custom Publishing

Reach a global audience in any language by creating a solution that will differentiate you from competitors, amplify your message, and encourage customers to make a buying decision.

- Apps
- Books
- eBooks
- Video
- Audio
- Webinars

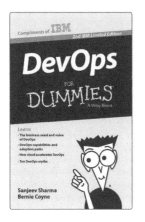
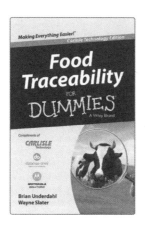
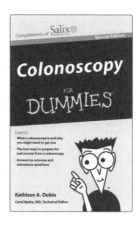
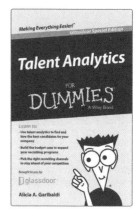

Brand Licensing & Content

Leverage the strength of the world's most popular reference brand to reach new audiences and channels of distribution.

For more information, visit dummies.com/biz

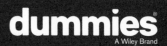

PERSONAL ENRICHMENT

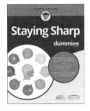
9781119187790
USA $26.00
CAN $31.99
UK £19.99

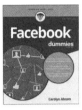
9781119179030
USA $21.99
CAN $25.99
UK £16.99

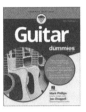
9781119293354
USA $24.99
CAN $29.99
UK £17.99

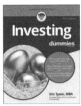
9781119293347
USA $22.99
CAN $27.99
UK £16.99

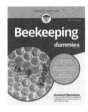
9781119310068
USA $22.99
CAN $27.99
UK £16.99

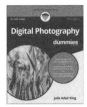
9781119235606
USA $24.99
CAN $29.99
UK £17.99

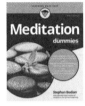
9781119251163
USA $24.99
CAN $29.99
UK £17.99

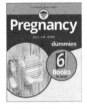
9781119235491
USA $26.99
CAN $31.99
UK £19.99

9781119279952
USA $24.99
CAN $29.99
UK £17.99

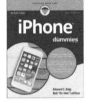
9781119283133
USA $24.99
CAN $29.99
UK £17.99

9781119287117
USA $24.99
CAN $29.99
UK £16.99

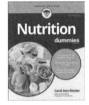
9781119130246
USA $22.99
CAN $27.99
UK £16.99

PROFESSIONAL DEVELOPMENT

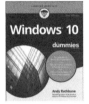
9781119311041
USA $24.99
CAN $29.99
UK £17.99

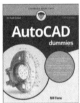
9781119255796
USA $39.99
CAN $47.99
UK £27.99

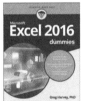
9781119293439
USA $26.99
CAN $31.99
UK £19.99

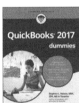
9781119281467
USA $26.99
CAN $31.99
UK £19.99

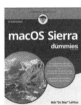
9781119280651
USA $29.99
CAN $35.99
UK £21.99

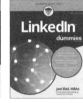
9781119251132
USA $24.99
CAN $29.99
UK £17.99

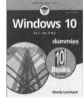
9781119310563
USA $34.00
CAN $41.99
UK £24.99

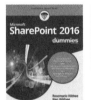
9781119181705
USA $29.99
CAN $35.99
UK £21.99

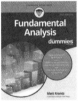
9781119263593
USA $26.99
CAN $31.99
UK £19.99

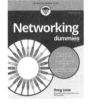
9781119257769
USA $29.99
CAN $35.99
UK £21.99

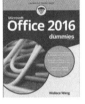
9781119293477
USA $26.99
CAN $31.99
UK £19.99

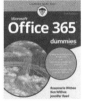
9781119265313
USA $24.99
CAN $29.99
UK £17.99

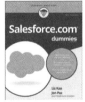
9781119239314
USA $29.99
CAN $35.99
UK £21.99

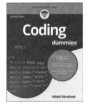
9781119293323
USA $29.99
CAN $35.99
UK £21.99

dummies.com

dummies
A Wiley Brand

Learning Made Easy

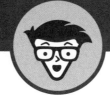

ACADEMIC

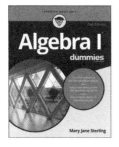

9781119293576
USA $19.99
CAN $23.99
UK £15.99

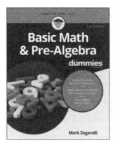

9781119293637
USA $19.99
CAN $23.99
UK £15.99

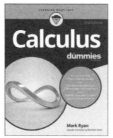

9781119293491
USA $19.99
CAN $23.99
UK £15.99

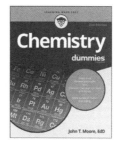

9781119293460
USA $19.99
CAN $23.99
UK £15.99

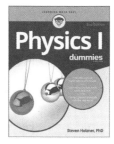

9781119293590
USA $19.99
CAN $23.99
UK £15.99

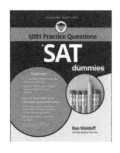

9781119215844
USA $26.99
CAN $31.99
UK £19.99

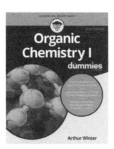

9781119293378
USA $22.99
CAN $27.99
UK £16.99

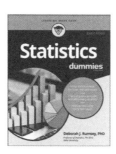

9781119293521
USA $19.99
CAN $23.99
UK £15.99

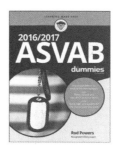

9781119239178
USA $18.99
CAN $22.99
UK £14.99

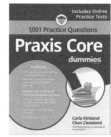

9781119263883
USA $26.99
CAN $31.99
UK £19.99

Available Everywhere Books Are Sold

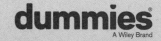

Small books for big imaginations

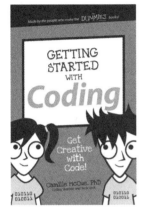

9781119177173
USA $9.99
CAN $9.99
UK £8.99

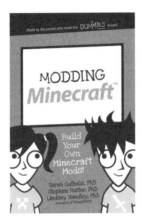

9781119177272
USA $9.99
CAN $9.99
UK £8.99

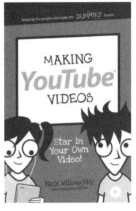

9781119177241
USA $9.99
CAN $9.99
UK £8.99

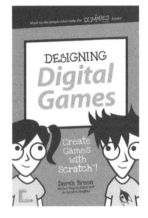

9781119177210
USA $9.99
CAN $9.99
UK £8.99

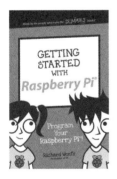

9781119262657
USA $9.99
CAN $9.99
UK £6.99

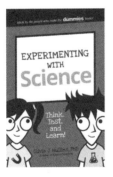

9781119291336
USA $9.99
CAN $9.99
UK £6.99

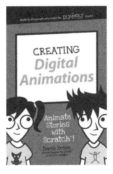

9781119233527
USA $9.99
CAN $9.99
UK £6.99

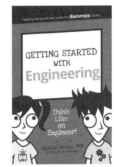

9781119291220
USA $9.99
CAN $9.99
UK £6.99

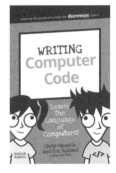

9781119177302
USA $9.99
CAN $9.99
UK £8.99

Unleash Their Creativity

dummies.com

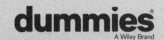